Tortoise Husbandry and Welfare

Tortoise Husbandry and Welfare

Jane Williams

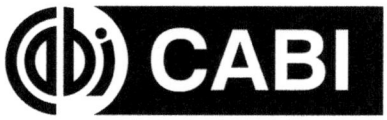

CABI is a trading name of CAB International

CABI
Nosworthy Way
Wallingford
Oxfordshire OX10 8DE
UK

CABI
200 Portland Street
Boston
MA 02114
USA

Tel: +44 (0)1491 832111
E-mail: info@cabi.org
Website: www.cabi.org

Tel: +1 (617)682-9015
E-mail: cabi-nao@cabi.org

© CAB International 2025. All rights, including for text and data mining, AI training, and similar technologies, are reserved. No part of this publication may be reproduced in any form or by any means, electronically, mechanically, by photocopying, recording or otherwise, without the prior permission of the copyright owners.

The views expressed in this publication are those of the author(s) and do not necessarily represent those of, and should not be attributed to, CAB International (CABI). Any images, figures and tables not otherwise attributed are the author(s)' own. References to internet websites (URLs) were accurate at the time of writing. CAB International and, where different, the copyright owner shall not be liable for technical or other errors or omissions contained herein. The information is supplied without obligation and on the understanding that any person who acts upon it, or otherwise changes their position in reliance thereon, does so entirely at their own risk. Information supplied is neither intended nor implied to be a substitute for professional advice. The reader/user accepts all risks and responsibility for losses, damages, costs and other consequences resulting directly or indirectly from using this information.

CABI's Terms and Conditions, including its full disclaimer, may be found at https://www.cabidigitallibrary.org/terms-and-conditions.

A catalogue record for this book is available from the British Library, London, UK.

ISBN-13: 9781800623712 (paperback)
9781800629561 (hardback)
9781800623729 (ePDF)
9781800623736 (ePub)

DOI: 10.1079/9781800623736.0000

Commissioning Editor: Alexandra Lainsbury
Editorial Assistant: Helen Elliott
Production Editor: Rosie Hayden

Typeset by Straive, Pondicherry, India
Printed and bound in the UK by CPI Group (UK) Ltd, Croydon, CR0 4YY

Contents

Introduction		vii
Biography		ix
Acknowledgements and Thanks		xi
1	What is a Tortoise?	1
2	How Tortoise Biology Affects Health and Behaviour	6
3	The Captive Environment	24
4	Artificial Lighting and Heat Sources	48
5	Tortoise Diets	61
6	Health Checks - Indicators of Good Health	79
7	Common Illnesses and Diseases in Tortoises	93
8	Tortoise Behaviour and Learning	118
9	Emotional States in Tortoises	132
10	Social Interactions in Tortoises	141
11	Breeding Tortoises	149
12	Tortoise Hibernation/Brumation	165
13	Mediterranean Tortoises	181
14	Tropical Dry Grassland Tortoises	198
15	Tropical Tortoises from Humid Forest Areas	211
16	Horsfield's (Afghan or Steppe) Tortoises	222
17	Egyptian Tortoises	230
18	What it Takes to Be a Tortoise Keeper	241
19	Health and Safety for the Tortoise Keeper and Tortoise	250
20	Tortoise Keeping – Past, Present, Future	257

Appendix 1: Example Tortoise Health Record	271
Appendix 2: Example Monthly Record Keeping of Tortoise Health	273
Appendix 3: Suitable Food Plants	275
List of Species	277
Index	283

Introduction

I remember having a tortoise for most of my childhood. Throughout the 1960s and 1970s, and into the 1980s, many UK families owned a tortoise bought from a pet shop for about 5 shillings old money (that's about 25 pence these days). They were sold from crates at pet shops, often stacked on top of each other, sometimes taken home in brown paper bags – which, if the tortoise urinated on the way, often meant that the bag fell apart, leaving the tortoise on the roadside or on a bus, its new owner completely unaware of its fate.

We had a series of tortoises that met various ends, largely due to being in captivity in a country where their needs, habits and welfare were not understood and where survival was not top priority, because you could always go and buy another the following year. We had two that died in hibernation, or shortly after – most tortoises were hibernated for 5–6 months at that time to allow them to sleep through the winter but also a lot of autumn and spring, which is much longer than in the wild. They were often described as garden tortoises and left to fend for themselves through the completely unsuitable British climate, not warm enough in summer, too cold and wet through the rest of the year.

Tortoises were a very popular pet in the UK and continue to be so. We were fascinated – they were so unusual and strange compared with the cats and dogs we all had as pets. Their longevity created the opportunity for very lengthy relationships with their owners, and many people express strong feelings of attachment towards their tortoise. Sadly, many tortoises did not survive to reach their natural lifespan of around 100 years, due to poor conditions in captivity. I was always captivated by the way ours moved and fed and lived through hibernation, but it was not until the late 1980s that I once again became a tortoise keeper, having been gifted five from my partner's mother as an interesting addition to the garden of our first home.

Tommy and Lucy were two North African Spur-thighed males. Lucy survived until the 2010s and Tommy is with us still. Matilda and Sappho, the two Hermann's females, lived until the 2000s. Sadly the very large Marginated male, Angie, died in 1994, ironically (in the British weather) due to overheating, from tipping over onto his back and being unable to right himself on a hot sunny day.

It was the opportunity to observe and engage with these five tortoises that really sparked my interest in this fascinating group of reptiles.

Tommy and Lucy developed a condition then called runny-nose syndrome (RNS) which, as the name suggests, means that the nasal passages run, the discharge sometimes becomes thick and infected. This can lead to pneumonia or other respiratory problems. Our local vet tried to help and put them on antibiotics. Of course, these only work when the tortoises are at a suitable temperature – around 30°C – so we had to line the bathroom floor with sheets of plastic for them to walk around on, and of course poo on, so that we could keep the area clean, and turn the heating up high to keep the smallest room nice and warm.

Eventually, when things were not improving our vet referred us to a Royal College of Veterinary Surgeons (RCVS) specialist he had been at college with, who not only helped with the condition (both tortoises survived) but also introduced me to the possibilities of improved health through better husbandry. Indoor accommodation, additional heat and light, shorter hibernations and improved diet were all introduced at home after this episode. Crucially, I started to realize the importance of trying to mimic the natural environment for any particular species. Without knowing that, how can we possibly meet their needs? How can we provide sufficient choice for the animal to find the conditions needed for good health and welfare?

Over the years my knowledge and experience grew, and I started a local support group at a time when there were very few. I gave advice to many other keepers, delivered workshops to vet staff and keepers and gave the tortoise husbandry lectures to students at the Royal Veterinary College in London for a number of years. I took into my care many tortoises needing help, support and homes and worked with a number of veterinary professionals to better understand the tortoises' complex needs.

Understanding has moved on tremendously from the early years, as you will see in this book. Tortoise keepers in Europe, Scandinavia and North America have developed extraordinary facilities and accommodation to try to mimic the natural environment for a range of tortoise species now kept in captivity. Zoos have also drastically revised their facilities. Many have become involved in training giant tortoises. The captive environment has been improved through enrichment, bigger enclosures, better lighting and diet, all of which have greatly improved welfare. A number of breeding programmes exist through zoos, and involving private collections, such as the European Studbook Foundation, to support critically endangered species. Programmes to reintroduce endangered species into their home territories with the cooperation of local people have begun.

It has been a privilege and a pleasure to have shared much of my childhood and adult life with tortoises and to contribute to a better understanding of their needs. Ideally of course, like other wild species, these animals would not need our support and could be left in their natural environment, to thrive without human interference. Sadly, that situation is unlikely ever to occur again, and we need to continue to question the ethics and welfare implications of keeping these animals as pets. We need to strive to do our very best for them while we have responsibility for their survival and welfare. This book brings together the understanding and experience I have gained over 30 years, much of that through collaboration with other keepers and veterinary professionals. Attending meetings, conferences and webinars, and making contact with others, has been an important part of my life with tortoises.

Biography

Jane Williams completed her first degree in Zoology from the University of Nottingham, and has a Post Graduate Certificate in Education from the same institution. She has an MA in Education from the Open University. She completed the Post Graduate Diploma in Companion Animal Behaviour Counselling at the University of Southampton, and a research MSc at the same institution. Her research topic was the husbandry and care of captive Mediterranean tortoises in the UK.

Jane is Animal Behaviour and Training Council (ABTC) Registered as a Clinical Animal Behaviourist, and an Animal Training Instructor. Jane was the ABTC Chair (2018–2020) and is currently a Trustee and its Secretary (2020–2024). She has been a full member of the Association of Pet Behaviour Counsellors since 2009, and was its Chair (2017–2020).

Jane has delivered Continuing Professional Development (CPD) for staff in veterinary practices and rescue centres and delivered seminars for owners, veterinary students, schools, colleges and rescue staff on tortoise welfare and behaviour. She has presented at the British Veterinary Nursing Association (BVNA) and written articles on reducing stress for reptiles during veterinary visits and treatment. She regularly presents at the European Turtle Alliance Conference.

Jane has a number of published articles in the field of reptile husbandry and welfare with a focus on tortoises.

Jane lives in Essex, UK, with 35 tortoises, six dogs, five tarantulas and another equally animal-mad human.

Acknowledgements and Thanks

Many people have contributed to this book, and I am grateful to them, along with all the tortoise keepers, helpers, volunteers and professionals I have had the privilege to encounter over the years.

The following tortoise keepers, breeders, friends and wildlife photographers have very kindly allowed me to use their photographs: Eleanor Lien-Hua Tirtasana Chubb, David Smith, William Lewis, Gary Franklin, Sian Bewick, Jackie Foulger, Janet Panter, Elizabeth Chapman, James Sullivan, Dillon Prest, Andy Lewis, Corrine Wayends, Andy Lane, Caroline Sumeray and Matthew Rendle. Chris Leon, Matthew Rendle, Dillon Prest and Andy Lewis have been generous with their time and provided me with very useful information.

Many of the photographs were taken at the rehoming centre of the Norfolk Tortoise Club, UK with Eleanor's kind permission. Special thanks to Eleanor and Jackie, and all the volunteers in Norfolk, for their work in rehoming tortoises for more than 10 years.

Sincere thanks to Frances Baines for allowing me to use her work on artificial lighting sources, including her diagrams of UV Index zones, in Chapter 4.

Martin Lawton, UK Veterinary Surgeon, very kindly reviewed the chapter on diseases and illnesses and is thanked for doing so (Dr M.P.C. Lawton BVetMed; CertVOphthal; CertLAS; CBiol; MRSB; DZooMed; FRCVS; RCVS Recognized Specialist; RCVS Advanced Practitioner in Veterinary Ophthalmology).

William Lewis BVSc, CertZooMed, MRCVS is thanked for allowing the use of his many photographs.

Jim Mackie, and his colleagues at the Zoological Society of London, London Zoo, are thanked for allowing the use of the photographs from their research with their Galapagos tortoises. Jim Mackie and Chris Michaels gave feedback on Chapter 8. Those involved in the research included: Luke Harding (Blue Iguana Conservation), Grant Kother (Animal Behaviour Consultant), Charli Ellis (ZSL), Joe Capon (ZSL), Jim Mackie (ZSL), Thomas Maunders (ZSL), Iri Gill (Chester Zoo), Laura Freeland, Chris Michaels, Matthew Rendle (RVN).

Tortoise South East is our local group, which we started in 1989 to support and advise tortoise keepers. In the early days, The Tortoise Trust was a huge inspiration in improving our husbandry methods. The British Chelonia Group has been supporting important conservation projects for many years, and continues to do so.

At Tortoise South East we have provided help to keepers, through telephone and e-mail support, webinars and workshops, together with local meetings. Myself, Debbie Savage and Sian Bewick have run the regular local meetings and workshops during that time – many thanks to them both.

European Turtle Alliance, of which I am a Board member, is a not-for-profit charitable organization based in the Netherlands. The organization has given me opportunities to meet with many UK, European and North American tortoise keepers, breeders and organizations – all committed to the welfare and conservation of Chelonians worldwide. I am grateful to Eleanor Lien-Hua Tirtasana Chubb for leading that work and inviting me to join the Board.

Anne McBride is thanked for her endorsement on the cover of this book.

Jackie Bingham is thanked for providing the IT skills needed to produce many of the diagrams included in this book.

Sian Bewick has been an editor and critical friend throughout the project. As my partner she has also endured the pains of writing a book with me, and is thanked for her patience and support throughout.

Final thanks go to the tortoises themselves – they are our inspiration and joy. I hope that the information in this book improves their lives while they live with us.

1 What Is a Tortoise?

Abstract

This chapter looks at the different groups of chelonians, or Testudines as they are sometimes called. The four main groups are defined in terms of environment and lifestyle: marine turtles; freshwater turtles; semi-aquatic turtles and terrapins; and terrestrial tortoises. The chapter outlines the features of the group of terrestrial tortoises, which is the focus of this book. Those species that are commonly kept as pets are introduced in photographs.

The chapters of the book are summarized. Meeting the needs of captive terrestrial tortoises by providing them with good health and care while giving the opportunity to show normal behaviours and so maintain their welfare needs is a challenge. The remainder of the book looks at how we can try to meet this challenge.

Introduction – how do we know what a tortoise is?

Most people would say that they know what a tortoise is and could easily recognize one; after all, they all have a shell. Identifying different species has always been contentious (Gerlach, 2012) with some species given several different names. If shown pictures that include not just types of tortoises but also turtles and terrapins, people may be less certain. Which of those pictured in Figs 1.1–1.4 are tortoises? (Vetter, 2002, 2004, 2005, 2006; Pritchard, 1979)

Aren't tortoises, turtles and terrapins just the same thing?

In some countries tortoises, terrapins and turtles are all referred to as 'turtles', while in other countries they are all called 'tortoises'. While tortoises, turtles and terrapins all belong to the classification group Chelonia (a word that comes from the Greek word for tortoise), they are not all the same thing.

Chelonians can be divided into the following subgroups, based on where they live and their lifestyle: (1) marine turtles; (2) freshwater turtles; (3) semi-aquatic turtles and terrapins; and (4) terrestrial tortoises.

1. Marine turtles

Marine turtles (as their name suggests) spend most of their life at sea, the females coming to land only to lay their eggs in holes dug on sandy beaches. Other than that, they roam the oceans, sleeping at the surface, searching for a mate and feeding on a variety of plants and animals, including jellyfish and sponges. Only seven species of marine turtle exist today. Some are very large indeed. The Leatherback turtle, for example, can grow to 3 metres in length and weigh up to 900 kg. For obvious reasons marine turtles are not common as pets, although some can be seen in zoos and aquaria. All are endangered because of human activity, some critically so, to the point of near extinction. They are killed for food or for their shells, which can be used for making jewellery, sunglasses and souvenirs. Their eggs are dug up and eaten. They become entangled in fishing nets and lines and drown, unable to reach the surface to breathe the air they need to stay alive. Loss of habitat, excessive hunting, coastal development and marine pollution are also factors that negatively impact populations.

2. Freshwater turtles

These are the freshwater equivalents of marine turtles, living in large bodies of water such as lakes and rivers, coming out only for egg-laying. Around 300 species of freshwater/semi-aquatic turtles have been identified and classified. Like the marine turtles, some are very large. The Yangtze Giant Softshell turtle (*Rafetus swinhoei*), for example, grows to 1.5 metres in length and weighs over 93 kg. Unfortunately, this turtle is likely to become extinct shortly. Only two

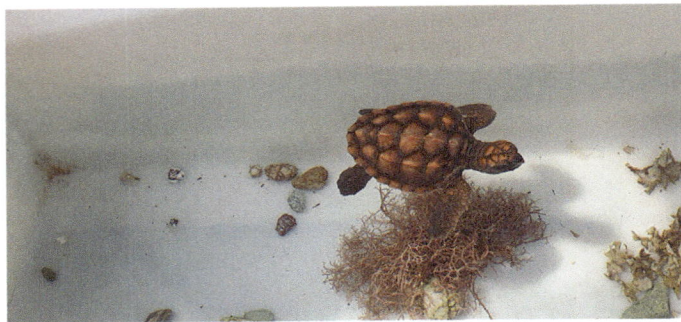
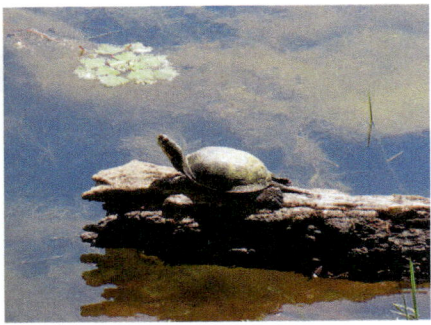

Fig. 1.1. Loggerhead turtles (Matthew Rendle).

Fig. 1.2. Freshwater turtles: European pond turtle *Emys orbicularis* (Janet Panter).

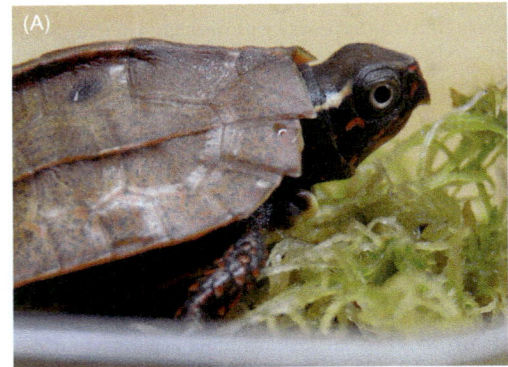
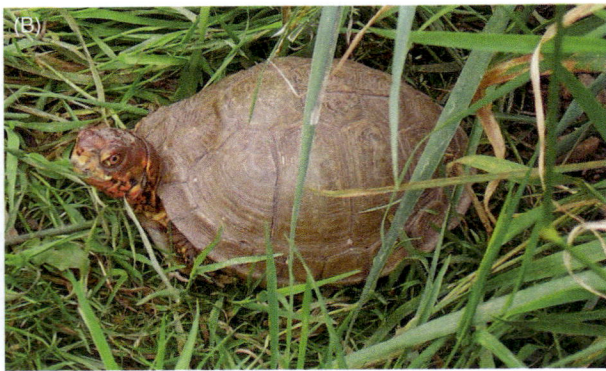

Fig. 1.3. Semi-aquatic turtles and terrapins: (A) Vietnamese leaf turtle *Geoemyda spengleri*. (B) American box turtle *Terrapene carolina*.

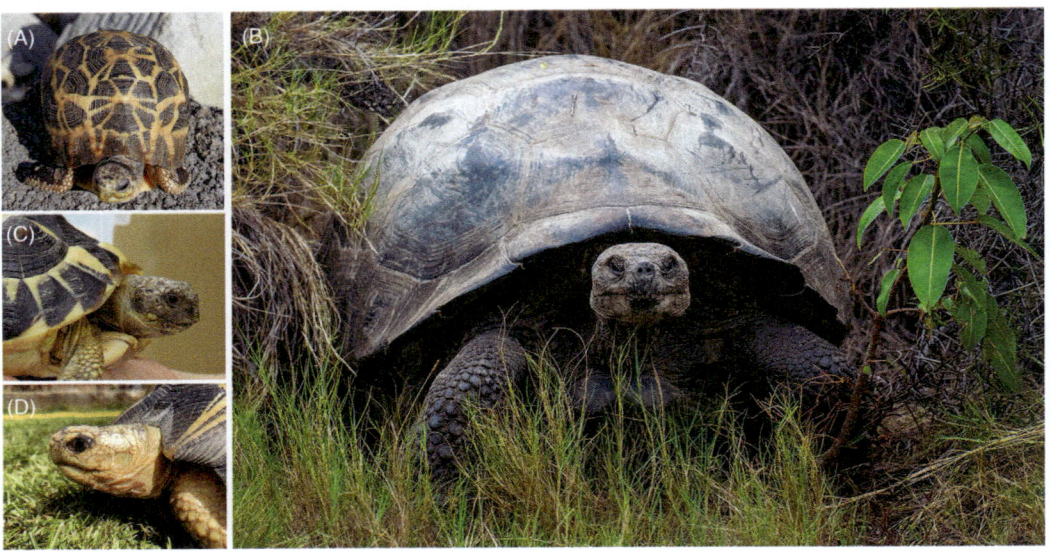

Fig. 1.4. Terrestrial tortoises: (A) Madagascan spider tortoise *Pyxis arachnoides*. (B) Galapagos tortoise *Chelonoidis nigra* (Gary Franklin). (C) Hermanns tortoise *Testudo hermanni*). (D) Radiated tortoise *Astrocehlys radiata*.

male Yangtze Giant Softshell turtles are known to exist, the last known female being found dead in May 2023. A valuable food source, freshwater turtles are particularly vulnerable to human predation and suffer too from habitat reduction. As with the marine turtles, larger species are rarely kept as pets. Smaller species can have very attractive shell colours and patterns and some are kept in captivity.

3. Semi-aquatic turtles and terrapins:

What makes these animals different is that they spend part of their time in water and part of their time on land. There are around 14 species referred to as terrapins. They are equally at home in both environments, as long as they can keep moist. While most generally seek freshwater and can be found in rivers and ponds, some species are capable of living in brackish (slightly salty) water, such as that found in estuaries. As well as swimming at the water's surface they are frequently seen sunbathing on rocks and logs or walking through wet and swampy vegetation. They tend to be a lot smaller than the freshwater and marine turtles. As with other chelonians, semi-aquatic turtles and terrapins are threatened by humans. Some are hunted for food, or suffer habitat loss, whilst others are targeted by the pet trade. The beautiful markings on the shells, heads and legs of some species make them very desirable. Because of this they are taken from the wild in unsustainable numbers.

4. Terrestrial tortoises:

What makes tortoises unique amongst chelonians is that they are adapted to live solely on land. Although they may wade into shallow ponds to drink, they do not permanently inhabit rivers, ponds or seas. More than 50 different species of tortoise have been identified, spread across the continents of the world except Australia (where only freshwater/semi-aquatic and marine species are found) and Antarctica.

The largest tortoises tend to live on islands, such as the Galapagos tortoise (Fig. 1.5), which reaches a length of up to 1.3 metres and can weight up to 400 kg when adult.

Others, such as the Aldabran tortoise (from the Seychelles) and the Sulcata (from Africa), are nearly as big, as shown in Fig. 1.6.

Most tortoises are considerably smaller than these enormous specimens, however. One of the smallest sometimes seen in captivity is the Egyptian tortoise (*Testudo kleinmanni*), which measures only 12 cm in length and weighs around 400 g when fully grown. The smallest tortoise species is the Speckled Padloper (*Homopus signatus*) from the South African Cape, which weighs in at 95–165 g and is only 6–10 cm in length. Some examples of tortoise species seen in captivity are shown in Fig. 1.7.

The fact that tortoises are land-dwelling and come in a convenient range of sizes and types has contributed to them becoming popular as pets. Some animals are specifically bred for the pet trade, but unfortunately many are still collected from the wild, severely depleting local populations. In some regions tortoises are still hunted for food or collected to turn into ornaments or jewellery (Fig. 1.8) for tourists, which has been continuing for hundreds of years (Young, 2003).

As with all chelonians, tortoises face the major problem of habitat destruction as more and more of their natural environment is removed to create farmland or housing. In Europe, for example, there is virtually no primary habitat remaining for Mediterranean tortoises (see Chapter 13 on Mediterranean tortoises). Much of the habitat has been destroyed by tourism, especially near the coast (Fig. 1.9).

Conclusion

Chelonians all have the same body pattern and basic features (Table 1.1). The differences between the terrestrial tortoises and other species are due to their need to walk, climb and dig on land. They also have differences in shell shape, size and patterning related to temperature regulation, camouflage and protection against predators, compared with their aquatic and semi-aquatic relatives.

This group of reptiles is superbly adapted to suit the environment. Their success is demonstrated by their evolution around 200 million years ago, and the degree to which different species have spread across the globe. Although restricted to warmer climates by the need for external body heat from the sun, as are reptiles generally, land-based tortoises are found across much of the Americas, Europe, Africa and Asia, including of course the island species such as the Galapagos and Aldabran tortoises.

In this book we will be focusing on tortoises, the chelonians most commonly kept as pets across the globe. We will:

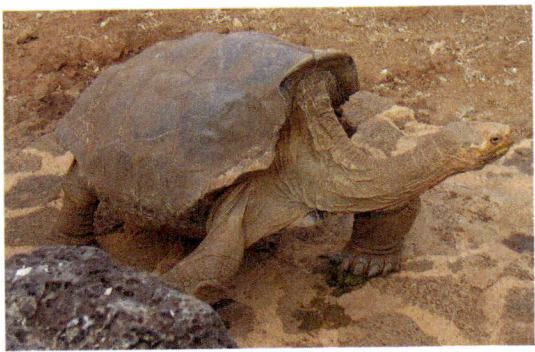

Fig. 1.5. Galapagos tortoise – Saddleback *Chelonoidis nigra* averages 250 kg in weight.

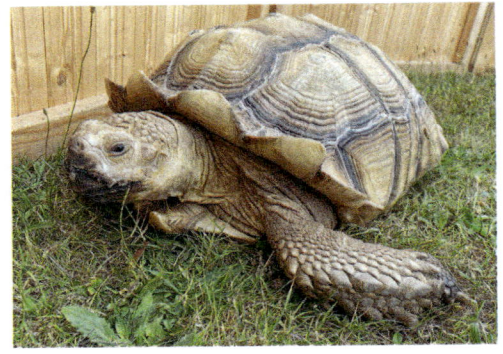

Fig. 1.6. *Geochelone* (more recently *Centrochelys sulcata*) Sulcata – can reach 100 kg.

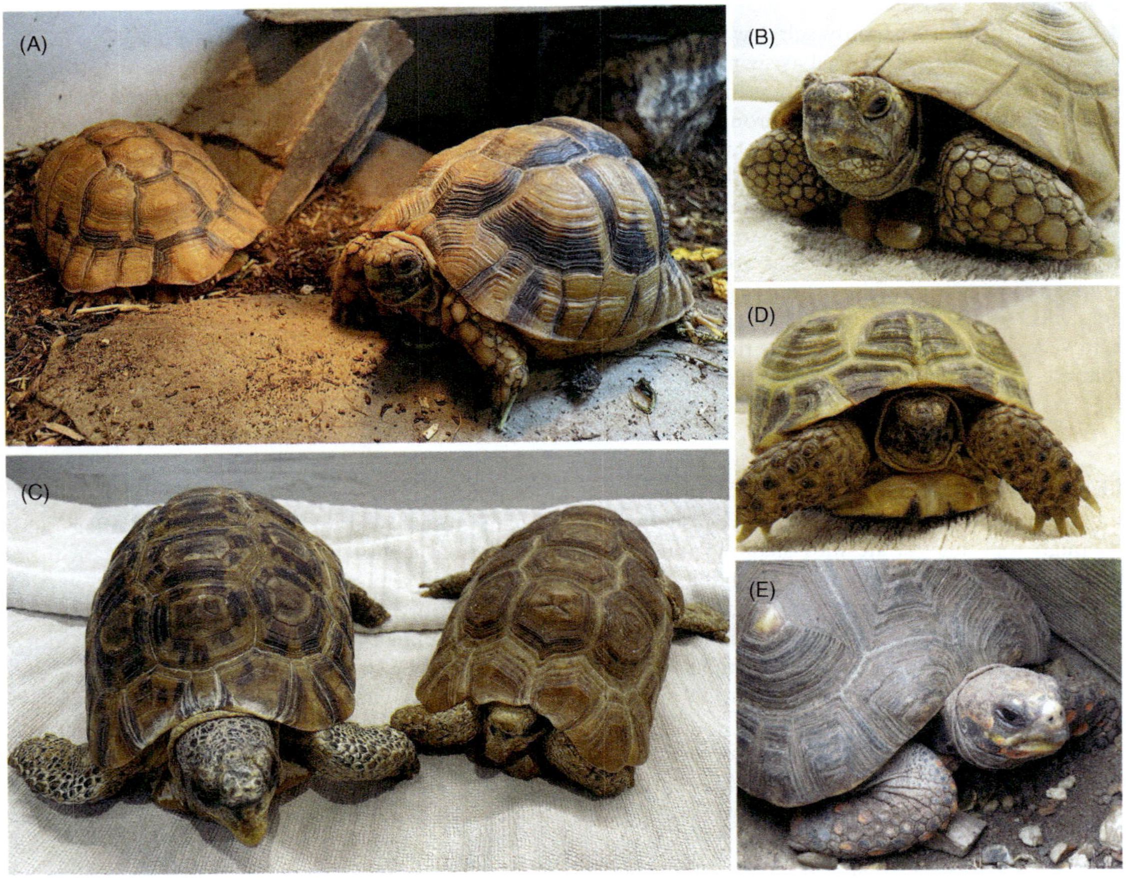

Fig. 1.7. (A) *Testudo kleinmanni* Kleinmann's – 200–400 g. (B) *Testudo graeca graeca* Spur-thighed – 0.5–3.0 kg. (C) *Kinixys belliana* Bell's Hingeback – averages 2 kg. (D) *Testudo horsfieldi* Horsfield's – averages 200 g. (E) *Chelonoidis carbonaria* Red-footed – large females can weigh 5 kg.

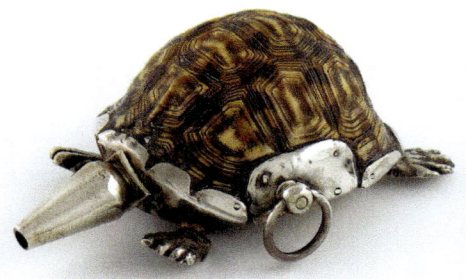

Fig. 1.8. Tortoise artefact – tortoiseshell silver-mounted powder flask c. 1850.

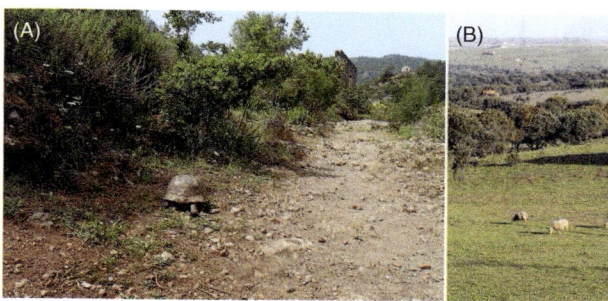

Fig. 1.9. (A) Before human development. (B) Farmed Mediterranean habitat with little grazing left.

Table 1.1. Chelonia classification (adapted from Rayment-Dyble, 2019).

Kingdom: Animalia – Animals	
Phylum: Chordata – Animals with a vertebral column (backbone)	
Class: Reptilia – Reptiles (scaly-skinned vertebrates)	
Order: Chelonia (Reptiles with a shell)	
Suborder – Pleurodira Side-necked chelonians	The head is withdrawn sideways (horizontally) into the shell. These are Southern Hemisphere freshwater turtles. Examples: African side-neck turtles; Spot-bellied side-neck turtles; Red-bellied side-neck turtles
Suborder – Cryptodira Hidden-necked chelonians	The head is withdrawn into an S-shape vertically into the shell. This is the majority of chelonians. Examples: Marine turtles; River turtles; Mud turtles; Musk turtles; Soft-shelled turtles; Tortoises

- look at tortoise biology and consider how that influences what we need to do to keep our tortoises healthy and to ensure that they can show all their natural behaviours;
- explore the history of keeping tortoises as human companions, examining how tortoise keeping has boomed in popularity since the Victorian age;
- discuss how good husbandry can promote good health, looking at the environmental, nutritional and management requirements of a range of the most commonly kept tortoise species;
- consider tortoise behaviour, both its individual and group aspects, and question to what extent tortoises can think, learn and be trained;
- investigate the practicalities and ethics of breeding tortoises in captive environments;
- describe some of the most common tortoise diseases and illnesses and consider causes and treatment with the emphasis on improving husbandry as well as more complex veterinary procedures;
- consider what skills and resources we need to be effective tortoise keepers and think about how best we can support captive tortoises to ensure that they are happy and healthy; and
- consider the future of tortoise-keeping going forward in the 2020s and beyond.

References and Further Reading

Gerlach, J. (2012) *The Great Survivors*. Phelsuma, Cambridge, UK.

Pritchard, P.C.H. (1979) *Encyclopedia of Turtles*. TFH Publications, Reigate, UK, and Neptune, New Jersey.

Rayment-Dyble, L. (2019) Ch 2 Reptile pet trade and welfare. In: Girling, S.J. and Raiti, P. (eds) *BSAVA Manual of Reptiles*, 3rd edn. BSAVA, Quedgeley, UK, pp. 26–35.

Vetter, H. (2002) *Turtles of the World Vol. 1, Africa, Europe and Western Asia*. Chimaira, Frankfurt

Vetter, H. (2004) *Turtles of the World Vol. 2, North America*. Chimaira, Frankfurt

Vetter, H. (2005) *Turtles of the World Vol. 3, Central & South America*. Chimaira, Frankfurt.

Vetter, H. (2006) *Turtles of the World Vol. 4, East and South Asia*. Chimaira, Frankfurt.

Young, P. (2003) *Tortoise*. Reaktion Books, London

2 How Tortoise Biology Affects Health and Behaviour

Abstract

This chapter sets tortoises in the taxonomic context of the animal kingdom as reptiles. The chapter examines the basics of tortoise biology – anatomy, structure, physiology and reproduction. The biological adaptations that have made tortoises so successful over the past 300 million years are described. Their ability to survive is greatly enhanced by their most obvious feature – their shell. The shell as a protective feature is described. The role of the skin and shell in camouflage and thermoregulation within this group of ectotherms is discussed. Tortoises are extremely well-adapted to live in a range of habitats, often in situations where there is limited water. The value of their waterproof skin and scales, together with an outline of how their senses function, makes up the main content of this chapter. They reproduce sexually using internal fertilization and are all egg-layers. Environmental sex determination is seen in tortoises, as a result of the specific temperatures experienced while developing in the egg.

What is a reptile?

Like all chelonians, tortoises belong to the larger classification group known as reptiles. Reptiles evolved from ancestral amphibians around 220–235 million years ago (Gerlach, 2012). Figures 2.1 and 2.2 are examples of modern amphibians. Rather than remaining water-dependent like amphibians, reptiles gradually became better adapted to living in dry habitats. This enabled them to spread far and wide, and so colonize many of the Earth's land masses.

The reptile group is a diverse collection of vertebrate animals. All reptiles possess an internal or endoskeleton, the spinal cord being encased within the vertebral column (spine) and the brain held within the skull. As well as chelonians, reptiles include a huge range of species (Table 2.1).

Tortoises are related to all these animals, having evolved from a common ancestor (Gerlach, 2012), see Table 2.2.

Reptiles are tetrapods with four limbs. Even the snakes, which have largely lost their legs, retain vestiges of this feature as part of their internal skeleton, which shows where the pelvis was originally located.

Reptiles breathe air, even those species that are aquatic or semi-aquatic, such as marine turtles and marine iguanas. They respire aerobically, breathing oxygen into their lungs and breathing out carbon dioxide as a waste product. Even those reptiles well adapted to aquatic life must access air in order to breathe through their paired lungs.

Many reptiles have the ability to produce a highly concentrated urine, which is the excretory product from protein metabolism. The nitrogen-containing waste products are urates. This is an adaption to living in dry and arid conditions, allowing them to survive on very little water.

In addition, they have a distinctive skin of scales and plates designed to retain moisture and to provide protection and camouflage, as shown in Fig. 2.12. The scales that cover the body are waterproof, helping them to retain water. The skin is adapted to form a hard protective shell in some species, e.g. tortoises Fig. 2.13.

Signalling and communication with humans, and each other, is often limited by the hard nature of these scales and plates, so identifying a reptile's emotional state is not easy (see Chapter 9 on emotional states).

Reptiles are ectothermic. This means that they are unable to generate heat internally like mammals and birds can. Because of this, reptiles rely on external heat sources like the sun for warmth. Without warmth their body's metabolic processes would stop functioning. Reptiles regulate their temperature largely through behaviour, basking when cold or hiding when they get too hot (Fig. 2.14). Chapter 8, on behaviour and learning, looks at a range of thermoregulatory behaviours, as do the chapters on health (Chapter 6) and specific species (Chapters 13–17).

Reptiles feed in a variety of different ways. Some, such as snakes and the Gila Monster, are venomous

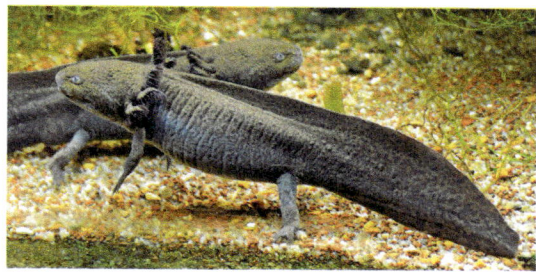

Fig. 2.1. Amphibian – Axolotl (David Smith).

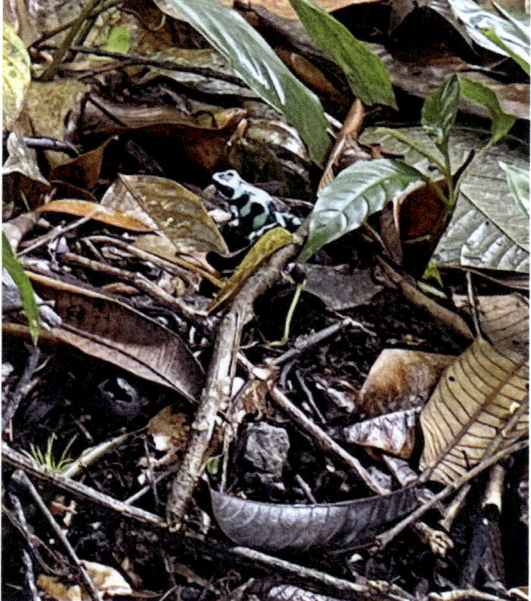

Fig. 2.2. Amphibian – Green and Black Poison-dart frog (*Dendrobates auratus*).

and kill their prey with poison. Other carnivorous reptiles include crocodiles and chameleons (Fig. 2.15). Some, like Red-footed tortoises, are omnivorous (Fig. 2.17), and eat a mixture of plants and animals. Many reptiles are completely herbivorous, including many of the tortoises (Fig. 2.16).

Reptile reproduction is sexual and involves internal fertilization. The males and females of different species may be very similar in appearance, as seen in the tortoises. Often the female is larger than the male, to allow for egg production within the body. Most reptiles produce eggs. Some, such as Pit vipers, produce live offspring. Where eggs are produced, they have a hard or leathery waterproof surface, or shell, to retain water (Fig. 2.18).

What types of chelonians (Testudines) are there today?

Living tortoises and turtles are grouped as two sub-orders according to the way in which they withdraw their heads as a response to danger (Table 2.3) (Gerlach, 2012):

Testudines can live in the sea, in freshwater or on land. Some combine their habitats to spend the majority of time in one habitat, but they all lay eggs on land in a nest. The marine turtles have to come ashore to lay eggs on beaches, for example. Freshwater terrapins and turtles lay their eggs in a nest dug into the soil substrate. Semi-aquatic species spend time in the water but often bask on logs and on the land, and may sometimes feed on the land. Figure 2.19 shows the regions of the world where tortoises are found.

Why are the chelonians (Testudines) special reptiles?

Chelonians are the only reptiles to have a shell. This large, bony structure encloses and protects the soft vital organs of the body, as seen in Fig. 2.20. The surface of the shell is usually very hard and covered in waterproof, pigmented scutes. (Aquatic soft-shelled turtles lack these scutes, so their bodies look and feel soft, see Fig. 2.21.)

As we focus on tortoises in this book, we now look in more detail at tortoise biology, examining how biology influences behaviour and how it might impact on tortoise health.

Looking at tortoises from the outside

The shell

All tortoises have a protective shell made up of the carapace (the domed top half) and the plastron (the lower flatter shell). The vertebral column, containing the spinal cord, is fused together as part of the carapace (Fig. 2.22). It is not possible for a tortoise to separate the rest of its body from its shell and run away, leaving the shell behind, despite what some cartoon illustrators might have you believe (Fig. 2.23).

The shell is essentially made of bone, but what we see is a very thin layer of epidermal tissue made of keratin (like the tissue that makes up our fingernails and hair). This forms individual plates or scutes over the bone (Fig. 2.24). The shells of very young tortoises are slightly flexible at first, but as the tortoises ages the shell quickly stiffens to become hard and dry (Fig. 2.25).

Table 2.1. Reptile groups.

Snakes	Iguanas	Geckos	Crocodiles
Green tree python (*Morelia viridis*) (Fig. 2.3, David Smith) 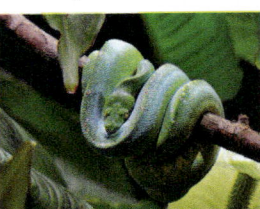	Green iguana (*Igunana igunana*) (Fig. 2.4, David Smith) 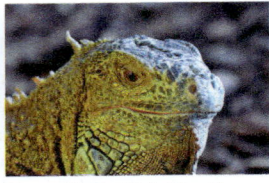 Emerald Basilisk (*Basiliscus plumifrons*) (Fig. 2.5) 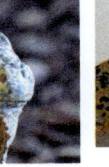	Leopard gecko (*Eublepharis macularius*) (Fig. 2.6) 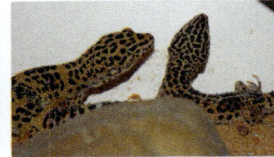	Cuban crocodile (*Crocodylus rhombifer*) (Fig. 2.7, David Smith) 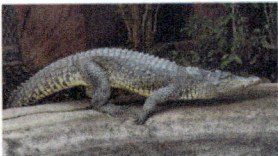
Lizards	**Chameleons**	**Tuatara**	**Tortoises**
Malachite Spiny lizard (*Sceloporus malatichicus*) (Fig. 2.8) 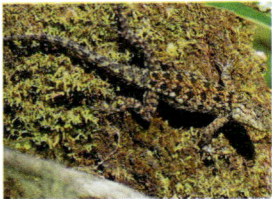 Komodo Dragon (Fig. 2.9, David Smith) 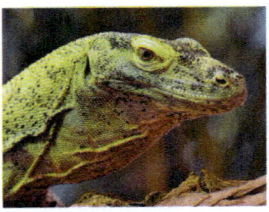	Veiled chameleon (Fig. 2.10, David Smith) 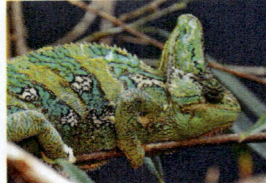	Order Rhynchocephalia Lizard endemic to New Zealand, all other examples now extinct.	Spur-thighed tortoise (*Testudo graeca*) (Fig. 2.11) 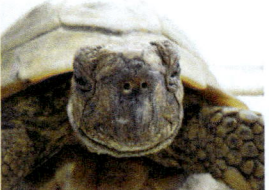

As the tortoise gets older new layers of plate form as part of the growth process. In younger tortoises this is visible as clear ridges and grooves on the scutes. In older tortoises the scutes can become flatter and shinier as the ridges are smoothed out over time (Fig. 2.26). In captive-bred tortoises the shell can be very shiny and takes on a more plastic appearance. This is because the shell is not subject to the wear and tear of the wild. Captive-bred tortoises that are growing very fast also have

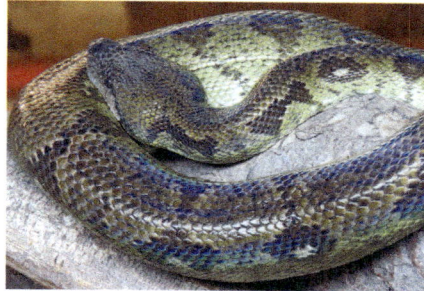

Fig. 2.12. Python scales and pattern.

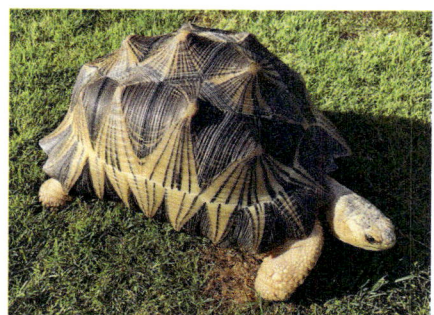

Fig. 2.13. Radiated tortoise shell, pattern and camouflage.

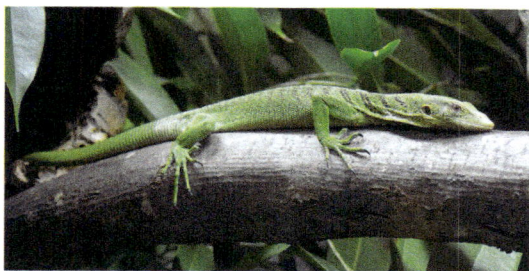

Fig. 2.14. Reptile – Emerald tree monitor basking (David Smith).

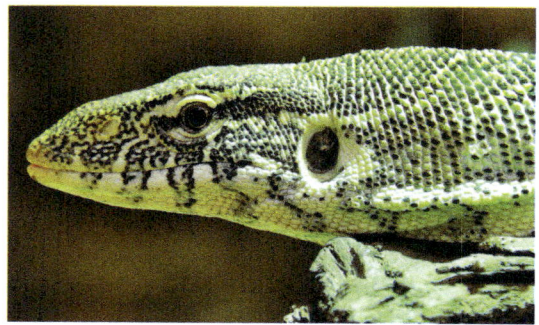

Fig. 2.15 Nile monitor, hunting (David Smith).

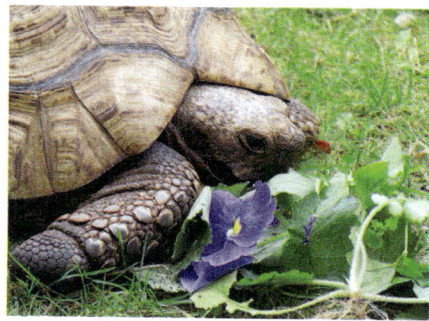

Fig. 2.16. Leopard tortoise *Centrochelys pardalis* grazing on grass and wild flowers.

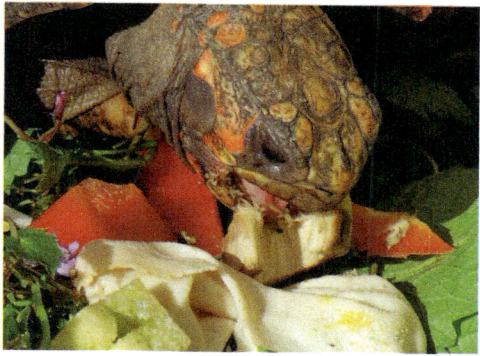

Fig. 2.17. Red-footed tortoises *Chelonoidis carbonaria* eating a mix of foods including weeds, mushrooms, fruit and chicken, supplemented with Nutrobal®.

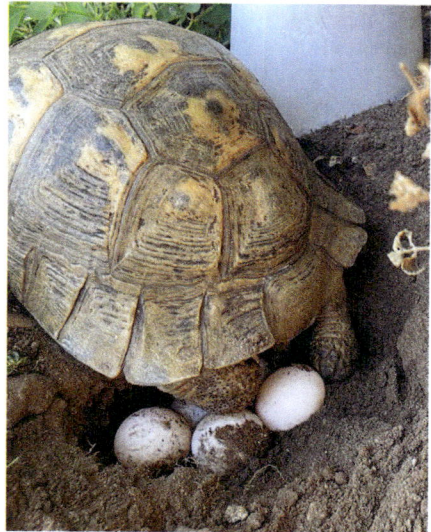

Fig. 2.18. Tortoise laying eggs in nest (Caroline Sumeray).

How Tortoise Biology Affects Health and Behaviour

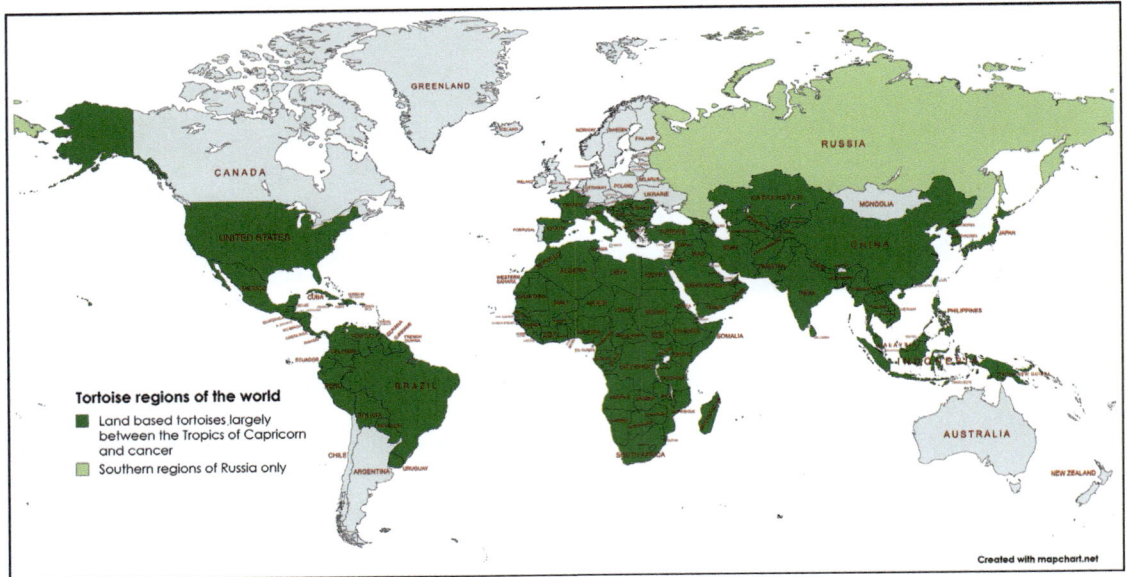

Fig. 2.19. Map of tortoise regions of the world. (source: https://www.mapchart.net/world.html)

Table 2.2. Tortoise classification or taxonomy.

Kingdom – Animalia (Animals)	Living organisms that can move
Phylum – Chordata (Vertebrates)	Animals with backbones
Class – Reptilia (Reptiles)	Reptiles have a scaly skin
Order – Testudinae (Testudines) (also called Chelonia) (Tortoises/Turtles/Terrapins = shelled reptiles)	Tortoises have a shell for protection and camouflage

Table 2.3. Sub-orders Pleurodira and Cryptodira.

Sub-order Pleurodira	Sub-order Cryptodira
Side-necked Testudines	Hidden-necked Testudines
Withdraw the head sideways into the shell	Withdraw the head in a vertical plane into the shell
Strong snapping jaw action	More powerful but slower jaw-closing action
Aquatic predators – carnivores	Includes carnivores, omnivores and herbivores

very sharply defined lines between the growth areas and the pigmented parts of the scutes. The more defined these lines are, the faster the growth that has taken place. Very rapid growth can cause significant health problems for juveniles (see Chapter 7 on common illnesses and diseases).

The shell provides protection to the soft internal organs. It also has a role in temperature regulation. Patterns on the shell provide camouflage. A tortoise might be easily seen against the background of a plain green lawn but will become almost invisible when in a more varied, natural habitat with a variety of plants (Fig. 2.27).

Any disadvantages of carrying around a weighty shell, and investing so many bodily resources into it, are greatly outweighed by the protection and camouflage it provides. In evolutionary terms, the shell has been a hugely advantageous adaptation to survival, which is why it has remained largely unchanged for around 220 million years. Tortoises are sometimes called 'living fossils' for this reason (Gerlach, 2012).

How does the shell affect behaviour and what do we need to look out for?

- Sensitivity to touch makes the shell a hugely important organ in terms of feeling and keeping safe. Tortoises can feel the heat from our hands if we touch them or pick them up – something that they find stressful. They like to have all their feet on the ground and will react if their feet are taken off a solid surface (see Chapters 8 and 9 on behaviour and emotional states, respectively).

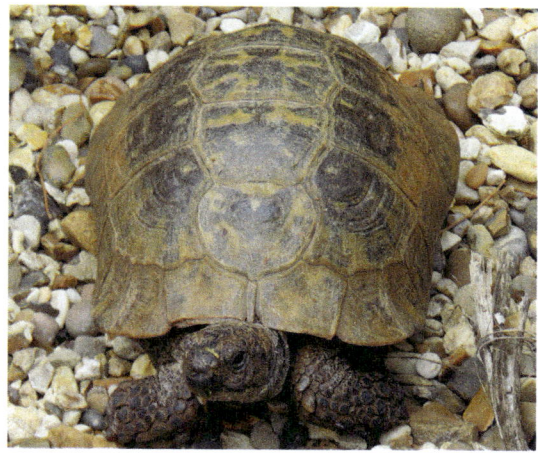

Fig. 2.20. Tortoise with hard shell.

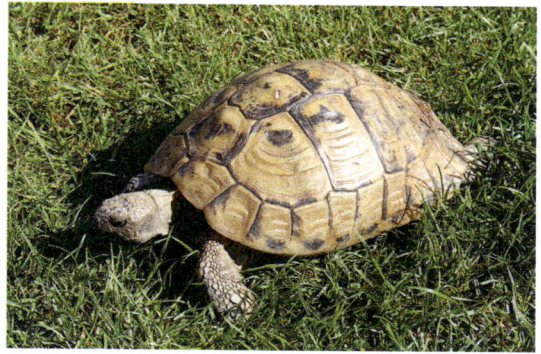

Fig. 2.23. Female Hermann's tortoise *Testudo hermanni* showing carapace and plastron, shell pattern, limbs and head. Sparta is a wild-caught tortoise imported into the UK before the ban in 1984.

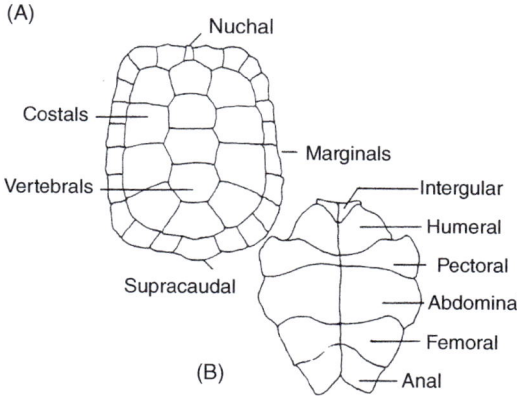

Fig. 2.24. Scutes of carapace (A) and plastron (B).

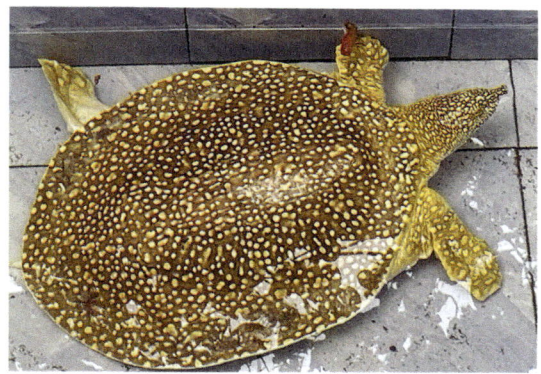

Fig. 2.21. Soft-shelled turtle *Trionyx triungis* (Matthew Rendle).

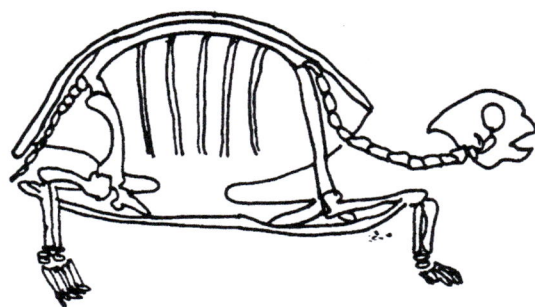

Fig. 2.22. Tortoise skeleton.

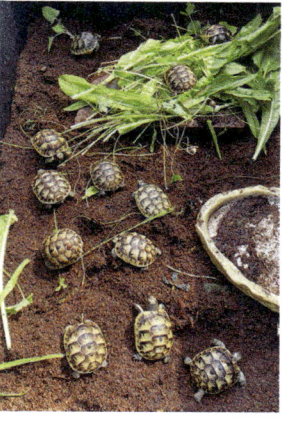

Fig. 2.25. Young tortoises – juvenile Spur-thighed less than 2 years old, with very clearly patterned shells.

How Tortoise Biology Affects Health and Behaviour | 11

This can often be seen during a visit to the veterinary practice, when the tortoise may be lifted up for examination. As reported in Williams and Beck (2021), this is very stressful for the tortoise.
- Thermoregulation – the shell acts like a large radiator, able to both absorb and give off heat as required during thermoregulation. This is a survival mechanism preventing the tortoise from overheating or being burned by excess heat. Tortoises are sensitive to even the slight changes in temperature when we hold them (Scheelings, 2019).
- Pulling body and limbs into shell for protection – this is an important survival mechanism to escape from predators. Once withdrawn, the tortoise is much more difficult to injure or eat. Even lions who live in the same areas as Sulcatas and Leopard tortoises are unable to bite through their thick shells (Fig. 2.28).

In male Leopard tortoises the gap between the plastron and carapace at the tail is very narrow, to prevent predators gaining access (Fig. 2.29). Female Leopard tortoises are more vulnerable. The gap is not so narrow, as the opening needs to be larger to allow eggs to pass. The scales on their front legs are very tough and strong to prevent access to the head when it is pulled in. The front legs create an effective seal and a smooth surface that makes it difficult for a predator to grasp any part of the leg.

If a tortoise has a deformed shell, or one that is too small for its body size, this protection is not effective (as shown in Fig. 2.30). An overweight or obese tortoise may find it impossible to withdraw fully into its shell. A hiss is often heard as a tortoise withdraws quickly into its shell. This used to be thought of as a sign of alarm but is in fact more likely to be caused by the sudden intake of breath caused by its lungs being suddenly squeezed and the breath expelled rapidly.

- The shell is strong but light enough to allow some species of tortoises to swim (for some time at least). Large Leopard tortoises have been observed swimming across lakes, but this is not the natural location for terrestrial tortoises (Highfield, 1996; Highfield and Highfield, 2009).

Tortoises have to be able to get out of any water they enter, using shallow slopes. If there is no escape (for example, the tortoise falls into a pond with no sloping edges), the tortoise will drown, because it has to breathe air and the shell and body weight ultimately weigh it down. Every year we hear of tortoises that have sadly fallen into a pond and drowned, even though they can survive for reasonable periods under water.

They achieve this by shutting down and reducing their demand for oxygen, similar to the method used during hibernation (McArthur et al., 2004). One year we were contacted by someone whose tortoise had been in a pond for 8 hours before being discovered and rescued. The owners were distraught and had tried to revive the tortoise, to no avail. They left it on the lawn for 24 hours but no change, so they buried it in their garden. Fortunately it was a shallow grave, because 3 days later much to their amazement the tortoise was out and about walking around the garden. The animal was very unwell, with eye infections and pneumonia due to the water in its lungs. With veterinary treatment, support and antibiotics the tortoise survived.

- The shell looks strong, and is strong in most natural situations, but when faced with some scenarios created by humans the shell is vulnerable to damage. For example, being dropped on concrete is likely to cause significant damage and may split the shell open. Lawnmowers, garden forks, spades and other garden implements can be serious hazards – all contain metal or moving parts that can break or split the shell. Being run over by vehicles on roads in their home countries is an all-too-common occurrence, but tortoises are also capable of surviving disastrous wounds. At times tortoises with big holes in their shell have managed to heal over time, and they survive and carry on as normal (Fig. 2.31).

Drilling holes in shells was once a common practice in the UK. A string was tied through the hole as an attempt to ensure that the owner did not lose the tortoise. This was at a time when secure tortoise gardens and enclosures were a distant tortoise dream. The hole was drilled through the bony shell itself, not just the dead keratin of the scutes (Fig. 2.32). This is enormously painful (equivalent to drilling a hole through your thumb, including the bone) and would cause bleeding and potential infection. Such practices cannot be justified as a humane way to keep a tortoise. The tortoise, if not supervised, then had the additional hazard of the string, which in some cases wound around legs, cutting off the circulation and leading to the loss of a limb.

- Painting of shells so that tortoises were easier to find, or to identify if they had gone walkabout, was once common as well. We have a tortoise that visits us for holidays whose shell was completely painted over with porcelain paint such as that used to repair sinks. The paint has now largely been removed.

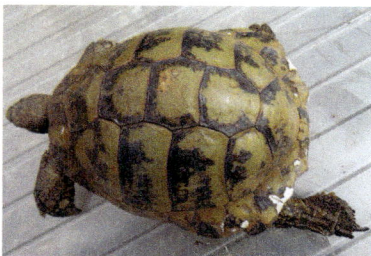

Fig. 2.26. Older tortoise – ancient Hermann's tortoise. Bony, a small male, one of mine taken in through rescue, was wild-caught into the UK before the 1984 ban. Very blurred, indistinct shell pattern and plenty of signs of wear and tear, with some old bone showing through from previous damage.

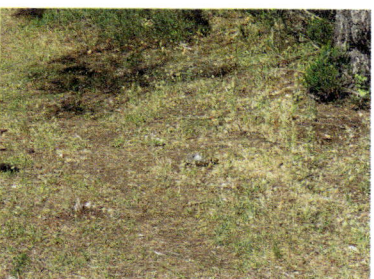

Fig. 2.27. Spot the tortoise! It is well-camouflaged in the natural habitat.

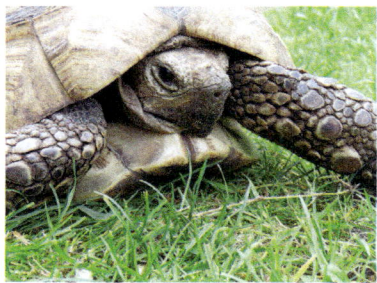

Fig. 2.28. Thick shell of a Leopard tortoise.

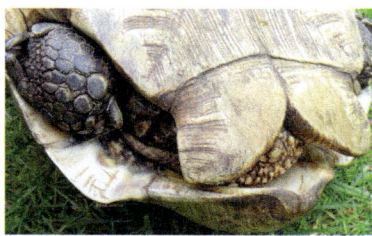

Fig. 2.29. Male Leopard tortoise (*Centrochelys pardalis*) with tail fully protected by the shell.

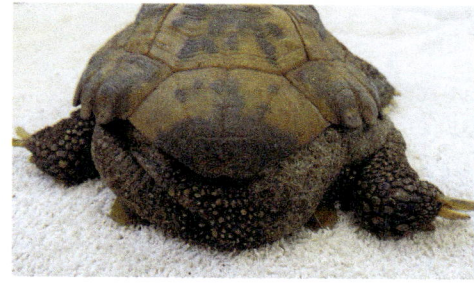

Fig. 2.30. Sulawesi tortoise *Indotestudo forstenii* with deformed shell and exposed rear legs and tail from poor diet.

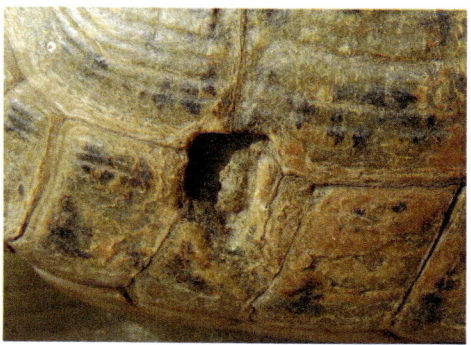

Fig. 2.31. Live tortoise with self-healed shell damage.

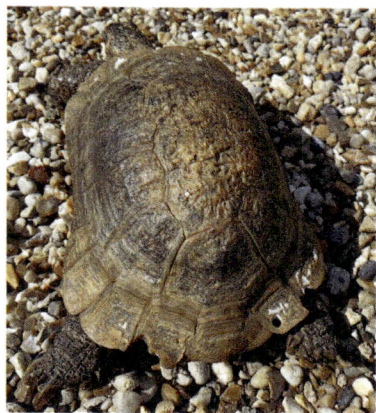

Fig. 2.32. Spur-thighed tortoise with a hole drilled in its shell, which was common at one time to avoid losing the tortoise rather than creating a safe enclosure. This poor tortoise, an elderly Spur-thighed, has had this done multiple times, as evidenced by the shell loss on the left where the hole has caused the shell to break. The hole has been lost so another has been drilled into the rear right side of the carapace, through shell and bone, causing great pain.

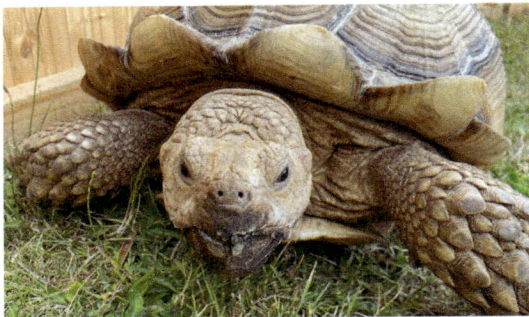

Fig. 2.33. Scales on head and legs of a Sulcata (*Centrochelys sulcata*) are strong and hard and very waterproof.

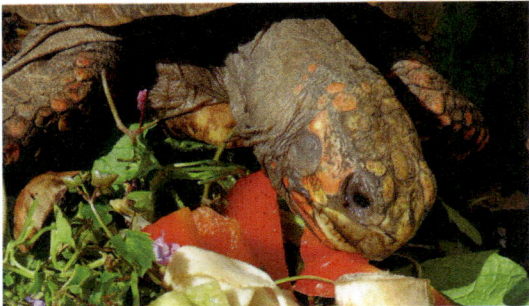

Fig. 2.34. Skin with smaller softer scales and moister, including around the eyes – Red-footed tortoise (*Chelonoidis carbonaria*).

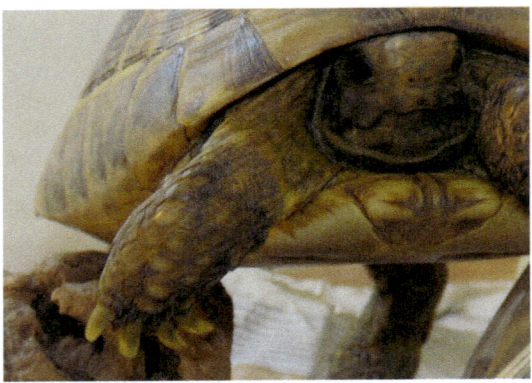

Fig. 2.35. Claws of normal length blunted by walking.

Putting olive oil onto shells to make them shiny was once thought to be good practice. It was believed that the oil would keep the shell clean and supple. In fact, it had the opposite effect. The oil makes the shell gather dirt and it sticks there. The oil also has a

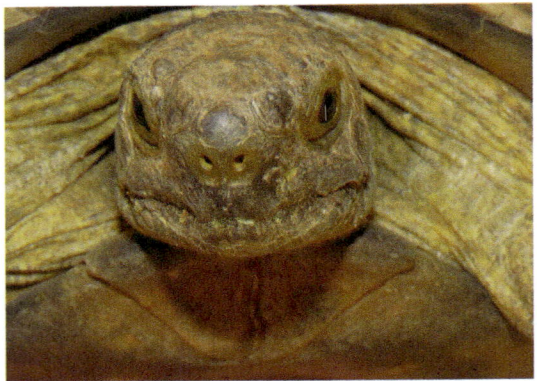

Fig. 2.36. Tortoise beak – normal length on Spur-thighed tortoise.

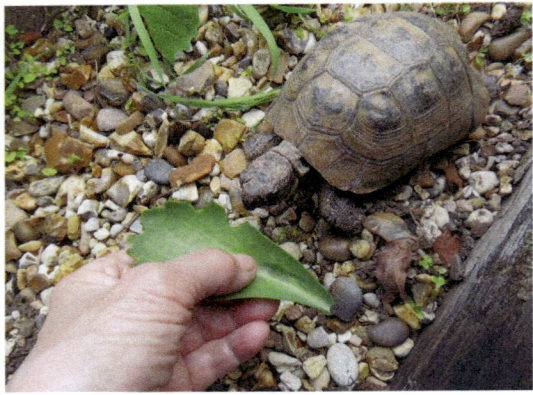

Fig. 2.37. Leaf with bite cut out from tortoise beak.

detrimental effect on the shell in hot sun (as it would if you sunbathed in olive oil). The effect would be like being roasted. Coating the shell in anything unnatural is potentially very harmful to the tortoise.

I once looked after a Spider tortoise (*Pixys arachnoides*) that had previously belonged to a nightclub owner, who had used it as a living ornament and entertainment for customers. Glitter had been stuck all over the carapace of the shell using glue, and then with a large piece of Blu Tack® in the middle of the shell, an open cocktail umbrella had been added. All of which would have been very damaging to the well-being of the tortoise.

- Nutritional deficiencies show up in shell growth – a shell can become too thick and may prevent the body from properly fitting into it. Pyramiding is the first sign of abnormal shell growth in juveniles, with the shell growing in a lumpy way rather than having a smoothly domed carapace.

Sometimes weak shells collapse along the vertebral column, or across the pelvis, pulling the back of the shell downwards, thus making the size of the body cavity within too small. The deformities can be enormous and affect the tortoise's ability to breathe, walk and reproduce (see Chapter 5 on diets and Chapter 7 on common illnesses and diseases).

- A normal loss of scutes with age is seen in older tortoises, along with chipping and slight scute damage. In some cases, previous damage allows the bone underneath to be seen, as in Fig. 2.26. New bone can also be seen showing through before the new scutes grow. Any looseness of the scutes indicates that infection from bacteria or fungi may be underlying. This is often called shell rot and can be quite extensive before an owner notices. Similarly any bleeding in the shell, or redness, may indicate infection and will need veterinary treatment (see Chapter 7 on common illnesses and diseases).
- Courtship rituals can involve shell-bashing by the male. The damage caused is usually to the back of the female's shell. In the wild the female might allow him to mate before she walks away. In captivity, if the female is trapped with a male in an enclosure that is too small or where she has no shelter, she is unable to escape. Prolonged shell-bashing behaviour under such circumstances can cause significant damage. Usually, it is best to keep female tortoises separately from males, for the majority of the time, in order to prevent stress and injury (see Chapter 11 on breeding). Some males may have to be kept entirely on their own as they will ram and batter other males too.

The Skin

A tortoise's head and limbs extend out from its shell. They are covered by an impermeable skin encased in scales. As this prevents the tortoise from drying out and dehydrating, it is an adaptation to life on land. Tortoises can feel vibrations through their skin and shell. This makes them aware of any approaching animal.

The skin will be flexible at points of articulation but may be very thick and scaled around the skull and along the legs. Where the tortoise lives in very rough and abrasive terrain, or walks through tough and prickly vegetation, the scales can be both large and closely set, with very little actual skin being exposed. This means that tortoises, such as Mediterranean tortoises or the larger grazers such as Sulcata and Leopard tortoises, are unlikely to suffer mechanical damage when moving through their environment (Fig. 2.33).

Tropical rainforest tortoises, on the other hand, have less need of such extensive protection from dehydration as their environment is more humid, so their skin appears to be softer and thinner, and the scales smaller and smoother. As they live in forests that are permanently wet, their skin is more sensitive to drying out and less adapted to resist dehydration (Fig. 2.34).

At the end of the legs are sharp claws, the number of which varies from species to species (four or five) and sometimes between the back and front feet within a species. These are usually shortened and blunted by walking. They are very strong and used for digging, climbing and scrabbling between obstacles like rocks and bushes (Fig. 2.35).

Tortoises do not have teeth. Instead, they have a beak, similar to that of a parrot (Fig. 2.36). The sharp edges of the beak cut effectively through tough vegetation (Fig. 2.37). The up/down action of the jaws produce a strong bite, as anyone who has ever been bitten by a tortoise (mistaking a finger for a foodstuff) will agree.

How does the skin affect behaviour and what do we need to look out for?

- There is a likelihood of tropical rainforest tortoises, in particular, wading into water as their skin needs to be kept moist and flexible. Indoor enclosures may need regular spraying, or use of a humidifier to keep the humidity levels at around 80%. Galapagos giant tortoises regularly sit in puddles, partly for thermoregulation and partly to keep skin moist.
- Thermoregulation – the skin is an area for heat loss and gain. It is thinner than the shell so it can absorb or lose heat quickly, but the surface area is relatively small and less exposed compared with the shell. Tortoises will splay their legs out to full length when basking to increase their body temperature.
- The skin can show signs of dehydration by being very dry, possibly discoloured, and with pinches and folds in the skin of the neck and at the leg joints. Infections can enter the skin if too dry, so good health requires suitably supple skin.
- Infections may also enter the skin because of mechanical damage due to injury from a predator such as bites or scratches, or from contact with

- hard objects such as metal or glass, if inappropriate objects are left in enclosures.
- Excessive flaking – all reptiles slough but in tortoises the amount of skin lost at any time is small. Flaking skin can indicate nutritional deficiencies such as a lack of minerals and vitamins such as vitamin C.
- In the wild, damage to the scales is a normal part of life as tortoises climb and walk over rough ground. Damage to scales can occur in captivity during attempts to escape through wire or fencing when unsuitable materials are used to build enclosures.
- Courtship rituals can involve biting the female's hind legs in Hermann's tortoises. In the wild the females may be able to get away from the male but in an enclosure in captivity she may be unable to escape. Wounds may be created, through which infection can enter.
- In the natural environment it is common for tortoises to carry parasites, such as ticks or mites, on the skin. Galapagos tortoises demonstrate a behaviour called the 'finch reflex'. When stimulated by finches pecking at their legs, the tortoises stretch out to extend their legs and neck. This allows the finches to pick off any parasites attached to their skin. Other species of tortoise will sit in water and muddy puddles as a way of reducing a skin parasite population.
- Nutritional deficiencies can show up as deformities in the beak. The upper beak often grows too long. This can make feeding difficult. A poor diet can cause the jaw to be either over-shot or under-shot, which can also affect the ability to feed.
- Damage to the beak can occur, such as a broken jaw. I once had a female Hermann's tortoise who had a broken lower jaw caused by an unknown event. Attempts to repair this failed and the two halves of the wired jaw separated again. Despite this handicap the tortoise ate normally for many years. She continued to have a very good appetite and seemed unaffected by the mobility between the two halves of her lower jaw.

The Senses

- Sight

Sight is very important to tortoises and damage to the eyes can cause significant changes in behaviour.

A tortoise's eyes are positioned at the sides of the head, as is common in prey animals. With the eyes on the sides (rather than front facing) they can see the maximum range around them and thus are more likely to note predators advancing upon them. Tortoises have eyelids to protect their eyes from the bright sun. Any overhead artificial lighting, therefore, must be pointed vertically downwards rather than at an angle.

Tortoises that come from the hottest, driest desert regions with little cover tend to have smaller eyes because light intensity is at its highest here. Those from more forested or wooded areas, where light intensity is lower and conditions are darker, have bigger eyes to pick up as much light as possible (Fig. 2.38).

How do the eyes affect behaviour and what do we need to look out for?

Behaviour – Tortoises with bigger eyes spend more time hidden away, or in the shade, particularly when the sun is hottest and brightest.

Behaviour – Tortoises can see in colour and have the ability to discriminate between different flowers and other food items.

Behaviour – A tortoise's vision allows it to see across reasonable distances and to focus for a close-up view when eating. The tortoise uses vision to select food items, along with other senses.

Health – Eye function may be damaged by the tortoise freezing during hibernation. If the tortoise's body reaches freezing point or sub-zero temperatures, the first affected parts of the body are those containing the most water. As the eyes are largely fluid, they are therefore one of the first parts to freeze. Freezing can cause blindness, which may impede the tortoise's ability to eat. Often the food must be cut up into small pieces, or made into a mash, to encourage feeding. The food should also be placed in a corner or some other small space so that it does not move. This makes it easier for the tortoise to find the food and eat. The tortoise must be placed very near to the food. This allows it to sense that it is there through smell and to pinpoint its exact location.

Health – Physical damage to the eyes caused by objects such as plant stems can occur but this is much less frequent than damage due to freezing. Similarly, predators like rats can cause physical damage. This is easily preventable with good husbandry during hibernation (see Chapter 12), and by the provision of secure enclosures.

Health – Puffy eyes, closed eyes or a discharge can be a sign of an infection. In addition, puffy or closed eyes can be a sign of nutritional deficiency, or other more systemic illness where the tortoise

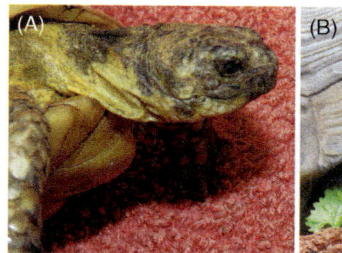 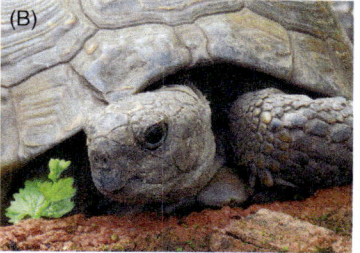 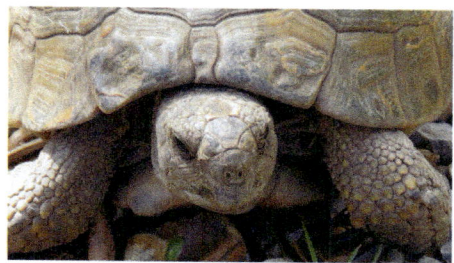

Fig. 2.38. Tortoises have smaller sized eyes in hot sunny environments such as deserts (A) compared with the larger eyes of darker more shaded habitats such as forests (B).

Fig. 2.39. Tortoise face with nares (nostrils) clear and open.

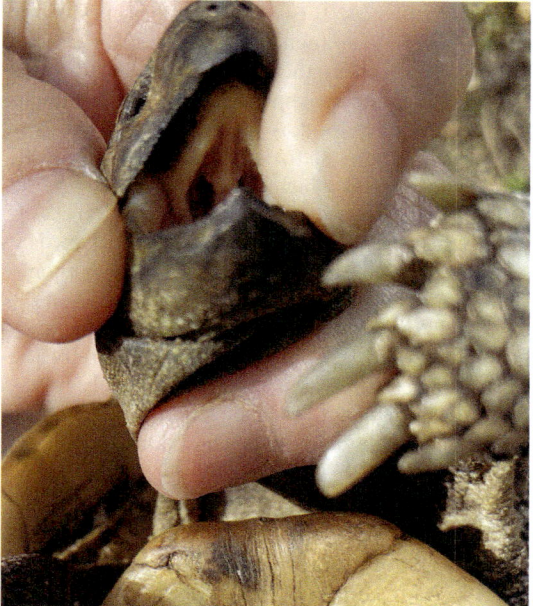

Fig. 2.40. Inside of mouth with internal structures of nose.

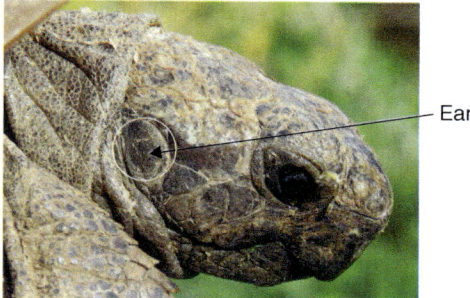

Fig. 2.41. Tortoise ear is a flat plate (scute behind the eye).

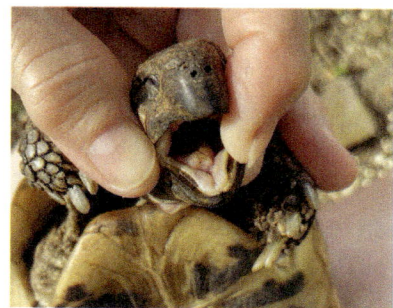

Fig. 2.42. Tortoise tongue.

just feels so unwell that it cannot open its eyes. Eye health can therefore be a sign of a number of health issues. Note that some species, such as the Red-footed tortoises, will produce tears as a normal function to maintain high humidity at the eye surface.

- Smell

A tortoise's sense of smell is very well developed, and it will usually spend time nosing at and sniffing potential food objects before attempting to eat them (Figs 2.39 and 2.40). Tortoises will also sniff other tortoises, particularly around the mouth and nose, when they first encounter them.

How does smell affect behaviour and what do we need to look out for?

Behaviour – Smell is an important sense in the finding and eating of food. Tortoises with loss of appetite, or suffering from blindness, can sometimes be stimulated to show interest in their food by using attractive-smelling foods. Favourites include cucumber, ice-plant (sedum), or berries such as strawberries. It is important to note that such foods should be used sparingly as an appetite

How Tortoise Biology Affects Health and Behaviour

stimulant only, and should not make up the majority or entire diet. They should not be fed on a regular basis (see Chapter 5).

Behaviour – Many tortoises live in an environment that smells strongly. This helps to explain the importance of the sense of smell. Creating a captive habitat that has aromatic plants such as herbs and scented flowers can contribute to a more natural setting for your tortoise.

Health – Any infection that causes blocked nostrils can reduce the sense of smell. Some species of tortoise, notably the North African Spur-thighed tortoises, can be prone to 'runny nose syndrome' where the nostrils discharge a clear fluid. The cause of this is likely to be a combination of environmental factors and infectious agents (viruses, bacteria) and will be covered more fully in the chapter on illnesses and diseases (Chapter 7). One or both nostrils may run with fluid, which may (with luck) resolve without need for intervention. The condition is often chronic, however, with symptoms seen as an episode that then clears, without any obvious ill-effects. In other situations, the fluid becomes thickened, cloudy and may become yellow, all of which could indicate a more serious infection requiring veterinary treatment. If in any doubt, seek the advice of an experienced tortoise veterinarian.

Health – It is not uncommon for one nostril to become blocked by a seed, blade of grass or other food item, which can cause discomfort and put the tortoise off its food. This needs to be removed, (with veterinary help if required) in order to prevent damage to the nostrils or it becoming a source of infection inside the delicate nasal passages.

- Hearing

Tortoise ears are seen as simply a flat plate or scute across the ear canal (Fig. 2.41). This is in fact the tympanic membrane or eardrum. Tortoises do not have visible ears and no ear canal can be seen, as it is covered by the membrane. It is relatively easily damaged, as it is exposed on the surface at the side of the head.

Hearing is thought to be much better in aquatic species than those on the land, because sound travels much better in water. For this reason, hearing is thought to be very limited in terrestrial tortoises.

How does hearing affect behaviour and what do we need to look out for?

Behaviour – People often tell me that their tortoise responds to their voice. When they call the tortoise by name it will hurry over to them. It is more likely that they can see their owner, or feel the vibrations on the ground from their footsteps. However, this is a little researched area. It was previously unknown whether tortoises could recognize individual humans. Recent training projects at the Zoological Society of London have shown that Galapagos tortoises are aware of familiar people, and that their training is more effective when carried out by familiar keepers within a constant environment (see Chapter 10 on social interactions).

Behaviour – Research into the ability of tortoises to learn shows that they can carry out taught training activities and remember them for up to 10 years (Gutnick *et al.*, 2020) (see Chapter 8 on behaviour and learning). When owners think that their tortoise is coming to see them, this may be true. The tortoises may be associating the approach of a familiar human with the arrival of food. As they are unlikely to recognize their own name (or even hear it being called), it is this memory to which they are responding.

Health – Ear abscesses are a relatively common health problem because they are part of the skin surface. The ear is usually seen to swell at first and maybe become red. Over a very extended period (possibly years if unnoticed), the abscess caused by infection will gradually increase in size. Due to the hard nature of the infected material, surgical removal is usually necessary, before treatment of the infection can begin (see Chapter 7 on common illnesses and diseases).

- Touch

As described in the sections about the importance of the shell and skin, tortoises are very tactile and use their body surface as a way of perceiving their environment. Tortoises are aware of being touched or handled by people. The presence of skin parasites can be detected too, and the tortoise will take action to try to remove them.

How does touch affect behaviour and what do we need to look out for?

Behaviour – The sensation of being scratched or rubbed can be an enjoyable experience for tortoises. Rubbing the back legs of giant species will stimulate a rocking movement side-to-side (sometimes called twokking), which the tortoise appears to enjoy. Certainly giant tortoises will stand still and engage in this rocking motion for extended periods of time.

Behaviour – Some tortoises appear to enjoy a head rub and will stay in position for extended periods.

This implies that they enjoy the sensation. If a tortoise does not wish to be touched it will pull away and walk away. Being over-handled by humans can be a cause of stress in tortoises. For example, when they live with families, children may want to interact with the pet tortoise more than it would like. Repeated picking up can be stressful, as tortoises feel most secure when all four feet are on the ground. Tortoises are in no way domesticated and are therefore unable to tolerate some of the more intense interactions many people might like with their pets.

Behaviour – Tortoises are stimulated in courtship rituals through tactile sensations such as leg-biting and shell-bashing, even if this does not seem very pleasant to us and may indeed cause damage. These physical sensations are an important aspect of the breeding process (see Chapter 11 on breeding).

- Taste

Tortoises have a good sense of taste and can discriminate well between food items using sensory cells on the tongue (Fig. 2.42).

How does taste affect behaviour and what do we need to look out for?

Behaviour – Tortoises can be very fussy feeders in captivity (see Chapter 5 on diets). Tortoises will spit out foodstuffs that they do not like. Taste is a very important sense in tortoises.

Behaviour – Tortoises will also refuse oral medication that has an unpleasant taste. They will try to avoid ingesting it, and claw at the side of the mouth with their front legs to try to remove it. An oral antibiotic called Baytril® has an unpleasant taste because it is very alkaline (the opposite of acidic). When Baytril is given orally, these behaviours are often seen, as the taste sensation from the drug is unpleasant. The tortoise will remember what has happened during a course of treatment and so become more and more difficult to handle in its attempts to refuse medication.

What you can't see – inside your tortoise

The soft vital organs

Tortoises have all their major organs enclosed and protected by their shell (McArthur, 1996; McArthur *et al.*, 2004). The simple diagram in Fig. 2.43 shows the internal layout, as does Fig. 2.44 of the actual organs.

The following body adaptations can be seen in tortoises (McArthur *et al.*, 2004):

- Tortoise ribs are fused with the shell. This means that breathing movements cannot take place using the ribs, as they would in most vertebrates. In order to move air in and out of the body, tortoises must instead use movements of their front legs. This is not as efficient as using the diaphragm and rib muscles as we do. Because of this the tortoise's ability to move air in and out of the lungs efficiently is reduced (Fig. 2.45).

- The trachea opening can be clearly seen at the back of the mouth with the protective flaps of the epiglottis clearly visible. The trachea splits high up into the two bronchi, left and right, leading to the respective lungs (Fig. 2.47).

- Tortoises have no diaphragm, which means that the digestive and reproductive systems are not separated from the lungs. The result is that the higher pressures necessary for the most efficient exchange of respiratory gases (oxygen and carbon dioxide) cannot be achieved. The mechanism for breathing and exchange of gases is therefore much less efficient than in a mammal. The overall effect of this is to lower the rate of metabolism generally, and slow down all tortoise physiology. The lungs are large structures to give a greater surface area for gas exchange (Figs 2.45 and 2.46).

- The heart is three-chambered. It has two smaller chambers at the top (the atria) but only one ventricle at the bottom. This makes the blood circulation less efficient, as the system does not completely separate oxygenated and deoxygenated blood. It also reduces the efficiency with which oxygen, nutrients and wastes move around the body within the blood. Again this makes body processes slower, so that everything happening within the body is at a much slower rate than in a mammal. The tortoise takes a long time to become ill, for example, and then takes a very long time to get well again.

- The liver is a large organ responsible for many chemical processes. The liver processes digested food. If the diet is poor, as with too much protein or fat for example, the liver can be damaged. Tortoises can get 'fatty livers' if they are given high-protein/high-fat foods over many years. The liver also has a role in reproduction and hormone metabolism. If it is not working properly, reproduction can be prevented and many illnesses can result.

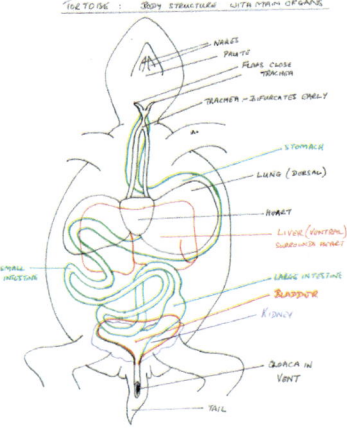

Fig. 2.43. Tortoise's internal structure showing main organs.

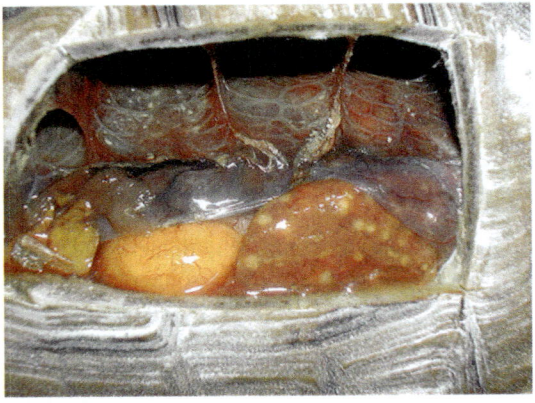

Fig. 2.46. Normal lung exposed under the carapace, with intestines and liver (with white spots showing disease) below the lungs.

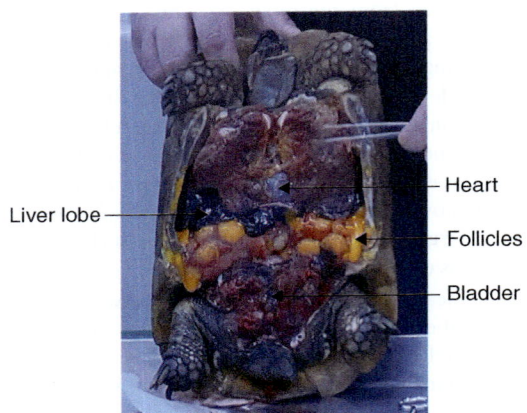

Fig. 2.44. Internal organs during a post-mortem examination.

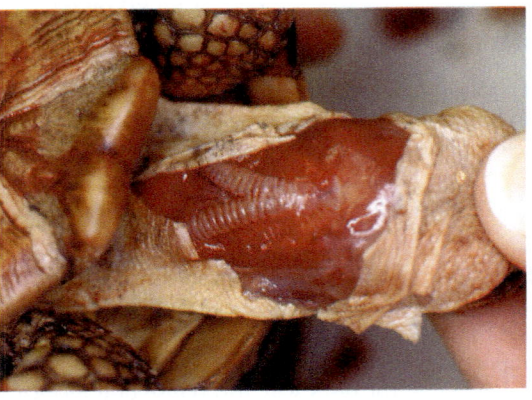

Fig. 2.47. Trachea splitting high up in the neck, into the right and left bronchi leading into the lungs (William Lewis).

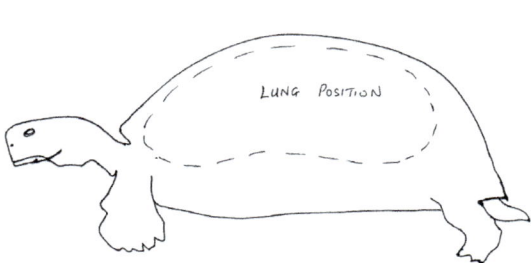

Fig. 2.45. Diagram of lung position from the side.

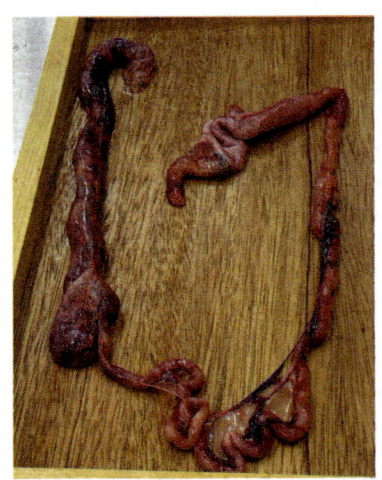

Fig. 2.48. Gut when removed post-mortem.

- The kidneys regulate water levels in the body and remove toxins, such as the nitrogen-containing wastes from protein metabolism. Water is needed to store and get rid of toxic nitrogen wastes.
- Tortoises living in drier arid environments with less available water need to get rid of their waste efficiently using the least amount of water. Because of this, tortoises from dry areas usually excrete uric acid as urates, seen as a white milky fluid when the tortoise is bathing. Often the tortoise will release these toxic wastes into the bath as a way of removing them. The advantage is that the tortoises can replace lost water by drinking at the same time.

The higher the amount of protein in the diet, the more nitrogen wastes there will be. Tortoises that eat animal protein, therefore, need greater access to water in order to be able to get rid of the waste. They must replace the water very quickly or they may dehydrate, so water must be freely available at all times. It is likely that excretory products and their proportions may change in response to environmental conditions relating to water availability (Table 2.4).

- Digestive organs are shown in Fig. 2.48, and the gut is relatively long (McArthur *et al.*, 2004). You would expect this in herbivores, as digestion takes longer because there are less nutrients in the food. A healthy diet produces healthy faeces, usually dark and fibrous. The smell is not unpleasant.

The results of a poor diet are soon noticed in the faeces being produced. They may be more liquid, discoloured, often yellow and often have a strong unpleasant smell.

The gut can contain internal parasites such as roundworms and tapeworms. Sometimes roundworms can be seen in the faeces. Worms may need treatment to remove (see Chapter 7 on common illnesses and diseases).

- The reproductive organs differ between male and female tortoises, as would be expected in animals that reproduce sexually (Fig. 2.49). During mating, the male inserts his penis and passes sperm to fertilize the eggs, inside the female's body. This internal fertilization process is essential for land-dwelling organisms, particularly so for those living in areas where water is scarce. Males have a longer tail than females because the penis emerges from it. The female will lay fertile eggs from which the offspring will hatch after incubation. Figure 2.50 shows a large number of follicles and some calcified eggs

Table 2.4. Four types of chelonian excretion (McArthur *et al.*, 2004).

Type of excretion	Products and adaptations	Environments
Uricotelism	= uric acid + urates (more energy efficient for water conservation)	Arid dry desert or grasslands with limited water
Ureo-uricotelism	= uric acid + urea combined	With adequate water supplies
Ureotelism	= urea	Aquatic freshwater
Amino-ureotelism	= ammonia + urea combined	Aquatic freshwater and marine

in this female Spur-thighed tortoise. (For things that can go wrong, see Chapter 7 on common illnesses and diseases.)

How do the internal organs affect behaviour and what do we need to look out for?

Behaviour – If any of the vital organs are not working properly the tortoise's behaviour will change. It may become less active and seek quiet, sometimes cool, places. Generally, the tortoise may become withdrawn and spend more time pulled into its shell. Often the tortoise will keep its eyes closed for much of the time and may appear to be asleep. It will not be seen basking or showing any of the other daily behaviours expected of a healthy tortoise. It is likely to become lethargic and may be unable to walk or move. If left untreated, eventually the body will shut down and death will follow. This may take many weeks, months or even years depending on what is causing the problem (see Chapter 7 on common illnesses and diseases).

Health – Without a diaphragm tortoises cannot cough, which makes it difficult for them to clear secretions and foreign bodies from their nostrils and nares. If straw or hay is used in hibernation, debris such as grass seeds and spores cannot easily be dislodged. This may lead to infection as described above. Respiratory infections can easily arise, leading to lung infections such as pneumonia. This may be fatal.

Health – Poor feeding often shows itself in damage to the liver or kidneys. This can occur over decades but eventually manifests itself as lethargy, failure to walk and puffiness due to fluid retention (Fig. 2.51). Bladder and kidney stones may result from dehydration or a diet that is too rich in protein and fat.

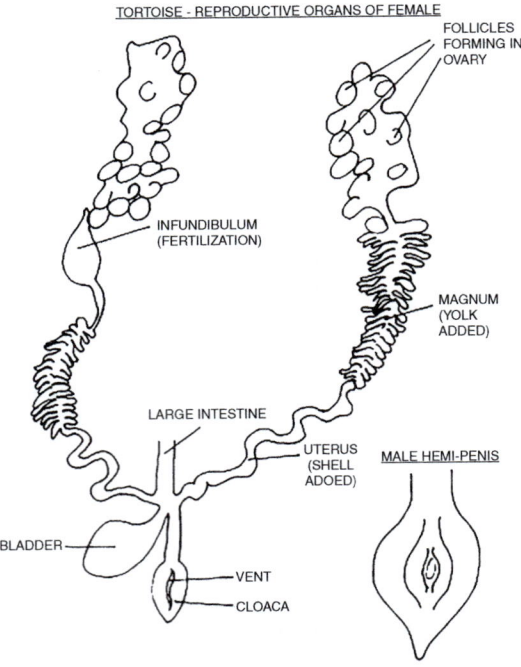

Fig. 2.49. Female reproductive organs diagram with male penis and opening to cloaca shown.

Health – Constipation can occur where the diet lacks fibre. A tortoise may choose to ingest foreign bodies that are not edible, such as small stones or soil. This may indicate a lack of minerals in the diet. For example, eating white-coloured stones may indicate a need for calcium (McArthur *et al.*, 2004).

Health – Abnormally coloured urates that are cream, yellow or even green indicate that there may be kidney or liver problems. If the urates become more paste-like, harder or gritty, the tortoise is becoming dehydrated. Access to water needs to be increased. As well as freely available water, sitting the tortoise in a shallow warm bath two to three times a week is very good practice. If the tortoise is unwell this may need to be increased to two to three times daily, as this is a very supportive and recuperative technique (see Chapter 7 on common illnesses and diseases).

What does this all mean for chelonians in terms of their distribution around the globe?

Tortoises, turtles and terrapins are distributed on land and sea, and in freshwater lakes and rivers over much of the warmer regions of the globe, as shown in Fig. 2.19.

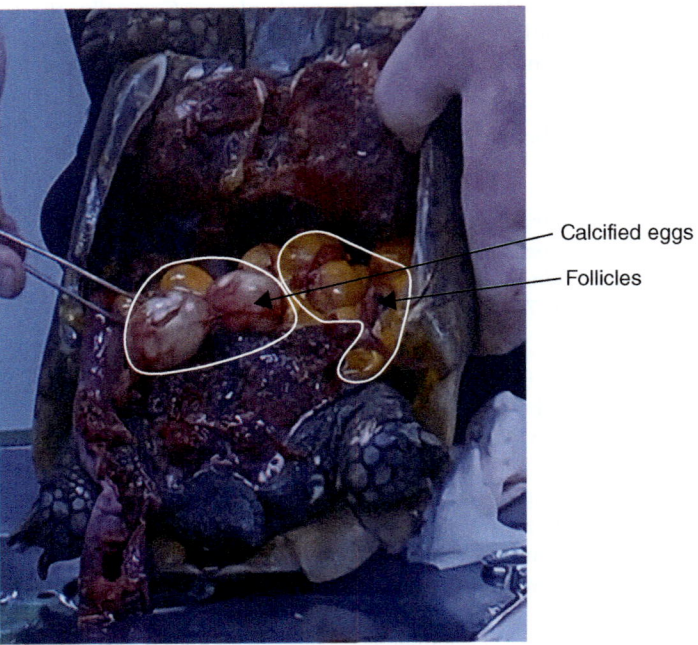

Fig. 2.50. Female reproductive organs are obscured by the large number of follicles (eggs and yolks) seen as yellow sacs, held within the body of this female tortoise post-mortem. This condition is called follicular stasis (see Chapter 7 on common illnesses and diseases). The eggs are not fully formed in most cases.

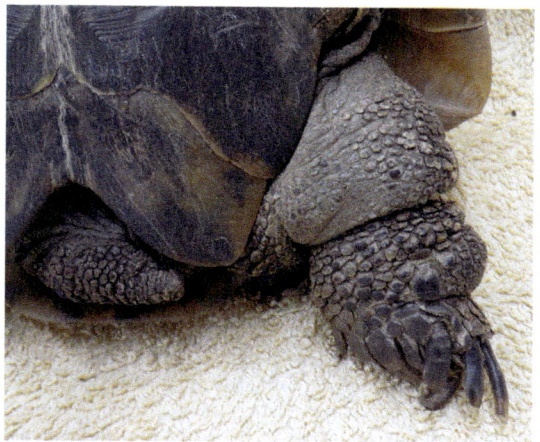

Fig. 2.51. Puffiness due to fluid-retention, or inflammation, can be an indicator of a number of illnesses, often related to infection or poor liver or kidney function. This large female Spur-thighed tortoise was diagnosed with gout. Gout is very painful and is due to a build-up of uric acid crystals in the joints (see Chapter 7 on common illnesses and diseases).

Restricted mainly by their need for warmth from the sun's rays, they have nonetheless adapted themselves to life in a huge range of habitats and situations. The variety of form, colour and habit is considerable in the 452 recognized subspecies (Gerlach, 2012). Taxonomy continually changes as a dynamic field of research and development.

The shell affords them great protection and has been a very successful biological adaptation over many millions of years. It does, however, reduce mobility and in many cases means that tortoises can be easily picked up and moved for collection by people. They can be damaged by human activities and developments where they cannot escape quickly, for example during fires or during habitat destruction for development. This means that their numbers have been drastically reduced by human activities in recent decades. They are valued for food, artefacts and products as well as in the pet trade (see Chapter 20 on tortoise keeping in the past, present and future).

Conclusion

Tortoises have been on Earth for around 220 million years. The adaptations that have helped them to survive have proved very effective until recently. Humans have had a huge impact on both their environment and their populations. The numbers of tortoises have declined dramatically as they have been collected for the pet trade, used to make artefacts and objects, and their habitat has been lost, leaving them without safe places to live.

Tortoise biology is an area that we have only recently started to understand fully. There is so much more to learn. Being aware of their basic body layout and the way in which their organs and systems function is vital if we hope to keep them alive and healthy in captivity. Problems arising from poor husbandry are covered in other chapters in this book. Common diseases and illnesses are covered, along with emotional well-being and mental health. The impact of health on behaviour has been introduced in this chapter and is looked at more fully in later chapters.

This chapter illustrates what a marvellously well-adapted group tortoises are and how fascinating their biology is. Understanding how their bodies work is an important aspect of our responsibilities as keepers. Without this basic understanding we cannot hope to provide the conditions that they need to thrive in captivity rather than to simply survive.

References and Further Reading

Gerlach, J (2012) *The Great Survivors*, Phelsuma Press, Cambridge, UK.

Gutnick, T., Weissenbacher, A. and Kuba, M.J. (2020) The Underestimated Giants: Operant conditioning, visual discrimination and long-term memory in giant tortoises. *Animal Cognition* 23, 159–167

Highfield, A. (1996) *Practical Encyclopaedia of Keeping and Breeding Tortoises and Freshwater Turtles*. Carapace Press, London.

Highfield, A. and Highfield, N. (2009) *Keeping a Pet Tortoise*. Interpet, Dorking, UK.

McArthur, S. (1996) *Veterinary Management of Tortoises and Turtles*. Blackwell, Oxford, UK.

McArthur, S., Wilkinson, R. and Meyer, J. (2004) *Medicine and Surgery of Tortoises and Turtles*. Blackwell, Oxford, UK.

Scheelings, T.F. (2019) Ch 1 Anatomy and physiology. In: Girling, S.J. and Raiti, P. (eds) *BSAVA Manual of Practical Veterinary Welfare*. BSAVA, Quedgeley, UK, pp. 1–25.

Williams, J. and Beck, D. (2021) Stress, anxiety, fear and frustration in different reptile species: How to reduce these negative emotional states during veterinary procedures. *Veterinary Nursing Journal* 36(7), 213–216.

3 The Captive Environment

Abstract
This chapter discusses the importance of trying to mimic the natural habitat of any given species of tortoise kept in captivity. The need to provide choice within the captive environment is central to maintaining health and welfare. The chapter sets out the factors that need to be considered in the construction of indoor and outdoor accommodation. The importance of suitable accommodation in maintaining good health and well-being is the central focus of this chapter. The chapter describes the importance of enclosure location, size, design, substrate, security and environmental enrichment to ensure that most natural behaviours are seen. The need for appropriate provision of light, heat and humidity is set out. Tortoises intrinsically know what conditions they need in order to stay healthy – the task of keepers is to provide sufficient options for the tortoises to find those conditions. There are many practical tips on designing and building enclosures.

Introduction

When setting up a home for tortoises it is important to try, as far as possible, to mimic their natural environment. If you are going to do this successfully you must first identify what type of tortoise you have and the environmental conditions for which the tortoise is adapted. Table 3.1 shows species of tortoises commonly kept in captivity.

Other species less commonly kept include:

- **Burmese Brown** (*Manouria emys*) – the largest tortoise species in Asia. Tropical rainforest species often at higher levels and can cope with damp and cool conditions but a tropical tortoise that does not hibernate. Feeds mainly on fruits, leaves and grasses.
- **Indian Star tortoise** (*Geochelone elegans*) – Found across Southern India, Pakistan and Sri Lanka. This is a very attractive tortoise. A tropical species that does not hibernate, living in arid and low woodland or forest. The diet is dry grasses, flowers and cactus pads. The species should not be mixed with other species of tortoise in captivity as they are susceptible to disease and are quite fragile as a species (Vetter, 2006)

Table 3.1 shows the natural environments for some of the different species of tortoise commonly kept in captivity and is illustrated with images that suggest the challenges we face when keeping these animals in captivity. We can mimic the natural habitat but never entirely recreate it.

What are Natural Habitats for Tortoises?

Tortoises can be found living wild over much of the globe. While some species live in temperate or subtropical areas, most species can be found in the tropics, between the Tropics of Cancer and Capricorn. Here there is sufficient sunlight to maintain tortoise body temperature at levels that allow activity for much of the year.

Tortoises are found in much of southern Europe, Asia, Africa, Australia, South America and in the southern parts of North America. Tortoises also inhabit tropical islands, such as Madagascar, the Seychelles (including Aldabra) and the Galapagos. They are also found in the Balearics and until recently colonised the Bahamas, the Greater Antilles (including Cuba and Hispaniola), the Lesser Antilles, the Canary Islands and Malta.

In Chapter 2, Fig. 2.19 shows a map of the world with countries where tortoises can be found.

The natural habitats in which tortoises can be found range from open grasslands and savannah to partially wooded hillsides, tropical and cloud forests, and temperate forest areas. When we try to accommodate these animals in captivity it can be quite challenging to try to recreate these natural habitats. Only if we can succeed in doing this can we provide for their physical, mental and emotional needs. Thus, when setting up a home for tortoises it is important to try, as far as possible, to mimic their natural environment. If you are going to do this successfully you must first identify what type of tortoise you have and the environmental conditions that it is adapted for.

Why is it so important to mimic a tortoise's natural environment?

As Table 3.2 below shows, natural environments and habitats may vary significantly from species to species. For example, the hot humid jungles from which tropical tortoises such as the Red-footed tortoise (*Chelonoidis/Geochelone carbonaria*) come are radically different from the barren steppes of Afghanistan, whose baking summer heat and freezing winter conditions provide homes for tortoises such as the Horsfield's tortoise *(Testudo/Agrionemys horsfieldii)*. Keeping Horsfield's tortoises in the type of conditions to which Red-footed tortoises are adapted, or conversely, Red-footed tortoises in environments more suitable for Horsfield's tortoises, would result in the tortoises suffering and becoming ill, and lead ultimately to the rapid death of the animals concerned. Hibernating/brumating tropical tortoises is another sure way to bring about their demise, as they have no mechanisms allowing them to adapt to very cold conditions.

I have had cases reported to me of Leopard tortoises that have died when they have been put in cold conditions during a Northern European winter and allowed to hibernate/brumate – they do not wake up.

What if I plan to keep just one type of tortoise?

If the geographical range inhabited by an individual type of tortoise is large enough, significant environmental differences between regions can also be seen. Allowances for this may need to be made, which will impact the type of habitats that need to be set up.

Spur-thighed tortoises, for example, can be found in countries all around the Mediterranean – Spain, the Balearics, Greece, Turkey, Bulgaria, Israel, Egypt, Tunisia, Libya and Morocco. As the environment differs (even if only slightly) across the range, the tortoises will show adaptation to the conditions in which they find themselves. Because of this, Spur-thighed tortoises show considerable variation – in size, colouration, physical features and behaviour. The variation in one species of Spur-thighed tortoises, *Testudo graeca* spp., can be seen in Fig. 3.7.

Amazingly it is even possible to tell the difference between Spur-thighed tortoises that come from one side of a valley and those that come from the other side, if the tortoises have been separated over time by an insurmountable physical barrier (e.g. a deep river). The slightly different environments of the two valley sides will create groups of tortoises that look notably different, if interbreeding between the two groups has been prevented.

If the environments differ radically, differences between Spur-thighed tortoises may be extreme. In countries like Greece and Turkey, for example, a higher rainfall and a narrower temperature range has produced habitats that include woodland and shrubby vegetation. These habitats are very different from the hotter, drier, more desert-like North African coastal regions. The appearance of Spur-thighed tortoises found in these different regions is so distinct that two subspecies can be recognised: *Testudo graeca ibera* in Greece and Turkey and *Testudo graeca graeca* in North Africa. There is a third subspecies found in Algeria: *Testudo graeca whitei*, a very large tortoise. As the DNA analysis continues, what are currently subspecies may be reclassified into separate species.

Some researchers suggest that the following additional subspecies exist (rather than just the three already mentioned) in particular geographical regions of North Africa (Vetter, 2002):

T. g. soussensis (South Morocco)
T. g. marokkensis (North Morocco)
T. g. nabeulensis (Tunisia)
T. g. cyrenaica (Libya)

Clearly there is a great deal more work to do on classification of this species, which is very varied across its range.

Spur-thighed tortoises live in a variety of habitats and are adapted to those habitats. Those living in sunny hot conditions have smaller eyes, and lighter shell and skin coloration. For *T. graeca ibera* (Fig. 3.7B), which live in more wooded areas with more vegetation and shade, the eyes are larger and the skin and shell coloration is darker.

Even within these three identified subspecies considerable variation still exists, the result of differences within more local environments. This makes it very difficult to pinpoint exactly where a tortoise has originally come from. Without this knowledge it is impossible to create an artificial habitat that precisely mirrors the one to which it is adapted. The more knowledge and understanding we have about our tortoises' origins, the better job we can do, and the more effective the artificial support we will need

Table 3.1. Tortoises and their natural environments (Vetter, 2002; 2004; 2005).

Tortoise species	Natural habitats
Mediterranean tortoises: Spur-thighed tortoises – *Testudo graeca* spp. Hermann's tortoises – *Testudo hermanni* spp. Marginated tortoises – *Testudo marginata* 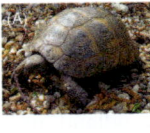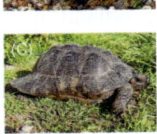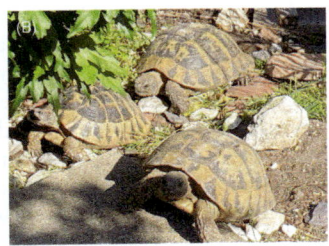 **Fig. 3.1.** (A) Spur-thighed *Testudo graeca ibera*. (B) Hermann's *Testudo hermanni*. (C) Marginated *Testudo marginata* (Dillon Prest).	Mediterranean maquis/garrigue vegetation 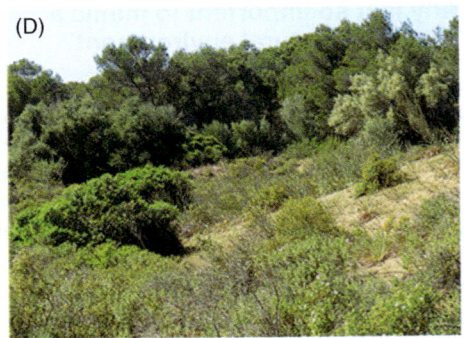 **Fig. 3.1.** (D) Mediterranean maquis/garrigue showing the mix of vegetation.
Yellow-footed tortoises – *Chelonoidis* (*Geochelone*) *denticulata* Hingeback tortoises – *Kinixys* spp. 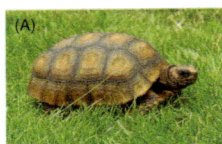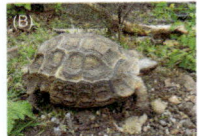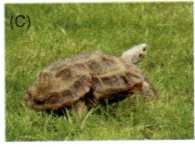 **Fig. 3.2.** (A) Yellow-footed (James Sullivan). (B) *Kinixys erosa*. (C) *Kinixys homeana* (James Sullivan).	Tropical rainforest and woodland. 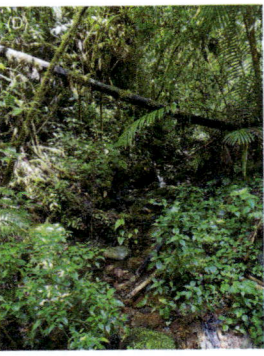 **Fig. 3.2.** (D) Tropical rainforest with plenty of vegetation cover and high humidity.
Red-footed tortoises – *Chelonoidis* (*Geochelone*) *carbonaria* Hingeback tortoises – *Kinixys* spp.	Drier forest, woodland and scrub

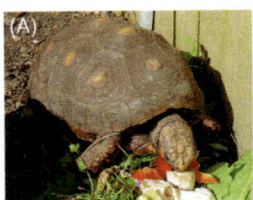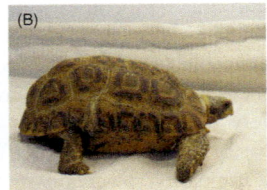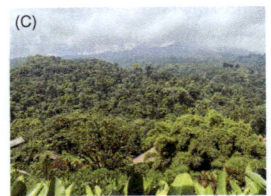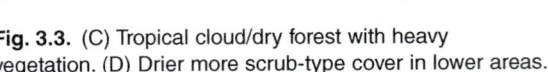

Fig. 3.3. (A) *Chelonoidis carbonaria*. (B) *Kinixys belliana*.

Fig. 3.3. (C) Tropical cloud/dry forest with heavy vegetation. (D) Drier more scrub-type cover in lower areas.

Table 3.1. Continued.

Tortoise species	Natural habitats
African Spurred tortoise – *Geochelone/Centrochelys sulcata* Leopard tortoise – *Geochelone/Centrochelys pardalis* Radiated tortoises – *Geochelone/Astrochelys radiata* 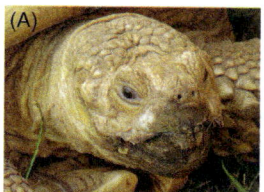 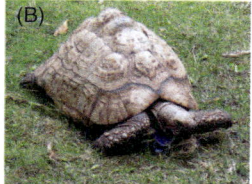 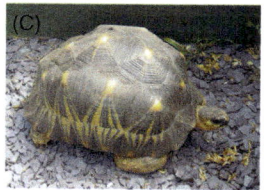 **Fig. 3.4.** (A) Sulcata. (B) Leopard. (C) Radiated.	Open grasslands and savannah 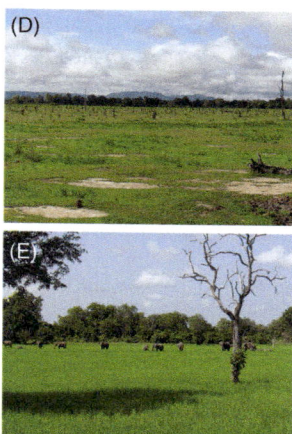 **Fig. 3.4.** (D) and (E) Savannah – open grasslands, with wet and dry seasons (Sian Bewick).
Egyptian tortoises – *Testudo kleinmanni* Californian/Mojave Desert Tortoises – *Gopherus agassizii* 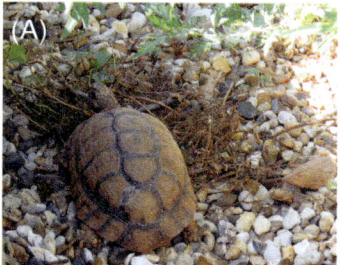 **Fig. 3.5.** (A) Egyptian tortoise.	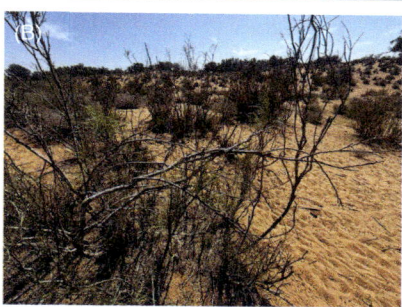 **Fig. 3.5.** (B) Dry desert with limited vegetation and cover (Corrine Weyands).
Horsfield's tortoise – *Testudo/Agrionemys horsfieldi* 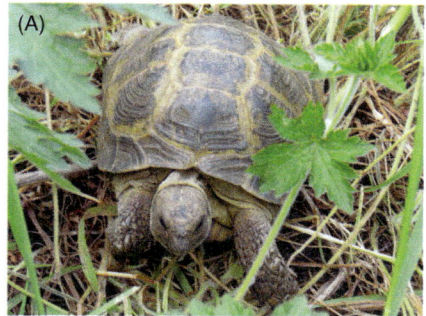 **Fig. 3.6.** A Horsfield's tortoise.	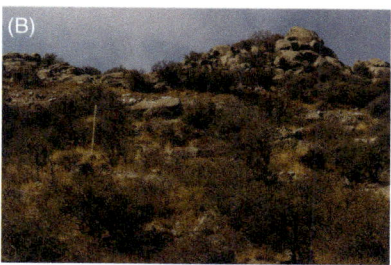 **Fig. 3.6.** (B) Rocky plains, hillsides of the steppes (Sian Bewick).

The Captive Environment

Table 3.2. Some commonly kept terrestrial chelonian species and their natural environments.

Common name	Latin	Countries of origin	Habitat	Habit Feeding
Mediterranean Spur-thighed tortoise	*Testudo graeca graeca/ Testudo graeca ibera/ Testudo graeca whitei*	Morocco/Tunisia/ Libya/Turkey/Spain	Terrestrial Desert, scrub, dry wooded	Solitary Herbivorous
Mediterranean Hermann's tortoise	*Testudo hermanni*	France, Italy, Spain, Greece, Balkans	Terrestrial Scrub, dry wooded	Solitary Herbivorous
Mediterranean Marginated tortoise	*Testudo marginata*	Greece	Terrestrial Rocky hillside, scrub	Solitary Herbivorous
African spurred tortoise	*Geochelone/ Centrochelys sulcata*	Sub-Saharan Africa	Terrestrial Dry desert, savannah	Solitary – males may be agonistic Herbivorous
Leopard tortoise	*Geochelone/Centrochelys pardalis*	South Africa, Tanzania, Kenya	Terrestrial Dry grassy savannah	Solitary Herbivorous
Radiated tortoise	*Geochelone/Astrochelys radiata*	Madagascar	Terrestrial Dry grassy savannah	Herbivorous
Horsfield's tortoise	*Testudo/Agrionemys horsfieldi*	Eastern Russia, Afghanistan, Pakistan, China	Terrestrial Dry, rocky scrub, steppe	Solitary Herbivorous
Egyptian tortoise	*Testudo kleinmanni*	Egypt, Libya, Syria, Israel	Terrestrial Desert	Solitary Herbivorous
Californian Desert tortoise	*Gopherus agassizii*	South-western United States	Terrestrial Desert	Solitary Herbivorous
Red-footed tortoise	*Chelonoidis (Geochelone) carbonaria*	Panama, Bolivia, Colombia, Venezuela, Guiana, Peru, Ecuador, Brazil	Terrestrial Tropical humid rainforest	Semi-social Share shelters Omnivorous
Hingeback tortoise	*Kinixys erosa*	Gambia, Uganda, Democratic Republic of the Congo	Terrestrial Tropical lowland humid forest	Omnivorous
	Kinixys belliana	Angola, Barundi, Central African Republic		
	Kinixys homeana	Benin, Cameroon, Democratic Republic of the Congo, Equatorial Guinea, Gabon, Ghana, Guinea, Ivory Coast, Liberia, Nigeria		

to provide in captivity will be. Tortoises will always need support, but the more like the natural conditions the captive environment is, the more likely they are to thrive.

How can we make our tortoises feel at home?

Later chapters in this book will examine the environmental set-ups needed for some of the most commonly kept species in more detail, but in general tortoises will need:

- Outdoor accommodation
- Indoor accommodation
- Hibernation/brumation accommodation (if the tortoise is a hibernating species)

Although the details of the accommodation that you provide will vary from species to species, it should always include the following (McArthur *et al.*, 2004; Highfield and Highfield, 2008, 2009; McArthur, 2012):

1. Appropriately sized, environmentally enriched, secure enclosures that allow most natural behaviours
2. A suitable temperature range to allow the tortoise to maintain its preferred body temperature (PBT).
3. Sunlight, or suitable artificial lighting, to provide appropriate daylength, intensity and UVB-levels
4. Suitable substrate composition and depth
5. Appropriate humidity levels, maintained through the creation of microclimates
6. An accessible source of water
7. A suitable diet
8. Allowances based on the tortoise's normal social structure. Does the tortoise usually live a solitary existence or as part of a small group? Do females and males need to be kept separately?
9. Suitable hibernation/brumation conditions and duration for those tortoise species that do hibernate

What do we need to think about when building an outside enclosure?

How much space does a tortoise need?

In general terms the larger the outside enclosures are, the better. Given that Hermann's tortoises may have territories as large as 7 hectares (17 acres) (Biedenweg and Schramm, 2019) in their natural environment as they search for food, clearly we can never give them enough space in captivity.

In the wild most tortoises walk several kilometres every day. The larger the species, the more ground they are likely to cover in order to find sufficient food. Walking, therefore, is an important part of natural behaviour. The opportunity to walk without continuously coming across impassable barriers reduces repetitive behaviours (such as walking round and round the same small path). The larger the enclosure, the greater the opportunity to provide variety and enrichment, reducing stress by making life more interesting for your tortoise.

Outdoor accommodation size varies in scale from huge fields many kilometres square for large grazers such as Sulcata and Leopard tortoises, to a few square metres for smaller species such as Egyptian tortoises (Kleinmann's tortoise). While little research has been carried out into the minimum size for tortoise enclosures, one suggestion (Divers, 1996) is that the minimum size should be based on 0.4 m^2 per 0.1 m (10 cm) of tortoise length. This is only the minimum, however; the recommended size is far larger: 1.0 m^2 per 0.1 m (10 cm) length of tortoise. More recently in the *BSAVA Manual of Reptiles* Varga (2019) suggested the area should be five times the animal's length squared.

For some commonly kept tortoise species enclosure sizes are suggested in Table 3.3 based on the above and my own experiences.

The degree of activity shown by the tortoise is also a factor – some species are livelier than others, while males may be more active than females at certain times of year. Age might also be relevant – young tortoises are likely to move around more than elderly ones. The more active the species, or individual, the more the space that is required. Observing your tortoise in the enclosure is important so that you can see if they are using the available space, or if repetitive behaviours, such as pacing in one area, are developing, which would suggest that more space is needed.

The ability to walk and generally move about to find the most suitable environmental conditions is essential to tortoise well-being. The fastest tortoise recorded (Guinness World Records, 2014, UK) is Bertie the Leopard tortoise, who walked at 0.28 m per second (1.0 kph, or 0.6 mph). If Bertie walks for around 12 hours per day, as would be usual, this would mean that he would cover around 12 km (7.5 miles) per day. In order to achieve this using the indoor enclosure size recommended above, he would need to walk around the edge of a 5 m × 3 m enclosure (= 15 m distance) around 800 times a day. To confine any tortoise in too small an enclosure can only result in them leading a stressed and unhappy existence, which is likely to lead to illness and will certainly have a negative impact on welfare. Figure 3.8A shows a large enclosure for a single male Spur-thighed tortoise with enrichment designed to break up the sight line and avoid repetitive circuits of the perimeter. Figure 3.8B shows a large enclosure for a group of Mediterranean tortoises. For a large grazing species such as Sulcatas, enclosures should be measured in acres/hectares.

Is it better to put my tortoise enclosure in a sunny or shady place?

As tortoises are ectotherms, they cannot make their own body heat as mammals and birds do. Because of this they are reliant on external heat sources such as the sun to keep them warm.

All tortoises have a preferred body temperature (PBT). Daytime temperatures must be high enough for them to achieve this. The preferred optimum

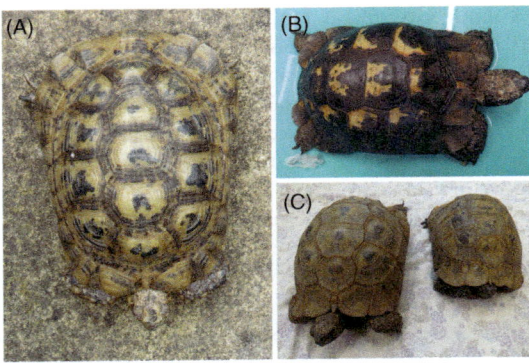

Fig. 3.7. Spur-thighed tortoises. (A) *Testudo graeca graeca*. (B) *Testudo graeca ibera*. (C) *Testudo graeca whitei*.

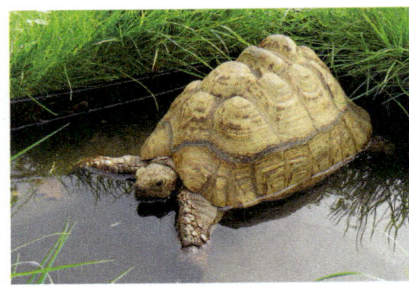

Fig. 3.9. Leopard tortoise sitting in a bath to cool and drink.

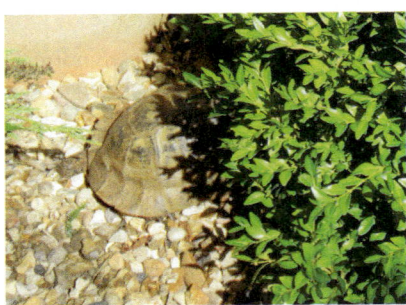

Fig. 3.10. Tortoise seeking shade using vegetation. This has the advantage that the tortoise can choose to be in complete or partial shade, depending upon the desired temperature.

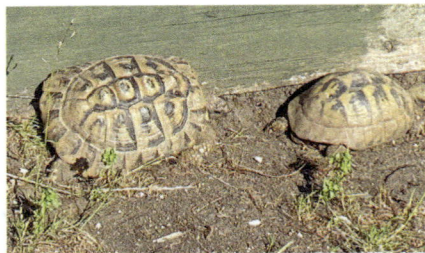

Fig. 3.11. Tortoises basking.

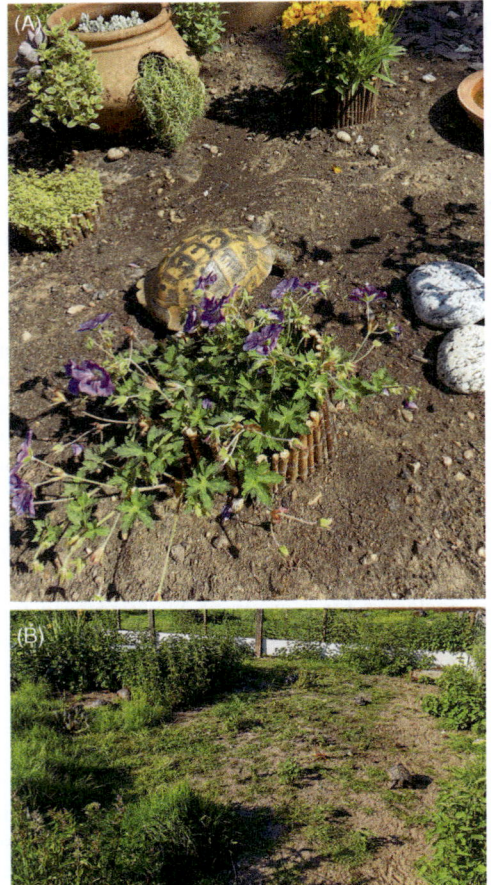

Fig. 3.8. (A) Enclosure for single male Mediterranean tortoise which is 6 m × 3 m. (B) Large enclosure for group of Mediterranean tortoises (Dillon Prest).

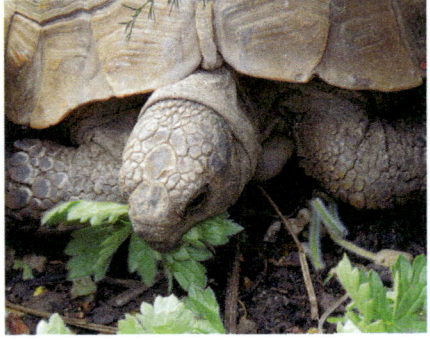

Fig. 3.12. Tortoise feeding.

Table 3.3. Recommended enclosure sizes.

Common name	Latin	Approximate length (adult)	Recommended indoor enclosure size m^2 (example dimensions)	Recommended outdoor enclosure size m^2 (example dimensions)
Mediterranean Spur-thighed tortoise	*Testudo graeca graeca/ Testudo graeca ibera/ Testudo graeca whitei*	0.3 m (30 cm)	9.0 m^2 (3m × 3m)	18.0 m^2 (6 m × 3 m)
Horsfield's tortoise	Testudo/*Agrionemys horsfieldii*	0.16 m (16 cm)	6.0 m^2 (3 m × 2 m)	10 m^2 (5 m × 2 m)
Egyptian tortoise	*Testudo kleinmanni*	0.12 m (12 cm)	6.0 m^2 (3 m × 2 m)	10 m^2 (5 m × 2 m)
Red-footed tortoise	*Chelonoidis* (*Geochelone*) *carbonaria*	0.3 m (30 cm)	9.0 m^2 (3 m × 3 m)	18.0 m^2 (6 m × 3 m)
Leopard tortoise	*Geochelone pardalis*	0.5 m (50 cm)	15.0 m^2 (5 m × 3 m)	600 m^2 (25 m × 25 m)
Sulcata (African Spurred tortoise)	*Geochelone/Centrochelys sulcata*	1.0 m (100 cm)	40 m^2 (8 m × 5 m)	1000 m^2 (0.2 ha) (0.5 acres) (32 m × 32 m)

temperature zone (POTZ) is the range that allows the tortoise to maintain its PBT (Chitty and Raftery, 2013). Daytime temperatures must be within this range, therefore, and must provide a temperature gradient (Varga, 2019) as suggested below. If tortoises are unable to maintain their preferred body temperature, then the normal metabolic processes (such as digestion of food), on which they rely, will be unable to take place. As a result, they will become unwell and, if this situation is allowed to continue, will die.

The PBT and POTZ values for some commonly kept captive species are shown in Table 3.4.

You might think that the best place for a tortoise enclosure is therefore in a really sunny spot. However, both sun and shade need to be taken into account.

Tortoises maintain their PBT by thermoregulating. If a tortoise (having reached its PBT) starts to overheat, it will move from a sunny position to one in the shade. If the enclosure has no natural shade, then it is important to create some shady areas by planting shrubs, for example. Moving into the shade allows the tortoise to cool down and reduce its body temperature until the PBT is restored. Figure 3.10 shows a tortoise using shade and Fig. 3.11 shows some basking Hermann's tortoises.

Other methods by which tortoises cool down include burrowing. Sulcatas will dig tunnels, which may be 3 m deep, in order to be able to find suitable cooler temperatures. Other ways of cooling down include sitting in water (such as puddles - Fig. 3.9), digging into the substrate, mouth gaping or fluttering the throat (gular fluttering), which works in a similar way to fluttering a fan to move air and so increase heat movement away from the animal.

Some species will seek cooler conditions in the summer if they live in a very hot climate. Horsfield's tortoises, for example, will hibernate in the winter when temperatures are around freezing; and also during very hot summer months, when temperatures may exceed 40°C, they will take a summer 'hibernation' (aestivation) to avoid this excessive heat. To aestivate means to hide and rest for long periods in cool spots, remaining dormant in a burrow or tunnel, while temperatures are above the POTZ.

Sulcatas will also use burrows for these dormant periods of aestivation in very hot weather, but they do not hibernate/brumate and cannot cope with cold temperatures.

Some tropical tortoise species have a much narrower range of temperatures to cope with, as tropical rainforests have a fairly constant temperature, day and night and throughout the year. They seek shade to thermoregulate, as the background temperatures are warm year-round. Other species, such as Galapagos tortoises, may adopt a crepuscular existence. This means they are most active at dawn and dusk when temperatures are within their POTZ. All of these are behavioural mechanisms for thermoregulation and are very much a part of the daily cycle of normal behaviours.

If, on the other hand, the PBT has not yet been reached, the tortoise will move into the sun to bask, allowing its body to heat up. Tortoises have a large surface area provided by their shell and can absorb heat, as infrared radiation. All exposed body parts can absorb heat. This can be achieved by the tortoise lying with its head and limbs stretched out, or posturing, angling its body to capture the sun's rays (Fig. 3.11). South-facing enclosures are best for tortoises kept by owners living in the northern hemisphere as these will provide the maximum available sunshine throughout the day. The opportunity to warm up each day is an essential part of their daily rhythm of activity. In the southern hemisphere the opposite would be true – the tortoise would need, at least in part, a north-facing enclosure.

Thus, the tortoise spends much of the day walking, not simply to find enough food to meet its nutritional requirements, but also for thermoregulation to achieve and maintain the preferred body temperature.

Tortoise keepers often observe a clear daily cycle of behaviour (Chitty and Raftery, 2013; Chitty, 2015; Williams, 2017). This cycle usually follows this sort of sequence, repeated throughout the day, to achieve physiological homeostasis (keeping all the main parameters for normal bodily functions within safe limits – temperature, levels of hydration, nutrients, waste products). The daily rhythms of tortoises are:

WAKE/WALK → BASK → WALK/FEED → BASK → SHELTER → WALK/FEED → BURROW → SLEEP

As we have seen, it is important to provide an enclosure that has a mixture of sun and shade. If the enclosure is in the blazing sun all day with no shade provided, or alternatively in deep shadow all day, the tortoise will find it impossible to thermoregulate and maintain its PBT. Only if its PBT is maintained, using a suitable temperature gradient, can a tortoise remain healthy and feed well (Fig. 3.12).

Will my tortoise try to escape from its enclosure and how can I stop this?

In the wild, tortoises wander over vast areas of land. We are unlikely to be able to replicate this, however large we make our enclosures. Every year thousands of tortoises escape from their garden. Some are found, often many kilometres from home; others disappear, never to be seen again by their original owner.

Enclosures must be made secure, as tortoises are great escape artists and are capable of surprisingly rapid turns of speed. They are also great diggers and climbers. Our large Leopard tortoise, Shaka, once used the side of a fence and the adjacent buddleia shrub to climb about a metre vertically upwards. He did this by scrabbling hamster-style, wedging himself between the flat surface of the fence and the thick middle branches of the plant. To prevent this, shrubs or ornamental grasses should not be planted too close to the sides of enclosures to prevent climbing, such as shown by this Horsfields tortoise in Fig. 3.13.

The corners of rectangular enclosures may need covers, as the easiest place for the tortoise to climb out is where two sides meet. The tortoise may be able to gain a purchase with two front legs in this way, and as they are so strong, be able to pull itself up using both sides. Triangles of board or Perspex® can be attached securely across the corners to stop tortoises wedging themselves and then pulling themselves upwards.

If they are not trying to climb over the enclosure sides, tortoises may try to dig under them. Some species are notoriously adept at this. One of our young Horsfield's tortoises managed to dig under a buried row of bricks, used to support a railway sleeper, positioned upright to make the enclosure sides. He almost made it out of his enclosure by digging a 25 cm tunnel (at a depth of 20 cm). Luckily, I noticed his excavations just as he was squeezing his body under the bricks.

Tortoises may continuously patrol the sides of their enclosure, or garden, looking for a way out. If

Table 3.4. Preferred body temperature (PBT) and preferred optimum temperature zone (POTZ) values for tortoises.

Species	PBT	POTZ daytime activity
Testudo graeca – Spur-thighed tortoise	28°C	20–28°C
Testudo hermanni – Hermann's tortoise	28°C	20–28°C
Testudo marginata – Marginated tortoise	28°C	20–32°C
Testudo/Agrionemys horsfieldi – Horsfield's tortoise	28°C	18–32°C
Geochelone/Centrochelys pardalis – Leopard tortoise	28°C	25–35°C
African Spurred tortoise (Sulcata) – *Geochelone/Centrochelys sulcata*	28°C	25–35°C
Red-footed tortoise – *Geochelone/Chelonoidis carbonaria*	26°C	21–27°C

they find one, they will return time and time again to the same spot even if it has been blocked up, scrabbling at whatever has been used to block it. Tortoises are very persistent in their behaviours.

To prevent escapes, enclosures need solid sides made of bricks/blocks or heavy wood, such as recycled railway sleepers as shown in Figs 3.14 and 3.15.

If tortoises can see out of their enclosure, they assume that they can get out. Solid sides are not just more secure, therefore; they also cause the tortoise less stress as it is unlikely to attempt to escape so frequently. Solid sides also help prevent tortoises from damaging their legs or necks, or ripping off scales or claws (which might allow infection to enter). This can easily happen if woven wire, such as chicken-wire, or welded fencing is used. Thinking that they can get through, tortoises will scrabble at the mesh, often injuring the more delicate parts of their bodies as illustrated in Fig. 3.16.

Will my dog or cat try to attack my tortoise?

Any predator can potentially cause injury to a tortoise. This includes our other pets, such as cats and dogs. Cats may scratch at the tortoise's head or legs as they move. Cats are very stimulated by small movements, which to them may resemble a prey animal, such as a mouse. Injuries to tortoises by cats are very rarely reported, however, and in most instances, cats are not interested in tortoises with whom they may share garden space.

Dogs, on the other hand, do injure tortoises and there are a number of reports of dog attacks every year. This is because dogs like to chew hard items such as bones. To a dog, a tortoise shell is very much like a bone in texture and structure. Given that the tortoise may not be moving that fast, the dog may pick up the tortoise or chew the edges of the shell, as seen in this small Horsfield's tortoise which has been chewed by a dog (Fig. 3.17). The larger the dog and the smaller the tortoise, the more severe the injury is likely to be.

Many dogs live in the same households with tortoises and never take any interest in them, as is the case for us. Our dogs have never shown any interest in the tortoises and they spend time in the garden largely uninterested in each other's presence. In that case they can cohabit without difficulty (although tortoises can pick up parasites from dog and cat faeces – see Chapter 7 on common illnesses and diseases). However, if a dog is being introduced to a tortoise household, careful supervision is needed in the early days to ensure that the dog does not show undue interest or is not stimulated by the tortoise's movements.

How should I set up my outdoor enclosure to make it interesting, and help keep my tortoise healthy?

The enclosures should be designed with lots of environmentally enriching features. This means that they will look as natural as possible and be a stimulating and interesting place for your tortoise to live. Tortoises are prey animals (even with limited predators in the modern era – largely humans) and choose to spend a good proportion of time in spots that provide cover and protection. Hatchlings and juveniles are more vulnerable than adults. They need cover and hiding places to an even greater degree, in order to feel safe and secure. Figure 3.18 shows the natural habitat of Mediterranean tortoises illustrating what we are trying to mimic for those species.

As previously discussed, there must be access to sunny areas for basking as well as shady places. The tortoise should also have the opportunity to burrow if it wishes to do so. This means that a uniform outdoor enclosure of grass alone (Fig. 3.19A), or one that is all concrete or patio (Fig. 3.19B), is not suitable, as neither of these provide enough choices for temperature regulation, types of substrate or humidity levels, or for tortoises to show the range of normal behaviours. The grass surface is unlikely to allow the tortoise to get warm enough even on sunny days. The hard surface of a patio would allow the tortoise to get warm enough, but does not provide opportunities to cool down, or hide. A uniform hard surface can also cause excess wear and tear on the legs, feet and the lower shell (carapace).

Providing a variety of substrates on which the tortoise can walk is a key element of enrichment. Tortoises also need to extend their legs and necks. They do this when stretching for food, or climbing over obstacles such as logs and rocks. Walking over and around plants and other objects provides your tortoise with interesting things to do. Figure 3.20 shows examples of enriched environments with opportunities for basking under Perspex® and using logs, rocks, stones, chalk lumps for a varied enriched substrate and surface for walking and climbing.

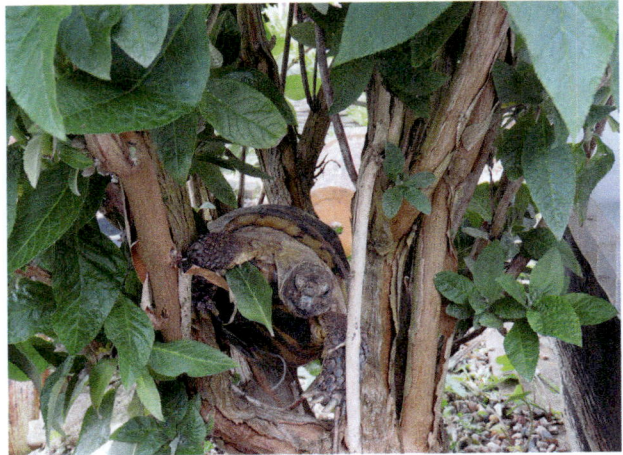

Fig. 3.13. Tortoise in a bush. Horsfield's tortoises are great climbers.

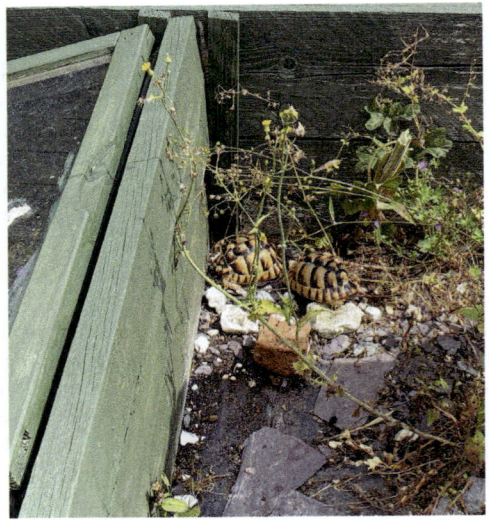

Fig. 3.15. Solid sides of wooden planks.

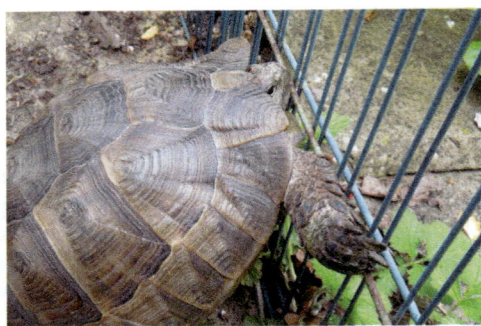

Fig. 3.16. Tortoises will scrabble at wire, with potential for scales to be damaged. Similarly, any barrier which they can see through means they are likely to try to climb out or to get through.

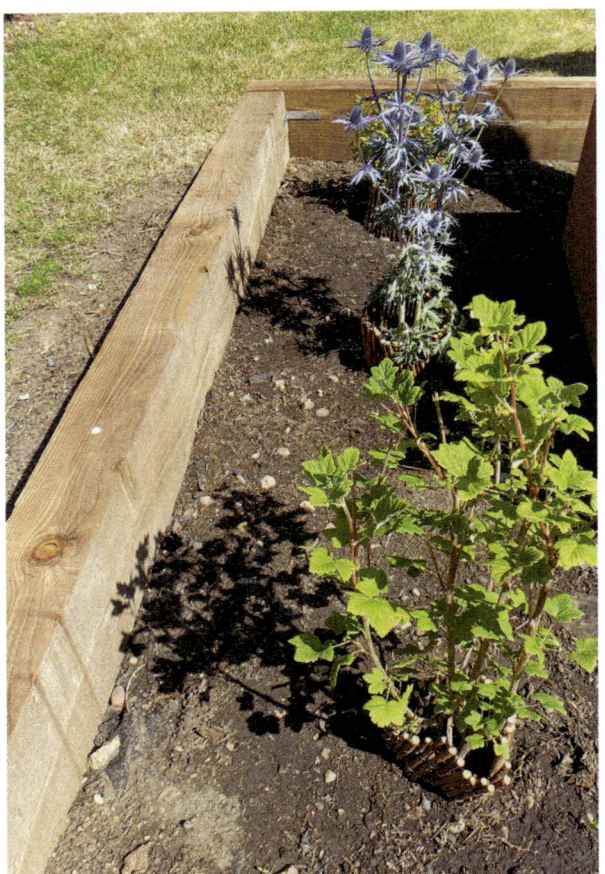

Fig. 3.14. Solid sides of wood such as railway sleepers.

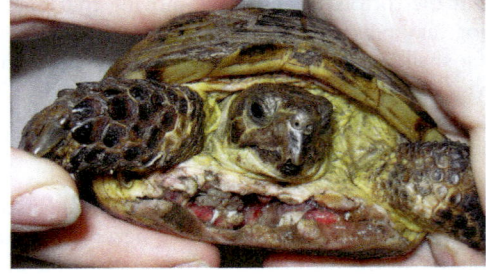

Fig. 3.17. Shell damage and injuries from a dog (William Lewis). This is a small juvenile tortoise, which is more susceptible to damage, receiving treatment for damage to the shell and underlying organs.

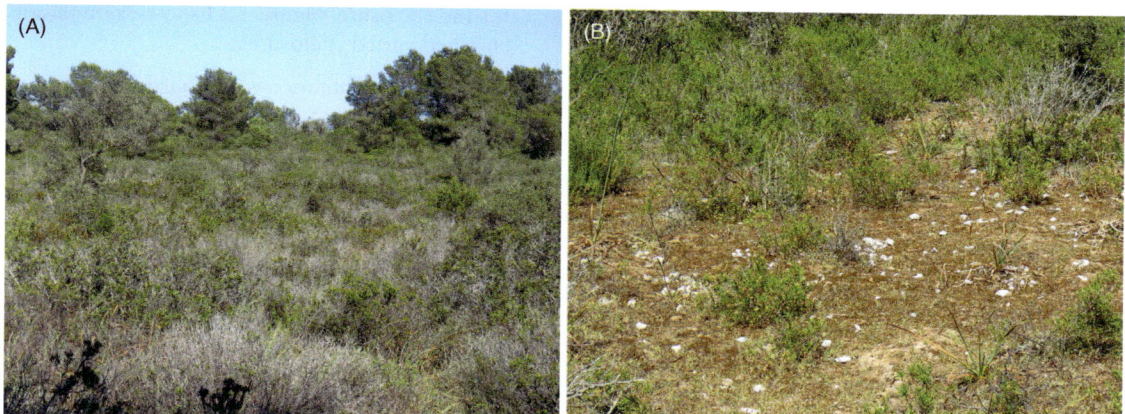

Fig. 3.18. Natural Mediterranean habitats.

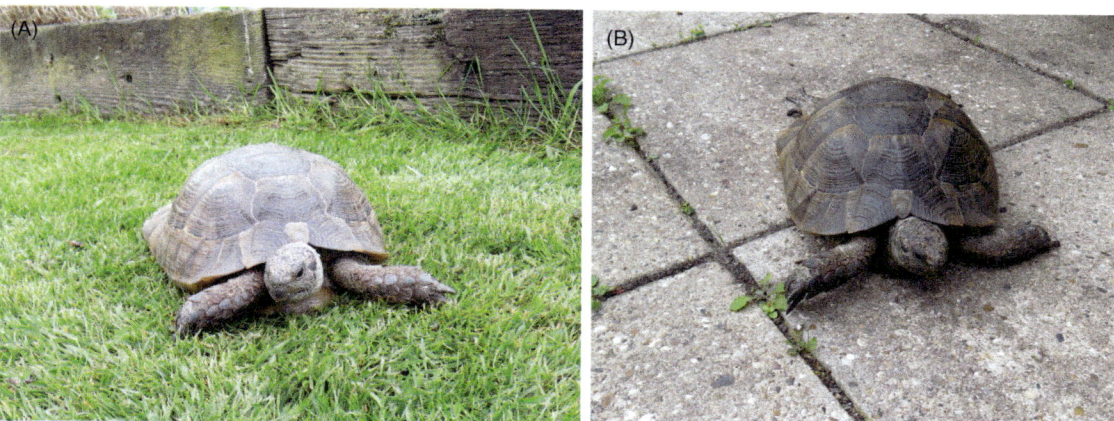

Fig. 3.19. Unsuitable outdoor enclosures. (A) Bare grass enclosure. (B) Patio enclosure.

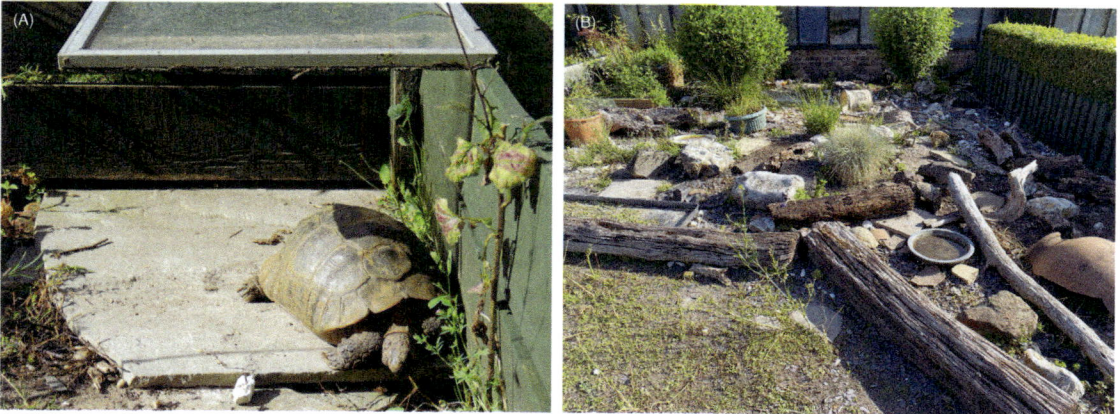

Fig. 3.20. (A) Using concrete or slabs combined with Perspex® for warming. (B) Using logs, rocks and stones for a varied enriched substrate and surface for walking and climbing.

The Captive Environment

The substrate also needs to be suitable for the humidity levels required. Mediterranean and Horsfield's tortoises need well-draining dry surfaces in the main to avoid damp conditions. Tropical tortoises from humid environments need softer, more absorbent surfaces, such as bark, compost or coco-coir (Fig. 3.21), which retain more moisture. Coco-coir can be used with soil to increase the moisture content in indoor enclosures, which can easily dry out as the depth of substrate may be only 8–10 cm.

The types of substrate provided within an outdoor enclosure, and the proportion of each type, will vary according to the species of tortoise and its original natural environment. In order to give a good variety of surfaces for warming, cooling, different humidities and enrichment, the following should be provided:

- Hard surfaces – concrete, slabs, slate, stone pieces
- Soil – bare soil that can be burrowed into (to a depth of around 15 cm), or where the tortoise can make a scrape for resting or sleeping. The soil in one area should be shaped into a mound with gentle slopes
- Gravel or loose stones – but large enough not to be eaten
- Larger rocks or boulders – for climbing, but positioned so that the tortoise cannot fall onto its back or use them to get over the enclosure sides
- Lumps of chalk/calcium carbonate – to provide added calcium to the soil and on which the tortoise can 'graze' as an additional source of calcium (as shown in Fig. 3.22)
- Enriching the soil with calcium allows food plants to take up good levels. This will then become available to the tortoise as a natural part of the diet. Supplementation of food plants with calcium can also be beneficial. This can be done by scattering calcium dust or limestone granules into the soil, or onto trays, where tortoise weeds are being grown
- Within the substrate a dish or tray of fresh water should be provided, sunk into the ground to allow the tortoise to walk in and out easily, without high risk of falling over upside down
- Vegetation – some suitable for grazing in season with larger shrubs for cover and shade. Seeds can be sown within the enclosure for grazing early in the spring (the amount of additional food provided should be reduced accordingly). Trays of weeds can also be grown for use later in the season when the first crop has been eaten. Suitable shrubs for cover and shade are those that are not poisonous and are of suitable size for the enclosure. Figure 3.23 show examples of enriched varied enclosures.

Research suggests that tortoises may build up a memory of training (for 10 years) and the layout of their environment (Gutnick *et al.*, 2020). This memory persists for a long time and enables them to return to known safe places to find refuge, for example when there are extreme weather events. One of our oldest tortoises, Tommy, a Moroccan Spur-thighed male, always finds his shelter every night. He has put himself to bed every evening for the 60 years he has been within our family. If the shelter is moved, he finds it within a couple of days and continues to go there to bed. This is very useful when I am looking for him in the evening when I need to move him into his overnight accommodation. Many other owners have reported the same behaviour over the years.

Places to hide are also very important to health and well-being, especially for young tortoises, who are more vulnerable to predation. Half-plant pots can be used for this purpose, as well as built structures (Fig. 3.24).

Planting of safe plant species, some of which can be grazed by your tortoise, is important (for suitable safe plants, see Chapter 5 on diet). Shrubs can provide shade and the tortoise can make a scrape – a shallow burrow at the base of the plant, to provide shelter from weather and predation. Provision of plants suitable for grazing is the most effective way to feed as naturally as possible, as long as a variety of species are available. Use of herbs and other aromatic plants can also help mimic the natural environment. For example, Mediterranean tortoises live in habitats with olive groves or fruit trees (Fig. 3.25A). Herbs and other aromatic low-growing plants such as lavender are common.

Suitable plants for enclosures include a range of small shrubs, herbs and some grazing food plants (Fig. 3.25B). (This is also covered in Chapter 5 on diets). Suitability of certain plants for growing outdoors will depend upon the country in which you live. Some plants will grow outdoors all year-round in warmer climates but are not hardy and will need to be put in a greenhouse or similar in colder climates. Figure 3.26 shows how an enclosure similar to that in Fig 3.25B may be set up.

There are also some plants that are toxic to tortoises and which should not be planted in enclosures. Tortoises generally do not eat toxic plants, but the risk is always there, particularly if they are hungry.

Toxic plants are listed in Chapter 5 on diets. If in doubt, before you plant, check a reliable source such as TheTortoiseTable app or www.thetortoisetable.

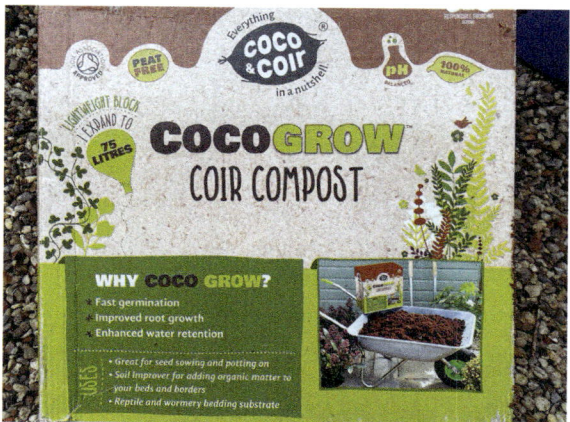

Fig. 3.21. Using coco-coir to increase moisture content of the substrate.

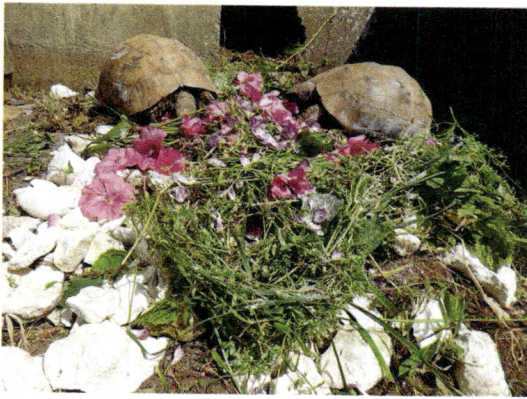

Fig. 3.22. Increasing calcium content in enclosures, so that growing feed plants take it up and so that the tortoise can gnaw and scrape the calcium source, can be achieved with limestone granules, chalk dust and lumps of chalk (Eleanor Lien-Hua Tirtasana Chubb).

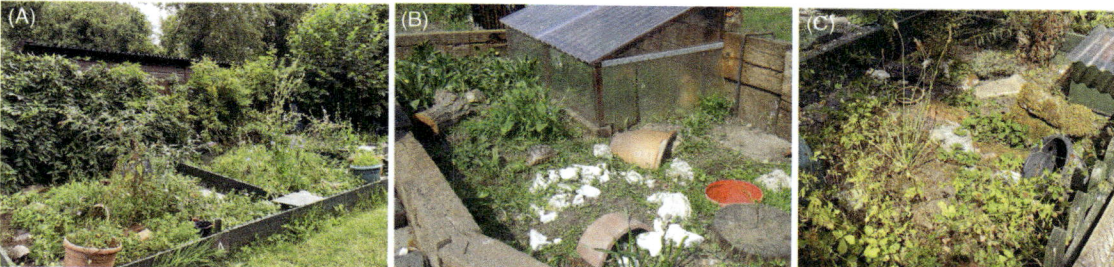

Fig. 3.23. Enriched enclosures: (A) Well-planted with forage foods, shade and sun. (B) Secure, solid high sides, chalk lumps, forage plants, varied substrate, access to large, warm enclosed area. (C) Smaller enclosure for juveniles, shallow water tray, varied food source plants, Perspex®-covered area for warmth, sun and shade.

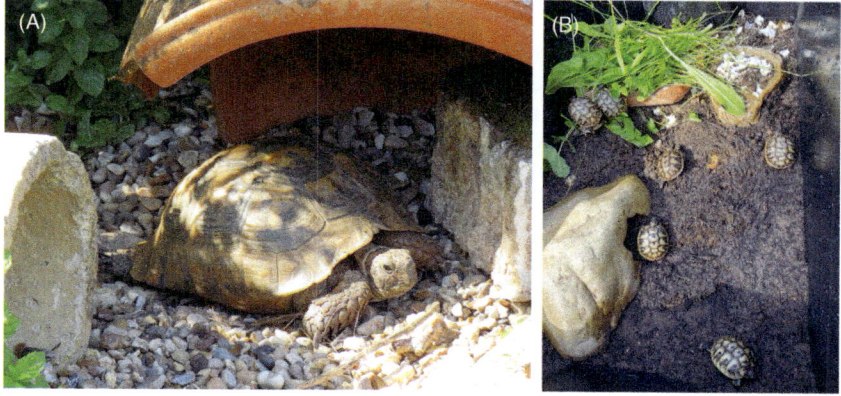

Fig. 3.24. (A) Half flowerpots/pipes provide covered areas for shelter and shade. (B) Shelter, security and retreats are especially important for young tortoises.

The Captive Environment

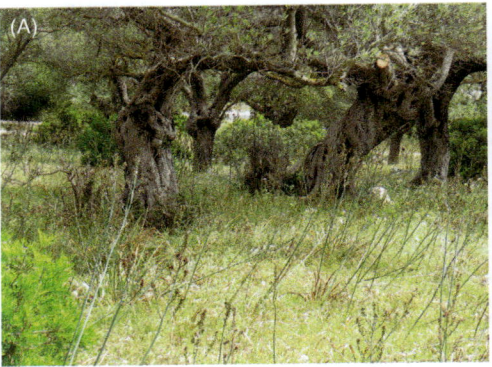
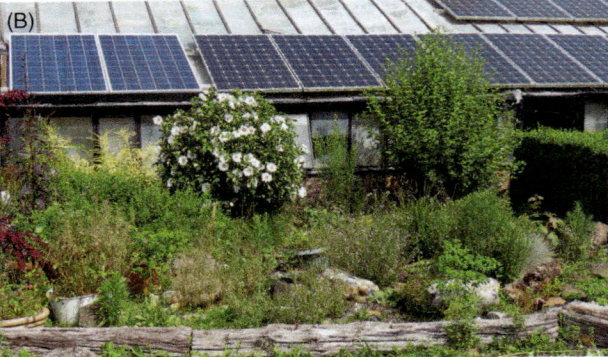

Fig. 3.25. (A) Mediterranean natural environment, aromatic hillsides with herbs and olives. (B) Well-planted enclosure including aromatic plants such as mallow, buddleia, chicory, evening primrose, snapdragons, plantains, dandelions, hawkbit, deadnettle and garlic mustard to provide a variety of larger shrubs, edible forage and low cover planting (Highfield, 1996; King, 2020).

org.uk where information about suitable weeds and flowering plants for tortoises can be found (see Chapter 5 on diets).

In colder climates an area where the tortoise can warm up even on cloudier days can be provided by covering parts of the enclosure with plastic sheet material such as acrylic (Perspex®), polyvinylchloride (PVC) or polycarbonate (Fig. 3.27). Inside these covered areas (especially if the substrate is concrete or paving slab) it can be up to 10°C warmer than the ambient temperature even when there is little sunshine. Cold frames or cloches with plastic covering can be adapted to provide shelters, which should have solid sides and an entrance/exit.

Should I leave my tortoise out in its enclosure at night?

Many tortoise keepers do not always understand that their tortoise cannot hold onto the heat gained from the sun for extended periods overnight. As the day cools into evening, the tortoise will also cool down.

Providing an outside shelter is no help at all in retaining a suitable temperature overnight. If the night temperatures go below the lower end of the preferred optimum temperature zone, the tortoise should be provided with warmer indoor facilities. For hibernating species, the temperature should stay several degrees above 10°C. This is the temperature at which hibernation begins (as discussed in Chapter 12 on hibernation). For tropical tortoises there should not be much variation in day and night temperatures, as the POTZ is around 22–30°C in many tropical species.

In addition, there is the potential for predators to cause injuries to sleeping tortoises. Although tortoises withdraw into the shell, the front and rear legs and the tail are exposed to some extent. The damage that can be caused is significant, and in some cases fatal. The wounds will always need veterinary treatment, even if the damage appears minor, to ensure that prevention or treatment against infection is provided. The teeth and claws of other animals have high levels of bacteria, which will have been transferred to the tortoise through the wounds.

Security from theft is also a consideration. In many countries tortoises cost a significant amount to buy. Some species have a very high monetary value. This makes them a potential target for theft and tortoise keepers are generally reticent when giving information about their animals to unfamiliar people. Security cameras, alarms and securing buildings in which the tortoises are kept can help. It is very difficult for security measures to be 100% effective against a determined thief, unfortunately (see Chapter 19 on health and safety), but most potential thefts can be prevented with sensible precautions. Being cautious about giving out information as to the location of tortoises is also a very good strategy, along with ensuring that people passing by cannot easily see the tortoises when outdoors.

Can I leave my tortoise out in the enclosure all year round?

The amount of time a tortoise can spend outdoors during the year will depend on the climate in the

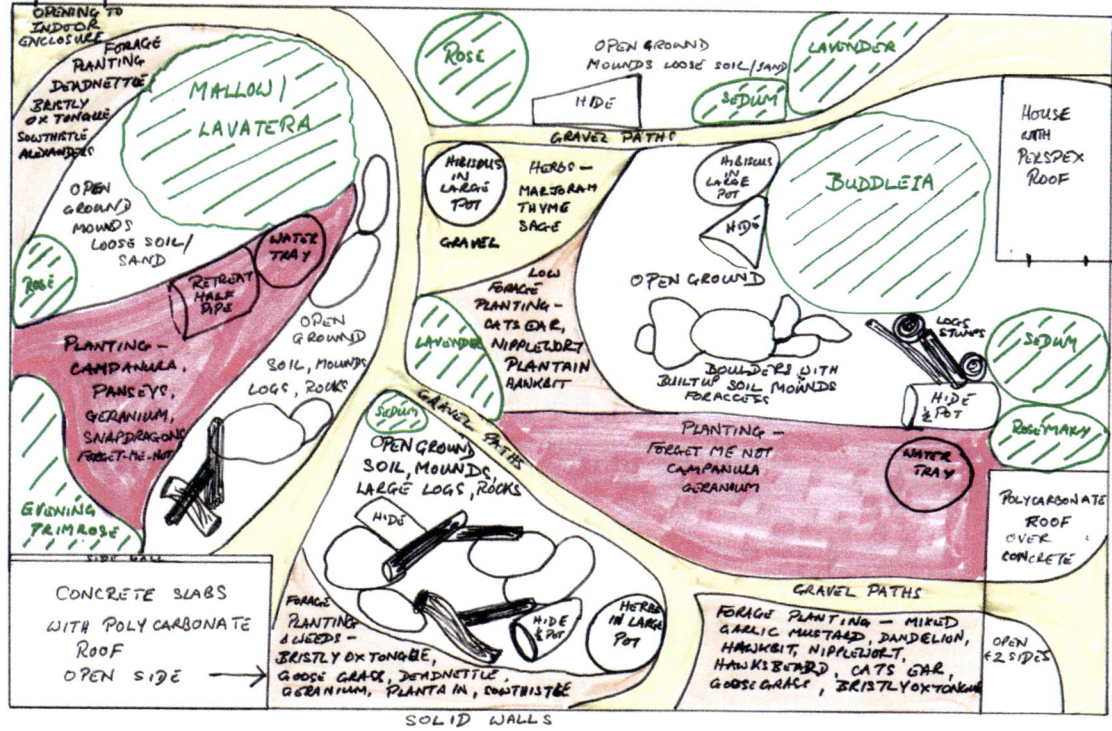

Fig. 3.26. Diagram of suggested outdoor enclosure planting in the UK or Northern Europe.

country of residence. The closer the temperatures and weather to the natural habitat, the more time can be spent outside. Tropical tortoises cannot tolerate the cold and are likely to spend more time in indoor enclosures than more temperate species. In general terms, tortoises can be outdoors on warm sunny days. Ideally the temperature will remain within the POTZ for that species. When the ambient air temperature is outside the POTZ, the tortoise will not be able to thermoregulate so effectively. Basking in the sun can of course raise the body temperature, but thermoregulation becomes more challenging when the ambient temperature is too low. Cold wet days provide little opportunity for the tortoises to raise their body temperature to anything near the preferred body temperature.

Larger tortoises will lose their body heat more slowly than smaller tortoises, which will cool quickly at low temperatures. Therefore, small species and young tortoises are likely to need more support to warm up.

In colder climates, tortoises will gradually lose heat as the sun goes down so that their body temperatures become that of the surrounding air. In spring and autumn, the tortoise will become very cold outside if not properly supported with additional sources of heat. Use of artificial heat sources (see Chapter 4 on artificial light and heat) is essential where the climate does not provide the POTZ for much of the year. For tropical tortoises, which do not hibernate, this means for all of the year in many countries.

Depending on where you live, some tortoises will spend far greater amounts of time indoors, with heat and light, than they do outside. For example, tropical species living in the UK may only spend a few hours each day outside, even during the summer. Mediterranean tortoises living in northern climates may spend most of their days outside from April to September in an average year, with a shorter number of hours outside in March and October. In some years they may be outside only from May to August. In all cases, additional support is needed for part of the year in countries where tortoises are not endemic.

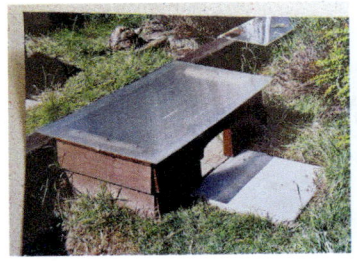

Fig. 3.27. Polycarbonate and Perspex® roof shelters.

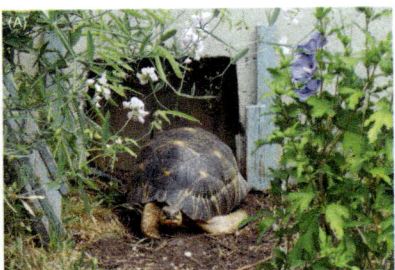
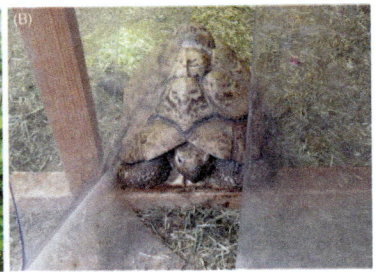

Fig. 3.29. (A) Heavy-duty plastic strip curtains covering a small opening (this also has a door which can be shut overnight) for this Radiated tortoise. (B) Heavy-duty plastic strip curtains can cover a much larger opening for Leopard tortoises or Sulcatas, as a means of access for the tortoise to get in and out without losing too much heat in the indoor set-up.

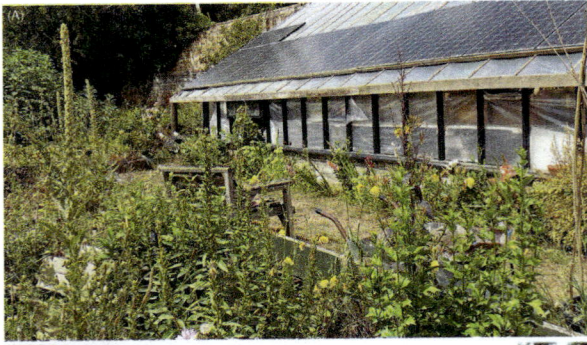
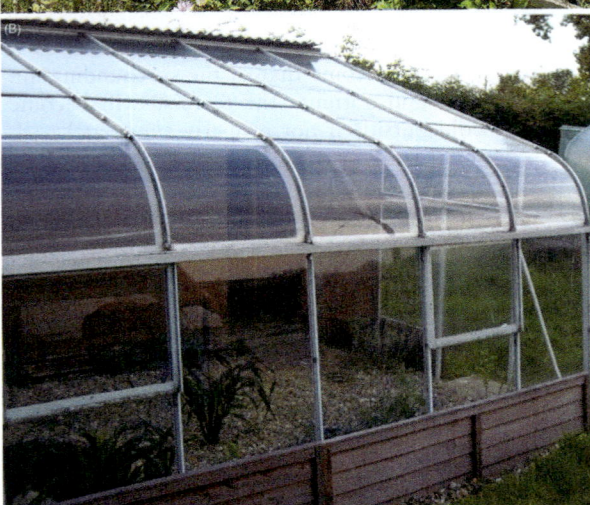

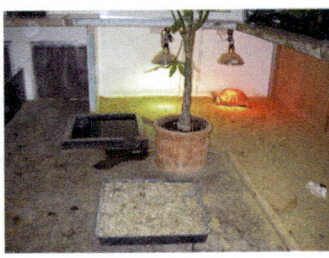

Fig. 3.30. Indoor set-up for large tortoises such as Sulcatas (Eleanor Lien-Hua Tirtasana Chubb).

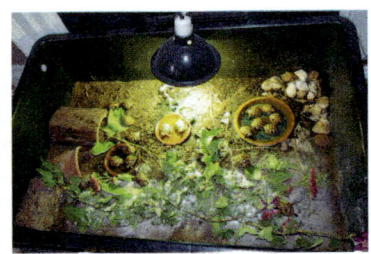

Fig. 3.31. Large plastic fish boxes can make easy-to-clean, effective indoor set-ups for juveniles and smaller adult tortoises (Eleanor Lien-Hua Tirtasana Chubb).

Fig. 3.28. (A) Large combined indoor and outdoor enclosures with free access in and out are by far the best option, giving tortoises the greatest choice of environmental options, particularly temperature.
(B) A greenhouse with solid sides at tortoise level, into which overhead lights can be added and access to the surrounding outdoor enclosure provided.

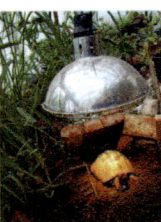

Fig. 3.32. Indoor set-up with overhead heat and light (Eleanor Lien-Hua Tirtasana Chubb).

Where should I build my indoor enclosure?

The ideal tortoise set-up will have the indoor and outdoor enclosures linked, as shown in Fig. 3.28. This ensures that the tortoise can access indoor enclosures with artificial heat and light, as well as being able to venture outdoors when the weather is warm and sunny.

The ideal solution is to build the tortoise garden (enclosure) around a greenhouse, conservatory or shed, so that the tortoise has somewhere to go and get warm on cool days (Fig. 3.29). Obviously when the outside temperature drops below the tortoise's preferred optimum temperature zone for any length of time then the tortoise will need to be moved into the indoor enclosure until the weather improves. This might be for several days, or it may be for weeks or months.

If it is not possible to provide this 'combined enclosure', the indoor enclosure will need to be located inside a building. This could be in the house, or in an insulated greenhouse or in a purpose-built shed. Garages are not suitable if cars are being parked there. They will get too cold when the garage doors are opened; additionally, the tortoise will be exposed to poisonous exhaust fumes.

It will be necessary to heat at least part of the indoor enclosure to a daytime temperature of around 30°C. Temperatures outside could well be 0°C or less. Raising parts of the indoor enclosure to a temperature of 30°C may well be easier, and less costly, if a room in the house is used. Central heating is likely to contribute background warmth, so less heat is needed to raise the temperature in the indoor enclosure to around 30°C under the basking light or heat source. Central heating will not be the sole source of heat; more localised basking light/heat sources are also necessary.

Outside buildings like greenhouses or sheds, if used, will need to be very well-insulated to reduce heating costs. Many tortoise keepers use solar panels and other renewable sources of energy such as heat exchange pumps to reduce their energy bills (Fig. 3.28A). If outside sheds, greenhouses or garages are to be used, it is also important to ensure that they are rodent-proof. Rats, in particular, have been known to inflict considerable damage to tortoises, or even kill them (see Chapter 7 on common illnesses and diseases).

How big should my inside enclosure (terrarium) be?

As large as possible is the basic answer. As shown in Table 3.3, the more space available, the greater is the opportunity for walking and seeking suitable environmental conditions. Unlike other reptiles, where the available space can be increased because the animal uses three dimensions, including climbing branches and other structures, the only important feature for tortoises is the floor area. This is where the tortoise will spend its time, walking around the enclosure, or terrarium (as indoor enclosures, in particular, are often named).

The indoor enclosure needs to provide light and heat gradients (see Chapter 4 on artificial light and heat), so that tortoise can thermoregulate. The ability to move around and to have an enriched environment becomes more of a challenge on a smaller scale (Fig. 3.33). The larger species, such as Leopard tortoises and Sulcatas, will need extremely big indoor facilities, such as insulated sheds, available all year around (Fig. 3.30), even though they will spend time outdoors in the summer. As they are tropical species and so do not hibernate/brumate, they need to be kept warm all year round.

What does an inside tortoise enclosure look like?

Examples of indoor enclosures include tortoise tables, or partially enclosed open tables with sides, large plastic holding tanks (Fig. 3.31) (usually used for fish) or custom-made spaces within greenhouses or sheds (Fig. 3.32). Making an indoor enclosure to fit the space is often the best option. The image in Fig. 3.34 shows how this can be done using suitable materials.

Glass fish aquariums or snake/lizard terrariums are not suitable as indoor accommodation. They are not big enough and do not have a large enough surface area for the tortoise to walk about. Also, as the tortoise can see through the glass it will spend the whole time crashing against the sides trying to escape. These materials can also cause very high humidity levels, which may not be helpful for good health. Humidity within the substrate is helpful as described but levels that are very high are not recommended. There is also a danger from breakage of the glass.

As with outdoor enclosures, security is important, as the tortoise will try to escape. The sides of tortoise tables and other similar enclosures should not be see-through, or be made of mesh. Equally the enclosure needs to be made of an easy-to-clean material in order to maintain good levels of hygiene, as illustrated in Figs 3.31 and 3.33.

Wood is a useful material from which to build indoor accommodation, especially where this is to be created to fit the available space. It is, however, of limited value unless enclosed in a waterproof material such as a pond liner, lino or thick plastic layer (Figs 3.34 and 3.35). An alternative is to use wood surfaced with a waterproof material such as melamine, or painted with a waterproof varnish that is non-toxic once hardened (Highfield and Highfield, 2008). Without one of these protections the wood will rot fairly quickly from contact with a damp substrate and some humidity.

How do I build my indoor enclosure or terrarium?

The cost of setting up and maintaining indoor enclosures is considerable.

The terrarium should not be small – use as much space as you can, to allow the maximum available walking area (Biedenweg and Schramm, 2019). The height of the terrarium should be sufficient to allow the safe fixing and hanging of overhead lights and heaters. There must be a suitable distance between the overhead lights and heaters and the top of the tortoise's shell. This distance will be determined by the types of lights and heaters used. The lights must allow the tortoise to access the relevant UVB and UVA light wavelengths, while the heaters must be used to create suitable thermal gradients (see Chapter 4 on artificial light and heat). The tortoise should be able to reach its preferred body temperature under the basking lamps but not get too hot.

The sides of the terrarium will be solid so that the tortoise cannot see out, but you will need to access the enclosure for feeding, cleaning, etc. Good ventilation is essential, but you will decide, based on your own situation and location of the enclosure, how best to set up the overhead light and heat to create light intensity and temperature gradients. Open-top tables with overhead fittings give good ventilation but require more heat to maintain temperatures, depending on the background temperatures. Setting up a tortoise table or terrarium in a cold space such as an unheated garage will cost much more to run in energy costs, for example, than one set up in an insulated heated shed or outbuilding or in the room of a house.

The terrarium could be created from wood, glass or plastic materials or a combination. Plastic and glass are easier to clean but have some disadvantages, as described in Table 3.5. Wood can be used but needs protection from water.

When using wood to create the terrarium, the whole base should be covered in waterproof material in one sheet, and be folded up the sides of the terrarium to the height of the substrate (10 cm minimum). The sheeting must be pushed carefully into the corners and up the sides, and then firmly attached to the side walls. It should be sealed at the edges with silicone. If a waterproof sheet is not to be used an alternative is waterproof varnish, epoxy resin, or a liquid rubber liner which can be painted onto the wooden surface, making it waterproof.

As tortoises are very strong the whole set-up should be firmly fixed in place to avoid damage. Any area which tortoises can access is likely to be disrupted or dislodged, causing potential damage to the set-up, equipment and of course the tortoise.

How should I set up my indoor enclosure to make it interesting, and help keep my tortoise healthy?

Creating the variety of microclimates essential for good health, and the necessary enrichment, becomes even more of a challenge in smaller-scale indoor enclosures than it does with outdoor enclosures. This applies particularly when creating gradients for heat and light with sufficient range and variation.

The substrate used should be as close to that of the outdoor enclosures as possible. Providing a variety will increase both interest and enrichment. A minimum depth of around 10 cm of substrate is recommended. An area with slates or flat rocks is useful for basking purposes, particularly if it is positioned beneath a lamp (Highfield, 1996; Highfield and Highfield, 2008, 2009). Gravel or small pebbles can also provide variety. Soil mixed with compost can be used to provide burrowing areas and places for natural planting.

Another very useful material is coco-coir, which holds moisture very well, allowing humidity to be maintained and providing a soft substrate for burrowing and hiding. Coco-coir can be used with soil to increase the moisture content in indoor enclosures, which can easily dry out as the depth of substrate may be only 10 cm. Coco-coir can hold very high volumes of water - Fig. 3.21.

Other materials can be used depending upon the species being kept. Sand and soil mixtures can be used for desert species, while coco-coir or bark

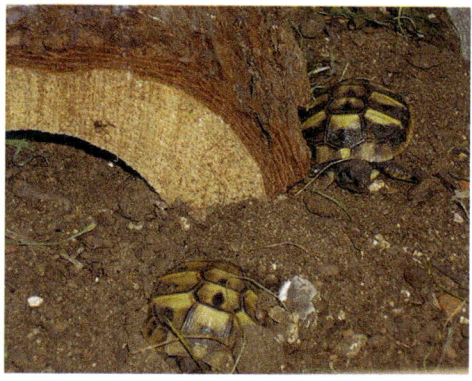

Fig. 3.33. Indoor set-up with soil/sand/compost substrate allows more natural behaviours such as burrowing, seen here, and use of microclimates (Eleanor Lien-Hua Tirtasana Chubb).

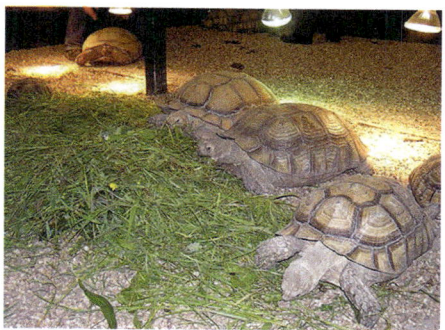

Fig. 3.36. Sulcatas on a dry surface with grazing.

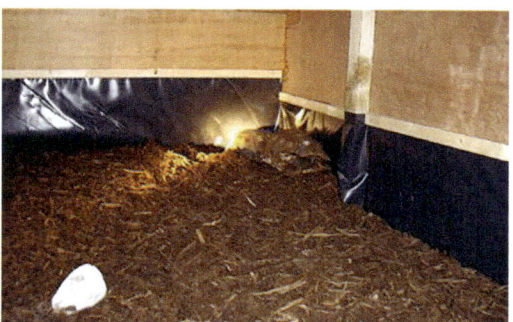

Fig. 3.34. Indoor tropical set-up with pond liner covering the base of the wooden structure, allowing use of a deep soil-based substrate (Eleanor Lien-Hua Tirtasana Chubb).

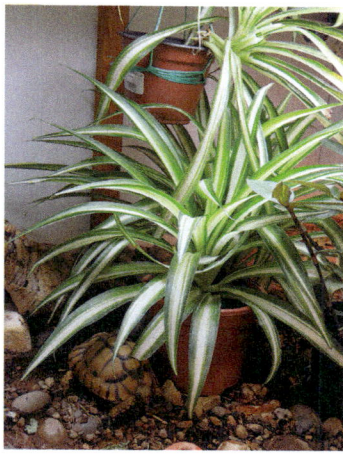

Fig. 3.37. Indoor enclosure with planting to create microclimates, provide forage and increase humidity (Dillon Prest).

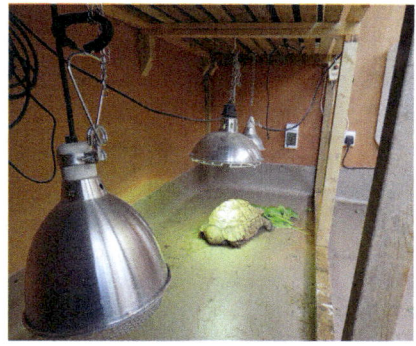

Fig. 3.35. Indoor accommodation being set up with lino covering the wooden floor and sides of this insulated shed. The substrate has not yet been added. Overhead heat and lights are in place, with a thermostat for temperature control.

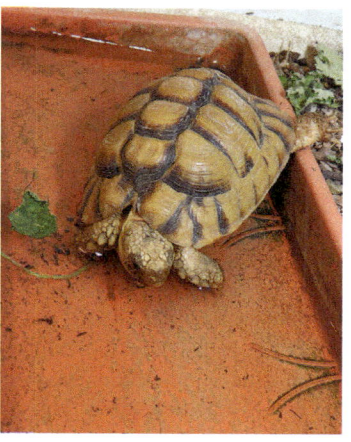

Fig. 3.38. Tortoise with free access to water indoors sitting in a shallow water dish.

The Captive Environment

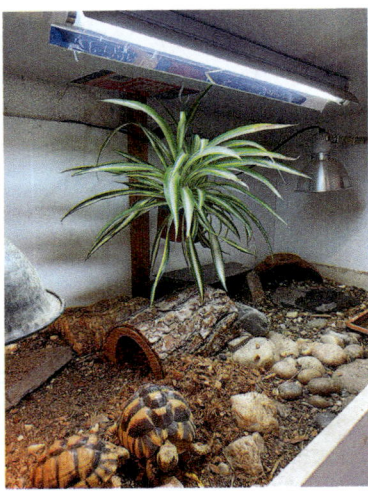

Fig. 3.39. Indoor lights and heat.

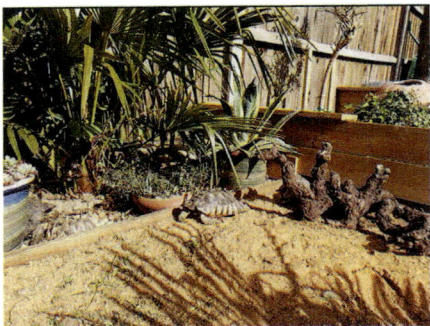

Fig. 3.40. Marginated tortoise in enriched enclosure (Dillon Prest).

chips are ideal for tropical rainforest dwellers, as they hold moisture and mimic the forest floor. Note that products made from pine or other conifers should not be used, as they can produce harmful oils when warm (Highfield, 1996; Highfield and Highfield, 2008, 2009).

The large tropical grazers such as Leopard tortoises and Sulcatas can be housed on a part-soil/compost substrate with a dry hay-like surface covering (Fig. 3.36). Readi-Grass® or similar grass-based products can be used for this. This product is dry and can be eaten by these grazing species. You should not try to substitute grass clippings from mowing your lawn for this product. The damp material can harbour mould and mildew and may present a health hazard to your tortoise.

Planting can really help to improve the microclimates created in smaller indoor enclosures and help produce a more natural looking environment (Fig. 3.37). Edible plants can be used as food sources. They also provide shade and shelter and increase variations in humidity levels. Indoor plants often have to be grown in pots, some of which can be hanging to avoid the tortoises eating them completely or flattening them (Fig. 3.39). Water should always be accessible (Fig. 3.38) and Figs 3.39 and 3.40 show varied enclosures.

Note that it is important to position the tortoise enclosure on something very solid and secure, particularly if you are creating a tortoise table or similar. The set-up is likely to be very heavy if substrates like soil/compost/stones, gravel etc. are used. Enclosures can be stacked on top of each other, as long as there is good ventilation and access for cleaning and feeding. The materials used to build the tortoise tables must be strong enough to hold a significant weight, depending upon the substrate used.

Besides enrichment, what else do we have to consider when setting up an indoor tortoise enclosure?

Humidity

Tortoises need an environment with varied humidity in order to ensure that their respiratory system does not become stressed by over-drying. They also need to avoid their shell and skin drying out.

In outdoor enclosures the depth of soil means that moisture tends to be retained for a long time, so humidity remains at an acceptable level. Maintaining suitable humidity levels indoors is more challenging. As the depth of substrate is limited (usually to only around 10 cm) it dries out more quickly, especially with overhead lights and heat. Water will need to be added to the substrate in significant quantities, in order to raise humidity levels. I often add a watering can of water to a terrarium every couple of days to prevent drying out and the creation of too much dust for the tortoises. Additional spraying of the enclosure is usually a daily necessity, while any plants in the enclosure will also need to be watered and sprayed.

Optimum substrate humidity levels are around 70% for many terrestrial species, and could be higher (80–90%) for tropical rainforest species such as Red-footed tortoises. Drying out is a particular problem for hatchlings and juveniles, as the drying out of the peritoneum is considered a major

Table 3.5. Comparison between materials used to create indoor accommodation.

Material and potential uses	Pros	Cons
Glass – for tropical tortoises needing high humidity. Many more cons than pros. Not recommended	Easy to clean. Allows natural light into the terrarium, depending upon its location	Heavy. Can create excessively high humidity in enclosed space. Where the sheets meet at edges and corners, they should be sealed with silicone. Glass sides at tortoise eye-level means they will attempt to get through the glass, increasing stress and frustration. Potential for injury to face and front legs trying to get through a barrier which they can see through. Can create very high temperatures in direct sunlight. Does not hold heat very well and may be more expensive to heat if the terrarium is in a cold room.
Plastic sheet material – opaque such as PVC, acrylic and polycarbonate. Balance of pros and cons. Expensive compared with wood, so use when cost is not an issue. Can be suitable where high humidity is needed.	Hard, resistant, waterproof materials. Light weight. Easy to clean. Can be cut – flexible for different situations and available spaces. Easy for fitting lights and heat.	Where the sheets meet at edges and corners, they should be sealed with silicone. Can create excessively high humidity in enclosed space. Expensive
Wood or composite material made of wood particles glued together such as plywood, made of thin laminated sheets of wood glued together, or oriented strand board (OSB), made of glued timber strands. In both cases the wood is bonded with heat and pressure. Plywood very suitable material recommended. OSB very suitable material recommended. MDF not suitable material, not recommended	Light weight. Holds heat more effectively than glass. Easy to cut – flexible for different situations and available spaces. Easy for fitting lights and heat. Plywood aesthetically pleasing. Plywood is more moisture resistant. OSB is less expensive.	Where the sheets meet at edges and corners, they should be sealed with silicone. Base needs to be made waterproof for contact with substrate, to avoid rotting, using pond-liner, lino, thick plastic liner, waterproof varnish. OSB is less attractive to the eye. Plywood is more expensive. Medium density fibreboard (MDF), also known as chipboard, is heavier. MDF less moisture resistant than either plywood or OSB.
Composite material made of wood, or wood particles glued together and with melamine resin to create a waterproof plastic surface. Balance of pros and cons. Expensive compared with wood so use when cost is not an issue. Can be suitable where high humidity is needed.	Easy to cut – flexible for different situations and available spaces. Waterproof if sealed at the edges and joins. Easy for fitting lights and heat.	Heavy. Expensive. Where the sheets meet at edges and corners, they should be sealed with silicone. Can create excessively high humidity in enclosed space.

factor leading to metabolic bone disease and shell pyramiding (McArthur et al., 2004).

Tortoises should always have access to fresh water (Fig. 3.38). It should be possible for the tortoise to walk into and out of the water container with ease. Shallow plastic or terracotta trays are useful water containers, especially if they are large enough for the tortoise to sit in, and deep enough to cover the base of the shell. This allows the tortoise to simply extend its neck to drink.

Plastic is particularly easy to keep clean. Terracotta is heavier and so sits better within the substrate without being disturbed by the tortoise. As adult tortoises are often strong and heavy, everything within the enclosure must be robust and solidly fixed. If this is not the case, it is likely to be dislodged, emptied or moved, or at worst damaged or destroyed as the tortoise moves around the enclosure.

Light and heat

Outside sunlight provides both heat and light. In the indoor enclosure, any available natural daylight must be supplemented by artificial sources (see Chapter 4 on artificial light and heat). These should simulate natural daylight as far as possible. This is particularly the case in northern climates where additional light (and heat) sources are needed in the spring and autumn.

While tortoises are awake and active, they need 12–14 hours of light daily. Shortening of daylength is the key trigger for hibernation/brumation in non-tropical species (McArthur, 2003). If we keep tortoises from temperate regions and do not give them the required amount of daylight there is a risk of jumpstarting the hibernation/brumation process. This is likely to lead to hibernation/brumation being too long.

Detailed information about setting up lights and heat effectively in the indoor enclosure can be found in Chapter 4.

Taking account of seasonal changes

Mediterranean tortoises and those from other temperate regions experience natural seasonal changes. These seasonal changes impact dietary food plants, as well as climatic change. Such variations should be replicated in captivity as far as is practicable. Factors such as changing daylength as well as temperature variations and amounts of rainfall across the year should be reflected in the ways in which we keep tortoises in captivity.

Daylength is the key environmental trigger for hibernation/brumation in species that naturally have this rest period. One of the reasons for hibernation/brumation is the lack of food available through the winter. Temperature is also crucial in the hibernation/brumation process – the temperature at which normal metabolism shuts down is 10°C. Above this temperature hibernation will not be completely in place; below this temperature hibernation/brumation begins, with the optimal temperature range for most species to avoid freezing but maintain a hibernation/brumation is 4–8°C (see Chapter 13 on Mediterranean tortoises).

In summary, considerable thought, time and effort are needed when creating indoor and outdoor enclosures. Having identified the species of tortoise, you should be in a position to provide the sort of natural conditions which will most effectively maintain your tortoise's health and wellbeing. This can only be successfully achieved if the environments you create provide sufficient natural choice to allow the tortoise to find the conditions that suit it best.

When thinking about your own indoor and outdoor set-ups, ask yourself these questions:

- Tortoises know what temperature they need for their body to function well – can they achieve that in the set-up you have provided?
- Is the daylength suitable to keep them active and feeding?
- Are you providing an enriched environment for them to show most natural behaviours?
- Do they have easy access to water and are the humidity levels right?
- Is the substrate suitable for them to dig, climb, create a scrape or nest, and to use for humidity and temperature regulation?
- Are their enclosures well-constructed, safe and secure?

Conclusion

Tortoises are a fascinating group of reptiles, which provide hobbyists and owners with the opportunity for a rewarding keeper experience. They are not in any way domesticated, however, and we must be mindful of their needs, above our own, when taking on responsibility for their care. The captive environment must provide them with sufficient choice and options for them to find the environmental conditions which they need, on a daily, monthly and annual basis. This is difficult to achieve – the more we know, the more we have to consider in our environmental provision for them.

The important starting point is knowing the species of tortoise, understanding the individual tortoise and providing the very best enclosures that we can. Meeting their needs is always going to be a challenge and we have to accept that we are unlikely to faithfully duplicate the conditions found in the wild. We can, however, provide a reasonable approximation. This will allow our tortoises to remain in good health with their welfare needs largely met. We are aiming to ensure that our tortoises are thriving not just surviving with us.

References

Biedenweg, F. and Schramm, R. (2019) *The Egyptian Tortoise Testudo kleinmanni Lortet 1883. A Fascinating Little Beauty*. Tartaruga-Verlag Ricarda Schramm, Grebenhain, Germany

Chitty, J. and Raftery, A. (2013) *Essentials of Tortoise Medicine and Surgery*. Wiley Blackwell, Chichester, UK.

Chitty, J. (2015) *Latest Methods in Chelonian Treatment: Improving Standards for Captive Chelonia*. In: Proceedings of Tortoise Welfare UK Conference, 8 November 2015

Divers, S. (1996) Basic reptile husbandry, history taking and clinical examination. *Veterinary Record In Practice* 18, 51–65

Gutnick, T., Weissenbacher, A. and Kuba, M.J. (2020) The underestimated giants: operant conditioning, visual discrimination and long-term memory in giant tortoises. *Animal Cognition* 23, 159–167

Highfield, A. (1996) *Practical Encyclopaedia of Keeping and Breeding Tortoises and Freshwater Turtles*. Carapace Press, London.

Highfield, A. and Highfield, N. (2008) *Taking Care of Pet Tortoises*. The Tortoise Trust Jill Martin Fund. Available from: www.tortoisetrust.org

Highfield, A. and Highfield, N. (2009) *Keeping a Pet Tortoise*. Interpet, Dorking, UK.

King, L. (2020) *Edible Plants for Tortoises in the UK* (4th edn). Available from: books@tlady.clara.co.uk

McArthur, S. (2003) *Post hibernation anorexia (PHA) Testudo species*. BCG symposium, 29 March 2003

McArthur, S. (2012) *Chelonian Medicine: Improving Standards for Captive Chelonia in the UK*. Proceedings of Tortoise Welfare UK Conference 17 November 2012

McArthur, S., Wilkinson, R. and Meyer, J. (2004) *Medicine and Surgery of Tortoises and Turtles*. Blackwell, Oxford, UK. The Tortoise Table App: available from www.thetortoisetable.org.uk

Varga, M. (2019) Ch 3 Captive Maintenance. In: Girling, S.J. and Raiti, P. (eds) *BSAVA Manual of Reptiles*, 3rd edn. BSAVA, Quedgeley, UK, pp. 36–49.

Vetter, H. (2002) *Turtles of the World Vol. 1, Africa, Europe and Western Asia*. Chimaira, Frankfurt

Vetter, H. (2004) *Turtles of the World Vol. 2, North America*. Chimaira, Frankfurt

Vetter, H. (2005) *Turtles of the World Vol. 3, Central & South America*. Chimaira, Frankfurt.

Vetter, H. (2006) *Turtles of the World Vol. 4, East and South Asia*. Chimaira, Frankfurt.

Williams, J. (2017) Stress in Chelonia (tortoises, terrapins and turtles), *The Veterinary Nurse*, Vol. 8, No. 5.

4 Artificial Lighting and Heat Sources

Abstract
This chapter is a detailed and, in places, complex examination of the vital need to provide captive tortoises with as much natural sunlight as possible. Where these opportunities are limited by living in northern climates, additional artificial heat and light needs to be provided to extend the day in autumn and spring, following hibernation and on cold wet days in summer. The types of artificial heat and light must provide suitable sources of ultraviolet, visible and infrared radiation. The intensity of light is also important to ensure that the tortoise stays in good health, grows properly if a hatchling or juvenile and is able to show normal behaviours.

Much of the tortoise's metabolism is influenced by light and temperature, and its daily rhythms are controlled by these external factors. Suitable sources of light and heat are discussed along with the role of vitamin D3 in calcium metabolism in the presence of UVB radiation.

Introduction

Natural sunlight is the best form of heat and light source for any tortoise. Where we have to provide additional daylight hours, because the tortoise is being kept in captivity in a climate that is not sunny or warm enough to meet its needs, it is as well to understand the basic biology involved so that we can try to provide the best possible light and heat sources.

The types of artificial heat and light provided, along with access to natural sunlight, can have a profound impact on health and behaviour. For young tortoises in particular, suitable light sources are essential for normal growth and development. Along with a suitable diet that is high in fibre and calcium but low in protein and fat, appropriate levels of ultraviolet (UV) light in particular have a profound impact on health, growth and well-being.

This is a complex topic in terms of the biochemistry involved in the metabolism of calcium and vitamin D3, both being essential in normal bone formation and growth. When taking into account the impact of the many different artificial light sources available for reptiles, and for tortoises in particular, the topic becomes a minefield of potential misinformation.

Much of the information here comes from the UVGuide research project led by Frances M. Baines in the UK (Baines *et al.*, 2016), which has been developed into the BIAZA UV Tool (BIAZA RAWG, 2021), and thanks are extended to her for allowing the use of diagrams in this chapter. The original research of Holick *et al.* (1981) is also important. Holick pioneered the work that has led to our understanding of the role of vitamin D3 in calcium metabolism, which occurs in the presence of particular types of UV radiation – namely UVB radiation.

Natural sunlight as a source of heat and light for tortoises

Natural sunlight is made up from the whole electromagnetic spectrum provided by the sun, and so collectively sunlight provides the full range of light and heat needed for life on Earth. Light is provided by the visible and UV parts of the electromagnetic spectrum and heat from the infrared (IR) parts of the spectrum as shown in Fig. 4.1 below.

The daily rhythm of life for tortoises is completely in tune with natural daylight intensity and the number of hours of sunshine. Tortoises should spend as much time as possible with access to natural sunlight. Even in climates where the sun does not shine as brightly, or for as many hours, access to natural sunlight is still the best way to ensure that your tortoise benefits from all parts of the spectrum.

© CAB International 2025. *Tortoise Husbandry and Welfare.* (J. Williams)
DOI: 10.1079/9781800623736.0004

Ultraviolet UV	Visible light	Infrared radiation IR
UVC 200–280 nm Blocked by ozone Very harmful	Red end 740–625 Orange/Yellow 625–565	IR-A 700–1400 nm Deeply penetrates dermis and subcutaneous tissue
UVB 280–315 nm Needed for vitamin D3 synthesis	Green 565–520 Blue 520–435	IR-B 1400–3000 nm Absorbed by epidermis mainly but some penetration to subcutaneous tissue
UVA 315–400 nm Visible to some invertebrates, fish, reptiles, birds	Violet end 435–380	IR-C 3000 nm–1 mm Absorbed by epidermis

Fig. 4.1. The different parts of the electromagnetic spectrum.

Ultraviolet UV	Skin penetration
UVC 200–280 nm Blocked by ozone Very harmful	Penetrates Stratum corneum and epidermis
UVB 280–315 nm Needed for vitamin D3 synthesis	Penetrates Stratum corneum, epidermis and just into dermis
UVA 315–400 nm Needed for vitamin D3 synthesis Visible to some invertebrates, fish, reptiles, birds	Penetrates Stratum corneum, epidermis and well into dermis

Fig. 4.2. Three types of UV radiation (Baines *et al.*, 2016).

UV Index colour code		
	Typically occurs in:	WHO category
11+	Full tropical midday sun	Extreme
10 9 8	Full tropical late morning sun; full summer mid-day sun in subtropical areas	Very high
7 6	Full tropical mid-morning sun or under light cloud at mid-day	High
5 4 3	Full tropical early morning sun; light shade or overcast weather at mid-day	Moderate
2 1	Very early morning sun; shade at mid-day	Low
0		

Fig. 4.3. UV Index colour code and WHO category.

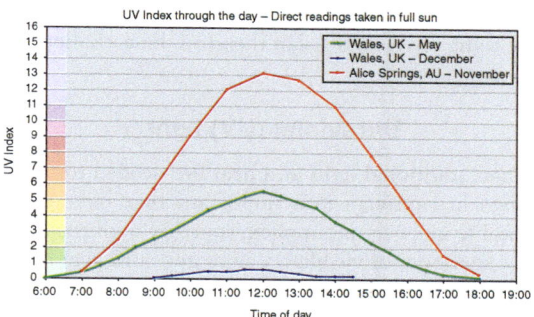

Fig. 4.4. UV Index daily fluctuations, compared for a summer day in Australia, a summer day in Wales and a winter day in Wales, UK. (Kind permission of Frances M. Baines.)

Visible and UV light are essential for normal growth and metabolism. Suitable temperatures from the IR end of the spectrum are also essential. The aim with tortoises kept in captivity should be access to sunlight for 12–14 hours a day. Mediterranean tortoises, for example, thrive on 14 hours of sunlight as this is similar to summer daylengths in their natural habitat. Tropical tortoises naturally live in areas near the equator, where daylength remains at a consistent 12 hours throughout the year. Shortening daylength in the autumn is the initial trigger which begins the process of hibernation (see Chapter 12 on hibernation/brumation), in those species that do hibernate/brumate.

Artificial sources of heat and light will always be limited compared with sunlight. Either they may not provide a high enough light intensity, or they may only provide part of the full spectrum. In some cases, there is the possibility that any imbalance causes the emission of too much of one part of the spectrum and an insufficiency of other parts.

UV, visible and IR radiation from natural sunlight all play a part in keeping tortoises healthy and well. Sunlight plays a part in many physiological processes, controlling body functions and activity levels (metabolism). Each process has a role to play in normal tortoise behaviour. For this reason, an inadequate provision of suitable heat and light sources may limit the tortoise's ability to show normal behaviours. This will have a potentially negative impact on welfare.

Light intensity

Light intensity is measured in lumens. These are a measure of the total illumination provided from a light source. For practical purposes light intensity is measured in lux, where 1 lux = amount of illumination from 1 lumen spread over 1 square metre:

$$1\,\text{lux}\,(\text{lx}) = 1\,\text{lumen}\,(\text{lm})\,\text{per}\,\text{m}^2$$

The higher the number of lumens (and therefore lux), the brighter and more intense is the light being emitted.

Tortoises are less active when light levels are below 20,000 lx. In the Mediterranean at midday, or when the sky is cloudless in the tropics, sunlight levels of 130,000 lx can be reached. In a bright office, artificial lights only generate around 700 lx. In an indoor tortoise enclosure using both a T5 UVB fluorescent and a tungsten halogen lamp, the maximum light generated is still only 5000 lx. Creating sufficiently bright artificial light levels, of the right wavelengths, can therefore be a challenge.

Ultraviolet (UV) light

When additional light and heat are needed for tortoises in captivity, it is important that light of a suitable intensity is supplied, together with the correct spectrum of visible/UV light and sufficient heat as IR radiation from the IR spectrum. The UV spectrum is particularly important for normal tortoise growth and for development, behaviour and good health.

The UV spectrum is divided into three parts of UV radiation, as shown in Fig. 4.2.

The UV index (UVI)

The UV index (UVI) is a measure of the photoreactivity of sunlight on human skin (Table 4.3). This is useful when considering suitable UV light ranges provided by artificial basking lamps for tortoises. For example, if you look at the solar spectra ranges that provide the UVI, a very weak early morning sun in the northern hemisphere would be around UVI 1, a strong summer sun would have a UVI around 6.4, while in extreme tropical sunlight the UVI might reach 14.7.

The role of sunlight in vitamin D synthesis

Calcium is an essential component of bone growth and development. In order for calcium to be taken up from food in the diet, vitamin D3 is necessary. Vitamin D3 cannot be synthesized without UVB light. (For a more detailed biochemical account explaining how vitamin D3 is synthesized, see Fig. 4.7 and Appendix I – Vitamin D3 synthesis.)

Once vitamin D3 has been synthesized using UVB light (a small amount is also taken up in the food) it is stored in the liver in an inactive form and then converted to an active form by the kidneys. When in this active form, vitamin D3 causes calcium to be taken up from the gut. (For more detailed biochemical accounts of these processes see Figs 4.8 and 4.9, and Appendix II – Calcium metabolism and homeostasis.)

Artificial lights

Thus, UVB light is essential, along with vitamin D3, for calcium uptake. Calcium is an essential component of bone growth and development. Unfortunately, UVB light is not easy to provide from artificial light and is only found at suitable levels in specialist reptile lights. While artificial UV lights have improved in recent years (through good, readily available T5 (tubular 5), halogen and tungsten lamps) many tortoise owners are still not providing adequate UV radation. As well as the health implications of this, increasing evidence suggests that reptiles can see in the UV spectrum in a way that we cannot. This probably has a behavioural benefit and makes the tortoise feel happier and less stressed (Baines *et al.*, 2016).

As described below, until recently the problem has been to provide enough UVB to ensure adequate vitamin D3 synthesis, through the use of artificial lights. With the development of LED UVB lights, we may find situations where too much vitamin D3 may be produced. This is due to some LEDs emitting wavelengths of light that prevent the natural buffering of vitamin D3 production (Baines *et al.*, 2016; Baines, 2021). This means that an excess accumulates, with potential damage to health. Further development is needed to provide tested, safe LED UVB lights for reptiles.

As LED lights are bright and provide visible light, they are helpful in providing high-intensity light. Reptiles need this to mimic the high levels of natural sunlight that they need. Unfortunately, LEDs do not emit UVA. As a consequence, they do not emit the full UV spectrum as is produced by sunlight. What we do not know (as this has yet to be studied) is whether reptiles change their behaviour under LED lights as compared with full-spectrum lamps like metal halides or fluorescent lamps. Unlike LED lights, these do emit UVA. We also do not know if reptiles actually have a preference for LED or full-spectrum lights.

When considering suitable types of lighting for your tortoise's enclosure, several products may be needed in order to meet intensity and spectrum requirements, as described below. Consider the following factors (Baines and Davis, 2005; Rendle and Calvert, 2019):

- Quality of light – which parts of the spectrum are emitted (this will vary over time and the manufacturer's guidance on replacements should be followed) and over what distance.
- Quantity of light – the intensity of light given out, which will be determined by the source and shape of the light beam produced, together with distance from the tortoise.

There is an extensive range of possible lighting products available, as shown in Table 4.1 below. Different manufacturers provide versions of similar products. Some examples are given here, based on my experience of their use and where data is available on their output (Baines *et al.*, 2016; BIAZA RAWG, 2021). There may be equally suitable products available in different locations. For the most up-to-date information, you are advised to check on suitable products to suit the purpose intended, at the time of purchase.

Some lighting sources emit UVB, including mercury vapour and metal halide lamps, fluorescent tubes and compact fluorescent lamps. Other sources do not, such as tungsten and halogen lamps. As described above, LEDs are now being developed to give out UVB, but this work is in the early stages of development. Newly developed products should therefore be treated with caution (Baines *et al.*, 2016; Baines, 2021) until their output has been further researched and deemed safe.

Where should artificial lights be placed?

Artificial lights should always be positioned so that they shine vertically down onto the tortoise. This ensures that the animal's eyebrow ridges and upper eyelids protect its eyes from direct light. The use of angled lights (such as fittings at 45 degrees) or clamp-on fittings set at an angle should be avoided. All lights should be positioned directly above the areas in which the tortoise will be moving around. The use of reflectors to help prevent light being

Table 4.1. Types of light source.

Lamps and tubes	Example products	Heat/Light	UVB levels emitted	Light beam features/Visible light
Mercury vapour lamps	Arcadia D3 Basking lamp ExoTerra Solar Glo Zoomed Powersun	Heat Light	High	Bright visible light in a narrow beam
Metal halide lamps	ExoTerra SunRay Lucky Reptile Bright Sun Zoomed Powersun	Heat Light	High	Bright visible light in a narrow beam
Fluorescent tubes	T8 (Reflector needed) Arcadia D3+ 12% UVB T8 ExoTerra Reptiglo Zoomed Reptisun T5 (Reflector needed) Arcadia D3+ Reptile 12% UVB T5 Zoomed Reptisun T5	Light	High	Low-intensity light High-intensity light
Compact fluorescent tubes	Arcadia D3 ExoTerra Reptile UVB Zoomed Reptisun	Light	High	Low-intensity light Narrow radius
Incandescent halogen/tungsten lamps	Any household supplier, e.g. Philips, Tungsram, Edison	Heat Light	None	Warm yellow visible light Narrow beam

lost to the upper parts of the enclosure can be very beneficial in providing additional intensity of light. Reflectors also increase the available UVB wavelengths reaching the tortoise.

In order to provide a tortoise with suitable artificial light, three things are crucial:

1. **The intensity of the light (the UVI).**
2. **The wavelengths of light provided.**
3. **The duration of the daylength.**

The picture is further complicated by the need to provide the tortoise with sufficient choice within its environment to allow it to access effective UV gradients. There must be an opportunity for the tortoise to bask near the light source, but it must also be able to move away from the light if required. This is essential to allow thermoregulation and also to regulate the exposure to light and to different wavelengths of UV light. This self-regulation can only be achieved when suitable environmental conditions are provided.

It is unlikely that one single light source will provide all necessary lighting requirements for your tortoise. Background light together with basking lamps will be needed, even where the tortoise rarely sits in direct sunlight, such as those in Ferguson Zones 1 and 2 (see Fig. 4.6). Opportunities to access suitable intensities and wavelengths of light must therefore be provided. When setting up lighting systems for tortoises in captivity, a UV light meter can be used to measure light intensities in different parts of the enclosure. Using a good-quality light meter, such as the Solarmeter 6.5® UVI meter, to check light intensities means that a UV gradient can be created.

A range of temperatures, light intensities and UVB levels creates gradients from high to low within the enclosure. These gradients allow the tortoise the opportunity to access suitable temperatures, light intensities and qualities around the enclosure (as long as it is large enough) to thermoregulate and vary its exposure to lights of different UV wavelengths.

The British and Irish Association of Zoos and Aquaria (BIAZA) has developed a tool that can be used to determine the most likely average UV exposure needs of captive tortoises. This tool is referred to as the BIAZA UV Tool (2021). The UV range for each species of tortoise can be identified and a UV gradient can be created in enclosures that is similar to that which the tortoise could expect to experience in its natural habitat. This gradient might range from full sunlight to full shade (as long as the enclosure is large enough) and so provide the tortoise with the best opportunity to self-regulate its exposure to UVB. This is turn will allow the best opportunity for 'natural' vitamin D3 production and regulation, which will lead to the most effective calcium uptake and metabolism for health and growth. The tool is in the early stages of development and although it provides invaluable information for the tortoise keeper, it is yet to fully elucidate all aspects of artificial lighting.

The BIAZA work also considers the natural biome in which the tortoise lives, as shown in Table 4.2, and the associated UVI information. Table 4.2 lists the world's 14 biomes – distinct major habitat types with specific climate, vegetation and animal life – as drawn up by the World Wildlife Fund (WWF) (Olson *et al.*, 2021). The WWF divided the Earth's land surface into eight biogeographical realms, which together contain a total of 867 smaller

Table 4.2. World Wildlife Fund (WWF) terrestrial biomes.

01 Tropical and Subtropical Moist Broadleaf Forests	Tropical and subtropical, humid
02 Tropical and Subtropical Dry Broadleaf Forests	Tropical and subtropical, semi-humid
03 Tropical and Subtropical Coniferous Forests	Tropical and subtropical, semi-humid
04 Temperate Broadleaf and Mixed Forests	Temperate, humid
05 Temperate Coniferous Forests	Temperate, humid to semi-humid
06 Boreal Forests/ Taiga	Subarctic, humid
07 Tropical and Subtropical Grasslands, Savannas and Shrublands	Tropical and subtropical, semi-arid
08 Temperate Grasslands, Savannas and Shrublands	Temperate, semi-arid
09 Flooded Grasslands and Savannas	Temperate to tropical, fresh or brackish water inundated
10 Montane Grasslands and Shrublands	Alpine or montane climate
11 Tundra	Arctic
12 Mediterranean Forests, Woodlands and Scrub	Temperate warm, semi-humid to semiarid with winter rainfall
13 Deserts and Xeric Shrublands	Temperate to tropical, arid
14 Mangroves	Subtropical and tropical, saltwater inundated

ecoregions. Each ecoregion was then classified into one of the 14 biomes.

In order to create the BIAZA UV tool for a number of different tortoise species, information from the following sources was used.

1. Biome – based on the WWF list of 14 major Biomes as shown in Table 4.2.

2. UV Index: Information and data gathered on the UV output of available lighting products (based on the work of Baines *et al.*, 2016). These images (Fig. 4.5, reproduced with the kind permission of Frances Baines) show how the UVI decreases the further away from the light the tortoise sits. The positioning of, and in particular the distances away from, the light source is an essential consideration in getting the best from the habitat. It is also important to ensure that the tortoise is not too close to the lamp, to avoid burns. (For further diagrams for other lighting products and information on the work of Frances M. Baines, see Appendix III.)

UVIs show the reduction in effectiveness with distance and the use of protective mesh across the light source. Different mesh screens will block different percentages of UVB and the reflectors make a huge difference to the output below the tubes.

3. Ferguson Zone: This categorization is based on the work of Gary Ferguson, who identified the likely UVB levels available to tortoises in their natural habitat from the UVI information and the animal's natural behaviour. As can be seen in Tables 4.3 and 4.4, the Ferguson Zones identify the maximum likely exposure to UVB and the need for those levels to be provided in a gradient down to zero (full shade), within the enclosure (Ferguson *et al.*, 2010).

Putting it all together

4. Lamp Indexes: The information collated from the work of Baines and Ferguson can be used to provide guidance on the suitability of background (Shade level) lights such as fluorescent lights and of basking light (Sunbeam) sources, for a given species of tortoise as in Table 4.5. The information can be used to select the best lighting options for the species as suggested in Table 4.6. Note that the Egyptian, Horsfield's and Hingeback tortoise are suggestions only. The other species have already been identified in terms of Ferguson Zones.

LED lighting

LED UVB lights have been developed for use with reptiles. These lights have a number of benefits – they are easy to use, small, lightweight and have easy fittings. They are also very bright and have a high intensity of visible light. This is important to reptiles. Also LED lights can be used to give a broad spread of light. This makes them useful for lighting larger tortoises or for groups of animals kept together. LED lights have a long lifespan and do not contain mercury. Mercury is risky to health because it is so toxic. Broken mercury lamps are dangerous both to human health and to the environment. Because of this mercury lamps are being phased out and are being replaced by LED lights.

While all this sounds very positive, research has shown that there may be a downside. LED UVB lights have greater intensities of certain wavelengths than is seen in intense natural light (Cusack *et al.*, 2017). The particular wavelengths found in greater intensity in LED UVB lights are damaging to DNA and the skin. LED UVB lights are also less effective in regulating the synthesis of vitamin D3. There is therefore a risk of vitamin D3 overdose amongst tortoises kept under these lights. Appendix IV has further detail regarding UVB wavelengths in LED lights.

Insufficient vitamin D3 and vitamin D3 overdose both produce similar symptoms in tortoises, so diagnosis of health problems related to the levels of this hormone is challenging (see Chapter 7 on common illnesses and diseases).

It is clear that the use of LED UVB lights has both pros and cons.

Sources of heat

Where artificial heat sources are used, they should be placed above the tortoise so that they mimic heat from the sun. Overhead heat sources may be provided without visible light wavelengths. This allows the tortoise a period of darkness, whilst still providing heat. As tortoises are ectotherms, they cannot make their own body warmth. They therefore rely of external sources (like the sun) to do this for them. This warmth is necessary for the effective functioning of all metabolic processes, including the conversion of vitamin D3 from its inactive to its active form.

Arcadia® deep heat projectors provide infrared-A and infrared-B. Both of these penetrate the epidermis and so reach the dermis and subcutaneous tissues, allowing the heat to be quickly dissipated throughout the body tissues.

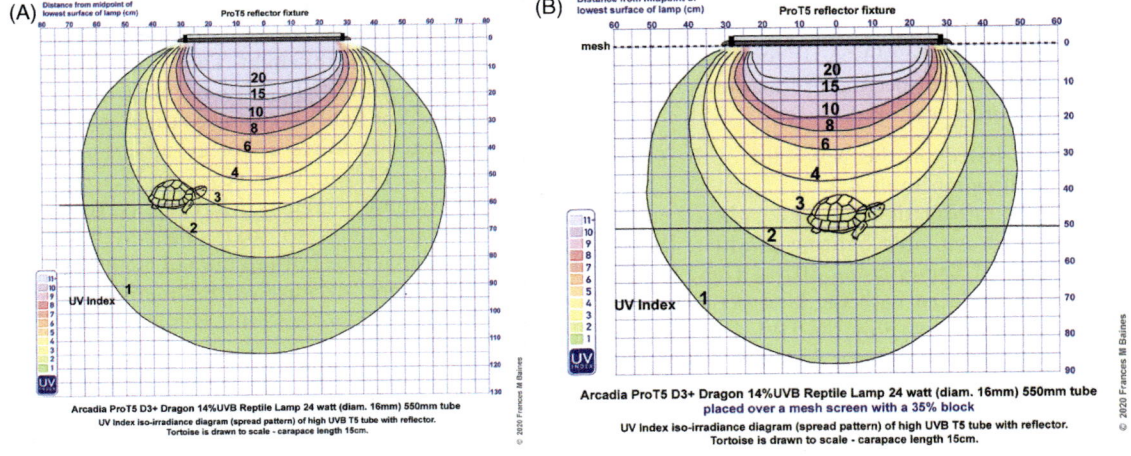

Fig. 4.5. (A) Arcadia D3 ProT5 14%. (B) Arcadia D3 ProT5 14% + 35% mesh. (Images used with kind permission of Frances Baines.)

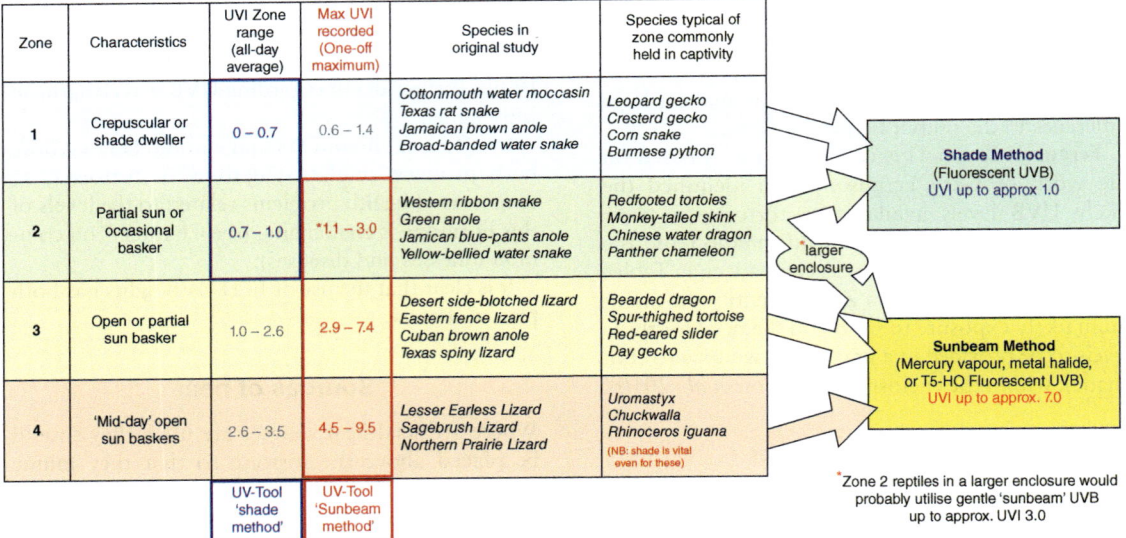

Fig. 4.6. Ferguson Zones showing UVI Zones and Maximum UVIs with detail of lighting and relationship with the Shade Method and the Sunbeam Method. (Image with kind permission of Frances M. Baines.)

Arcadia® recommends the use of four of its products as a way of providing suitable levels of infrared-A, infrared-B, suitable intensity of light with high lux levels, together with a source of UVB. These products are:

1. Deep Heat Projector® – provides infrared-A, infrared-B heat energy with the combined effect of heating rocks in the enclosure, giving infrared-C.

2. Tungsten or Halide Flood light – provides heat, brightness, infrared-A.

3. ProT5 High Output UVB tube – provides UVI, source of UVB.

4. Jungle Dawn LED bar – provides brightness, high lux.

These combined products provide heat, UVB, background and basking sources of light. There are

Table 4.3. Ferguson Zones and UVB gradients with tortoise species.

Zones	Characteristics	UVI Zone range/gradient	Example tortoise species
Zone 1	Crepuscular or shade dweller	0–0.7	
Zone 2	Partial sun/ occasional basker	0.7–1.0	Red-footed tortoise
Zone 3	Open or partial sun basker	1.0–2.6	Spur-thighed tortoise Hermann's tortoiseLeopard tortoise Sulcata tortoise
Zone 4	Mid-day sun basker	2.6–3.5	Marginated tortoise

Table 4.4. Ferguson Zones linked to suitable light sources and lamp indexes.

Zones	Characteristics	UVI Zone range/Gradient	UVI Ranges	Suitable lighting types
Zone 1	Crepuscular or shade dweller	0–0.7	0–0.7	Shade Method
Zone 2	Partial sun/ occasional basker	0.7–1.0	0.7–1.0 1.1–3.0 in basking zone	Shade Method Larger enclosure also Sunbeam Method
Zone 3	Open or partial sun basker	1.0–2.6	2.9–7.4 in basking zone	Sunbeam Method
Zone 4	Mid-day open sun basker	2.6–3.5	4.–8.0 in basking zone	Sunbeam Method

(From Baines *et al.*, 2016, BIAZA RAWG, 2021)

Table 4.5. Ferguson Zones and recommended lighting for tortoise species.

Species	Biomes	Ferguson Zone	Background/ambient temperatures (°C) DAY/NIGHT	Basking Zone substrate surface (°C)	Photoperiod (captivity) (hours)	Suitable lighting types
Red-footed tortoise *Geochelone carbonaria*	01 Tropical Moist Forests 07 Tropical Savannah	Zone 2	27–30/ 24–26	30–35	12	Shade Method Sunbeam Method in large enclosure
Leopard tortoise *Geochelone pardalis*	07 Tropical Savannah	Zone 3	28–32/ 24–28	40–50	12	Sunbeam Method
Spur-thighed tortoise *Testudo graeca*	12 Mediterranean Forests	Zone 3	20–30/22–24/ 10–15	35	14	Sunbeam Method
Hermann's tortoise *Testudo hermanni*	12 Mediterranean Forests	Zone 3	22–24/22–26/ 10–15/>12	35	14	Sunbeam Method ProT5 D3+ Reptile Lamp 12% UVB
Marginated tortoise *Testudo marginata*	12 Mediterranean Forests	Zone 4	28–32/ 20–24	35	14	Sunbeam Method
Egyptian Tortoise *Testudo kleinmanni*	13 Deserts and Xeric Shrublands	Zone 3	28–30/ 22–25	30–35	12	Sunbeam Method
Horsfield's tortoise *Testudo horsfieldii*	08 Temperate grasslands 10 Montane grasslands	Zone 3	25–30/20	35	14	Sunbeam Method
Bell's Hingeback *Kinixys belliana*	02 Tropical Dry Forests 07 Tropical Savannah	Zone 3	25–30/20–25	35	12	Sunbeam Method

Table 4.6. Example lights (mercury vapour lamps not included as may become less available due to legislation to reduce pollution from mercury; similar issues are to be faced for fluorescent tubes) giving suitable for provision of background shade and basking light sources for the Ferguson Zones (based on Baines et al., 2016; BIAZA RAWG UV Tool, 2021).

Ferguson Zone	Fluorescent/Shade background with Reflector	Basking/Sunbeam (with background fluorescent)
Zone 1	Arcadia Natural Sunlight Lamp 2% UVB	Arcadia Basking Lamp
Zone 2	Arcadia D3+ Reptile Lamp 12% UVB Narva BioVital T8 ZooMed Reptisun 2.0/ Naturesun Arcadia ProT5-SO Shade Dweller 7%UVB Arcadia D3+ Compact Lamp 10%UVB Zoomed Reptisun 5.0 Compact Lamp	Lucky Reptile Bright Sun UV Desert ZooMed Powersun
Zone 3	Arcadia ProT5 D3+ Reptile Lamp 12% UVB	Arcadia Basking Lamp
Zone 4	Arcadia ProT5 D3+ Dragon Reptile Lamp 14%UVB Reptisun 10.0 UVB T5-HO	Lucky Reptile Bright Sun UV Desert ZooMed Powersun

other products available as heat sources such as the Reptile Systems® Gold Infrared lamp.

Thermostats are recommended to control temperatures, to reduce risk of overheating. When buying a thermostat care must be taken to ensure that the wattage with which the thermostat can safely deal is consistent with the wattage of the heat source. For example, a 600 Watt dimming thermostat, from manufacturers such as Habistat® or Microclimate®, can be used to control heaters up to 600 Watts. A dimming thermostat gives the most effective control of temperature.

Underfloor heating is not advised as suitable for tortoises. This is because it does not allow for sufficient external heat to be absorbed through the shell and skin. In addition, radiant heat panels, heated cables and ceramic heaters provide only infrared-C. As this is the least absorbed part of the IR spectrum, it provides the tortoise with the least heat energy in terms of availability.

It is also easy for the tortoise to damage fittings that can be walked on, or with which the tortoise comes into physical contact. Liquids can easily be spilt from water bowls onto floor heaters, or they can be urinated on. This is also a potential electrical hazard (see Chapter 19 on health and safety).

The use of heat sources always comes with a potential fire risk, so every precaution must be taken to prevent such an outcome (see Chapter 19 on health and safety).

Environmental and climate change considerations

Many countries have introduced, or are about to introduce, restrictions on the sales of lights that give off heat. These are not environmentally friendly. To increase energy saving, the use of incandescent light bulbs has already been phased out in many countries, for example.

In addition, lights that contain toxic components, such as mercury vapour lamps and fluorescent tubes, are also being phased out. This has meant that LED lights giving out UVB have been developed. As indicated above, these may have the problem of creating a vitamin D overdose. These lights should therefore be used with caution.

Exemptions to the legislation controlling the sale of light sources will be needed to allow the use of appropriate sources of heat and light for reptiles in captivity. Without overhead heat and light, the metabolic and behavioural needs of reptiles cannot be met in captivity.

The environmental impact of keeping tortoises in captivity provides another dimension to our considerations of the suitability and ethics of keeping tortoises as pets. While we may have a positive impact on conservation by breeding endangered species, we may also have a negative impact on the environment by increasing CO_2 output because of our use of heat-emitting light sources. If our energy supply does not come from renewable sources, we contribute even more to our carbon footprint by keeping tortoises as pets. In 2023, it became increasingly common for tortoises to be given up for rehoming in the UK and Europe. A primary reason for this seems to be the owner's inability to fund their pet's heating and lighting needs, as the cost of living rises.

While we continue to keep tortoises as pets, we must do our best to ensure effective provision of light and heat in indoor enclosures. At the same time, it is essential to ensure maximum access to natural sunlight, given the prevailing climatic conditions in the environment in which they are kept. Setting up indoor habitats that meet health, welfare and behavioural needs will always remain a big part of our role as tortoise guardians.

Conclusion

Providing artificial lighting and heating presents a challenge for all tortoise keepers, as outlined here. There is much research to be done in this field, particularly in terms of the needs of individual species. There is some generic data becoming available. The work by Frances M. Baines and the BIAZA RAWG UVTool has been pioneering in taking forward the data gathered on light sources, and using that data to create useful diagrams of lamp indexes for lighting products. Setting up a terrarium, which is beneficial in terms of welfare, requires careful consideration of the information in this chapter and in further reading. Lighting and heating have a profound impact on behaviour and health in reptiles.

Nothing can replace natural sunlight and wherever possible access to sunlight should be given to captive tortoises. At times of the year when that is not possible, we have to try to provide the most suitable sources of artificial heat and light for our animals. The information in this chapter is very much an introduction to this topic, giving basic information. It is an ever-changing field and one that we all need to keep up with when providing the best environment for our tortoises.

Appendix I:

Vitamin D3 synthesis (Baines *et al.*, 2016; Rendle and Calvert, 2019 pp. 368–370; Baines, 2021)

Figure 4.7 explains how 7-dehydrocholesterol (7-DHC) and lumisterol use the shortest wavelengths 290–315 nm. Pre-D3 and tachysterol also use the longer wavelengths up to 340 nm. The shorter wavelengths are more likely to convert the molecule to pre-vitamin D3 and the longer wavelengths are more likely to convert the molecule to any of the other three substances (7-DHC, tachysterol, lumisterol).

Wavelengths of 290–310 nm lead to generation of vitamin D3 and wavelengths of 310–335 nm are part of the feedback loops to prevent too much vitamin D3 being produced and causing an overdose. Hence the self-regulation of vitamin D3 levels when the source is sunlight action on the skin and underlying tissues.

Holick *et al.* (1981) and Baines *et al.* (2016) refer to this continuous transformation between isomers 7-DHC, tachysterol, lumisterol and pre-D3 as a molecular 'dance' which is controlled by the wavelengths of radiation reaching the skin. This complex photo-regulation of the isomers is also controlled by the UVI as a measure of the intensity of light, which also affects the wavelengths of light.

Once pre-D3 has been synthesized, warmth is need for the conversion to vitamin D3 itself. The vitamin D3 is then taken up by vitamin-D-binding protein and carried away in skin capillaries to the bloodstream. The storage form of vitamin D3 is 25(OH)D3. As shown, some of this is stored in fat cells and the liver, but much remains in the bloodstream, reaching all parts of the body. The kidneys continually require small amounts 25(OH)D3 for conversion into the active form 1,25(OH)D3, which is essential for maintaining calcium homeostasis.

Appendix II:

Calcium metabolism and homeostasis (Baines *et al.*, 2016; Rendle and Calvert, 2019 pp. 365–368; Baines, 2021)

Once vitamin D3 has been absorbed by the reactions shown above, or from dietary sources, this hormone (as that is the group of substances to which it belongs) is stored in the liver as 25(OH)D3 and then converted to an active form 1,25(OH)D3 by the kidneys. This stimulates calcium uptake from the guts.

Figure 4.8 shows the route of vitamin D3 from the skin into the blood and its role in increasing calcium take-up from the guts into the blood and to the bones, where it can be used for mineralization.

The main role of vitamin D3 is to regulate calcium absorption and transport in the intestines and kidneys, as part of calcium homeostasis, which it does in conjunction with parathyroid hormone (PTH).

Figure 4.9 shows how calcium homeostasis takes place in simple terms to maintain required levels of calcium in the blood.

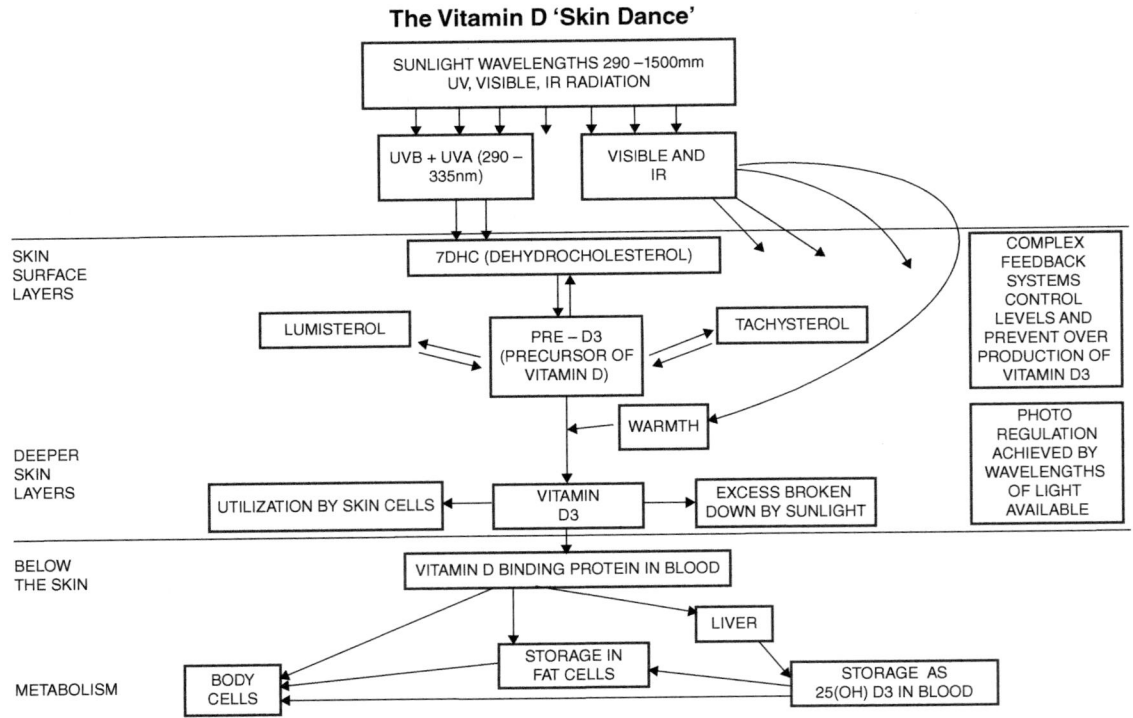

Fig. 4.7. More detail of the biochemistry involved in vitamin D3 conversions in the skin in the presence of sunlight.

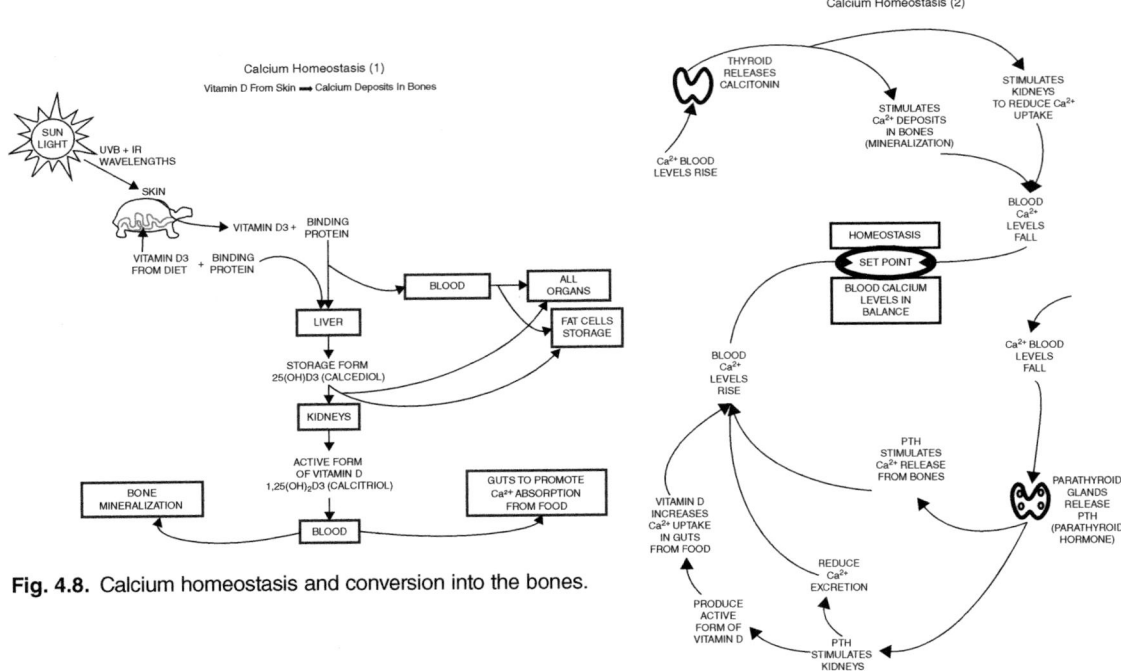

Fig. 4.8. Calcium homeostasis and conversion into the bones.

Fig. 4.9. Calcium homeostasis maintaining blood levels.

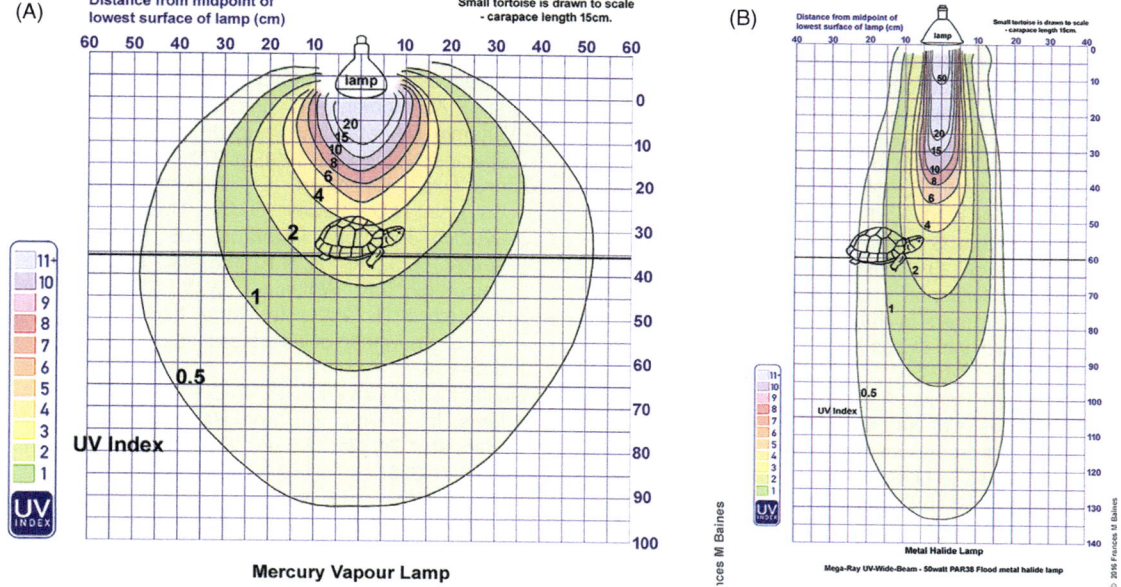

Fig. 4.10. Differences in UVIs for additional lighting. (A) Comparison of T8 sources Arcadia and Zoo Med: Arcadia T5 HO sources based on UVB% for fluorescent tubes. (B) Impact of mesh covering on Reptisun 10. (Images by kind permission of Frances Baines.)

Appendix III:

The work of Frances M. Baines

The diagrams in Fig. 4.10 show the UVIs for additional lighting and the differences between Arcadia T5 HO sources based on the UVB% for fluorescent tubes and the impact of mesh covering, which reduces effectiveness of the light source. The effect of a difference in wattage is also shown, and an end-on view. Figure 4.10A is for a mercury vapour lamp (Arcadia Reptile 100 W D3 basking lamp); Fig. 4.10B is for a metal halide lamp (Mega-Ray UV-wide beam). The diagrams include a small tortoise, drawn to scale, with a carapace length of 15 cm.

Appendix IV:

LED lighting (Frances M. Baines, 2021)

Research has shown that UVB LED lights have greater intensity in the wavelengths below 300 nm than is seen in intense natural light (Cusack *et al.*, 2017). These wavelengths are most damaging to DNA and the skin (see UVC above). The high levels of UV below 310 nm will allow synthesis of high levels of vitamin D3. In comparison, there is little UVA and UVB emitted from them (between 310 and 335 nm). The result of these two properties is that little regulation of the synthesis of vitamin D3 can take place. The natural feedback loops, which control the levels of pre-D3 available for conversion to vitamin D3, are not effective when these combinations of UV radiation are being emitted. There is therefore a risk of vitamin D3 overdose.

Given that insufficient vitamin D3 and an overdose of vitamin D3 both produce similar symptoms, diagnosis of health problems related to the levels of this hormone will be challenging. The LC-MS/MS chromatographic method of determining levels of 25(OH)D3, rather than immunoassay tests which may be very inaccurate (Hurst *et al.*, 2020), should be used in determining whether hypervitaminosis D or hypovitaminosis D is the cause of the symptom seen (see Chapter 7 on common illnesses and diseases).

References and Further Reading

Baines, F.M. (2021) *Vitamin D3 synthesis. A self-limiting process in natural sunlight.* Available at https://literatur.licht-im-terrarium.de

Baines, F.M. and Davis, C. (2005) Natural light in the vivarium. *Natterjack* [Newsletter of the British Herpetological Society] 127, 9–12

Baines, F.M., Chattell, J., Dale, J., Garrick, D., Gill, I., Goetz, M., Skelton, T. and Swatman, M. (2016) How much UV-B does my reptile need? The UV-Tool, a guide to the selection of UV lighting for reptiles and amphibians in captivity. *Journal of Zoo and Aquarium Research* 4(1), 42–63.

BIAZA RAWG (2021) UVTool Update (266 species)

BIAZA RAWG (2022) LEDs and Reptiles. Available at: BIAZA_RAWG_2022_LEDs_and_Reptiles.pdf

Cusack, L., Rivera, S., Lock, B., Benboe, D., Brothers, D. and Divers, S. (2017) Effects of a light emitting diode on the production of cholecalciferol and associated blood parameters in the bearded dragon (*Pogona vitticeps*). *Journal of Zoo and Wildlife Medicine* 48(4), 1120–1126.

Ferguson, G.W., Brinker, A.M., Gehrmann, W.H., Bucklin, S.E., Baines, F.M. and Mackin, S.J. (2010) Voluntary exposure of some western-hemisphere snake and lizard species to ultraviolet-B (UVB) radiation in the field: how much UVB should a lizard or snake receive in captivity? *Zoo Biology* 29, 317–334.

Highfield, A. (1996) *Practical Encyclopaedia of Keeping and Breeding Tortoises and Freshwater Turtles*. Carapace Press, London.

Holick, M.F., MacLaughlin, J.A. and Doppelt, S.H. (1981) Regulation of cutaneous previtamin D3 photosynthesis in man: skin pigment is not an essential regulator. *Science* 211(4482), 590–593.

Hurst, E.A., Homer, N.Z. and Mellanby, R.J. (2020) Vitamin D metabolism and profiling in veterinary species. *Metabolites* 10(9), p. 371.

Olson, D.M., Dinerstein, E., Wikramanayake, E.D., Burgess, N.D., Powell, G.V.N., Underwood, E.C., D'Amico, J.A., Itoua, I., Strand, H.E., Morrison, J.C., Loucks, C.J., Allnutt, T.F., Ricketts, T.H., Kura, Y., Lamoreux, J.F., Wettengel, W.W., Hedao, P. and Kassem, K.R. (2001) Terrestrial Ecoregions of the World: a new map of life on Earth. *Bioscience* 51(11), 933–938.

Rendle, M. and Calvert, I. (2019) Ch 22 Nutritional problems. In: Girling, S.J. and Rain, P. (eds) *BSAVA Manual of Reptiles*, 3rd edn. BSAVA, Quedgeley, UK, pp. 365–396.

Zheng, W., Xie, Y., Li, G., Kong, J., Feng, J.Q. and Li, Y.C., (2004) Critical role of calbindin-D28k in calcium homeostasis revealed by mice lacking both vitamin D receptor and calbindin-D28k. *Journal of Biological Chemistry* 279(50), 52406–52413

5 Tortoise Diets

Abstract

The diets of captive tortoises are described for both herbivores and omnivores. Land-dwelling tortoises are not carnivorous – the dietary needs of carnivorous turtles and terrapins are not described. The macronutrients and micronutrients required in the diet are described. The essential features of any tortoise diet being high in calcium and fibre, and low in protein and fat, are explained. The need to provide a diet as close as possible to that available in the wild is explained. Herbivorous tortoises often eat around 40 different species of plant on a regular basis. The value of using wild plant species (weeds), home-grown flowering plants and succulents as by far the biggest component of the diet is discussed.

Nutritional needs are best met with this approach, rather than through shop-bought foods. Lists of suitable food plants and those that are toxic are provided. Use of commercially available tortoise diets is covered, together with the use of dietary supplementation with vitamins and minerals to improve the availability of essential micronutrients.

The provision of food plants within the enclosures is discussed, so that tortoises can forage and graze when food plants are available, providing the opportunity for the natural behaviours of walking, seeking food items and feeding to be carried out.

What do tortoises eat?

Tortoises are either herbivores or omnivores. Herbivorous tortoises eat only plants while omnivorous ones will eat a variety of food, including both plant and animal material.

All tortoises are opportunistic feeders and will eat the majority of food items that they come across. Herbivorous tortoises walk several kilometres each day in order to find sufficient food in the wild. The food plants they seek are often few and far between, especially at ground level. Spur-thighed and other Mediterranean tortoise species will eat over 40 different types of plant on a daily basis. Rouag *et al.* (2008) identified only 16 species of plant in the faeces of *Testudo graeca whitei* in an arid area of Algeria, but this represented almost all of the available species. *Testudo hermanni* tortoises been found to eat between 134 plant species (Vetter, 2006) and 250 plant species (Celse *et al.*, 2014). The diet of herbivores includes the leaves, stems and flowers, and in some cases, the seeds, of the plant. Figure 5.1 shows a mixed diet of captive Mediterranean tortoises. They will also scavenge for bones, animal faeces and remains, but these are a very small proportion of the diet.

Grazing tortoises such as Leopards (*Centrochelys pardalis*) and Sulcatas (*Centrochelys sulcata*) eat a large proportion of grasses and succulents in their diet, with some flowering plants (Fig. 5.3). Kabigumila (2001) found that the diet of Leopard tortoises contained 47 species, over 50% of which were succulents and almost one-fifth were grasses, with Egyptian crowfoot (*Dactyloctenium aegyptium*) being the most common grass eaten. These data also showed a preference for some plant types, such as the herbaceous flowering plant, *Cissus rotundifolia* (grape or round-leaf ivy). This is in contrast to other areas, such as South Africa, where grasses are more predominant in the diet. Milton (1992) found 75 plant species in the faeces of Leopard tortoises studied in the arid South Karoo area. There is selection of food items, even taking into account prevalence of species in the environment, and some species are eaten more frequently. These herbivorous tortoises rely on digestion through fermentation in the lower gut achieved through symbiotic gut flora to digest the plant cell walls (cellulose) (Fig. 5.3).

Omnivorous tortoises will eat both plant and animal material, as shown in Fig. 5.2B. Bearing in mind that tortoises are not generally agile enough to move quickly to kill other animals, any animal material they eat will be from a carcass or will be small invertebrates such as insects, woodlice, snails, earthworms and slugs (Fig. 5.2B). They will also eat insect larvae and pupae. Some tropical tortoises will also eat mushrooms and toadstools as a protein source. The diet of Red-footed (*Chelonoidis carbonaria*) and Yellow-footed (*Chelonoidis denticulata*) tortoises studied in north-western Brazil (Moskovits and Bjorndal, 1990) was identified as varied, consisting of 'plant parts (grasses, leaves, vines, roots, bark, fruits, and flowers), fungi (several gilled and woody mushrooms), animal matter (vertebrate carrion, insects, snails), soil, sand, and pebbles'.

Although the best food choices are naturally growing weeds, flowering plants and succulents (see Fig. 5.4 where succulents are part of the diet), there are times of the year when it is difficult to completely avoid salad leaves as part of the diet. This should be kept to a minimum, as described below.

How much should I feed my tortoise?

In captivity it is very easy to overfeed tortoises. They often have a voracious appetite (Fig. 5.5). The fact that food in the wild is very limited means that they are designed to eat as much as they can, whenever they can. Figure 5.6 shows a Horfield's tortoise eating a suitable amount of weeds. When, in their natural environment, they do find suitable food items they will eat everything available, as they know that they will not necessarily be able to find food again quickly. They may go for very long periods without finding anything at all to eat. Because they do not always find food every day in the wild, their stomach has a large capacity. This allows them to eat more than they need to keep themselves alive. In the wild this rarely happens, and if it does (maybe due to a seasonal glut in the spring) there will be other times when there is little food available.

In captivity, food is generally provided on a regular basis. Tortoises have a very low demand for calories, which means that they need relatively little food compared with mammals like humans, cats or dogs. Tortoises should generally be hungry by the time their next meal is given. Overfeeding in captivity is one of the biggest problems for reptiles generally, and tortoises in particular.

Ideally, for at least part of the year, tortoises can feed themselves in outdoor enclosures planted with safe weeds as food plants, as shown in Fig. 5.7. This allows tortoises to show the natural searching and grazing behaviours they would carry out in their natural environment. If this is the case, in order to avoid overfeeding, the addition of supplementary food should be kept to a minimum.

Overfeeding can take two forms. The first is inappropriate feeding of unsuitable items. Tortoises will eat foods that are not their natural diet, and which are bad for them, as described in the section below. The second, feeding too much, can also cause problems, even if the food items are suitable.

Young tortoises that are growing and developing are very susceptible to the harmful effects of poor diet. Their growth can be too rapid, which then leads to deformities in both shell and limb growth, resulting in pyramiding of the shell, or a flattened, collapsed shell, both frequently seen. Similarly, weak bones in the legs can leave the tortoise unable to lift itself off the ground, or to walk properly. Chapter 7, on common illnesses and diseases, looks at these problems in more detail.

Adult tortoises can develop liver and kidney disease as a result of poor diet. Also, the complex reproductive systems and processes, controlled by hormones, can easily be disrupted (see Chapter 11 on breeding). Female tortoises, in particular, can have problems with egg production and egg-laying due to poor liver function, often linked to dietary issues.

Feeding can be daily, or on alternate days for herbivores, depending upon the amount of available foods in the enclosures. A healthy tortoise will be enthusiastic when presented with food, eat with vigour and devour everything given within about 20 minutes. This will give you an indication of how much to feed. If the tortoise leaves food, you have given too much (or there are other problems), and if the tortoise eats everything really quickly and is still seeking food, you may need to give more. For hatchlings and juveniles, a rough guide of food portion size for a varied mix of weeds is a small pile about the same diameter as the tortoise's shell, given once daily.

The feeding process involves the beak cutting food into pieces then swallowing whole as shown in Fig. 5.8. There is no chewing or breaking up the food in the mouth, as tortoises have no teeth. The food is swallowed in bite-sized pieces and digestion starts in the stomach. The process is slow. Food can take several weeks to pass through the gut. This is why tortoises fast before hibernation/brumation, to allow all food to pass out of the digestive system, preventing gas production through fermentation and decay of undigested food.

If natural eating behaviours are not seen, or if your tortoise is selecting particular foods, leaving food or largely disinterested in eating, you may be overfeeding or feeding too frequently. Of course, there may be other reasons for not eating, which might involve ill-health or disease. This makes it very

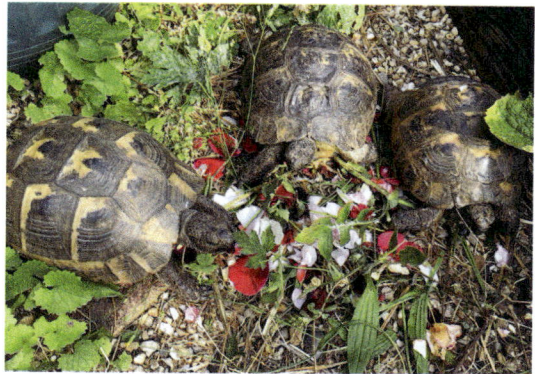

Fig. 5.1. Mediterranean Spur-thighed tortoises (*Testudo graeca*) feeding.

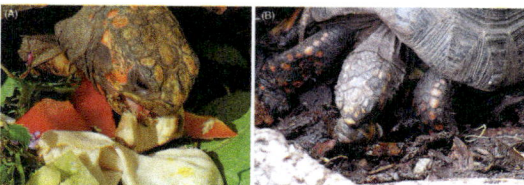

Fig. 5.2. (A, B) Red-footed tortoises (*Chelonoidis carbonaria*) feeding on plants and a snail.

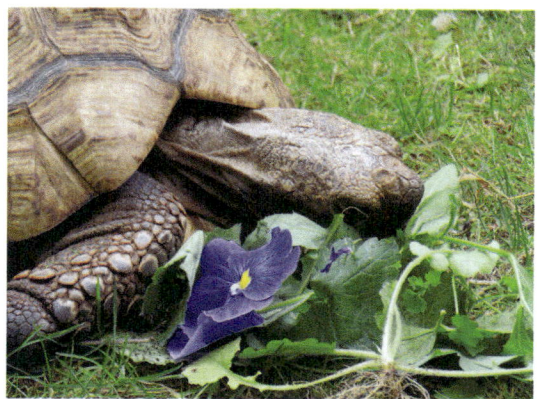

Fig. 5.3. Leopard tortoise (*Centrochelys pardalis*) feeding.

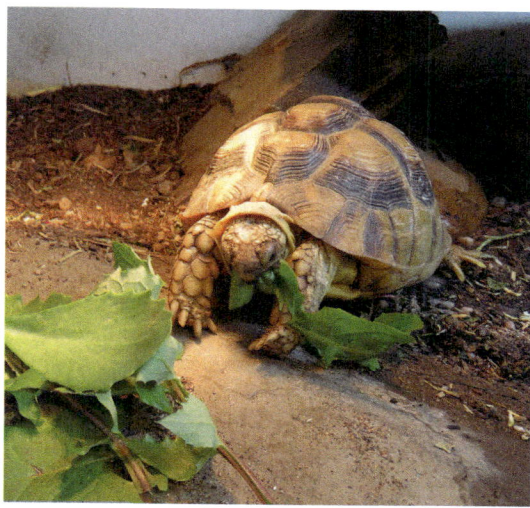

Fig. 5.4. Egyptian tortoises (*Testudo klienmanni*) feeding.

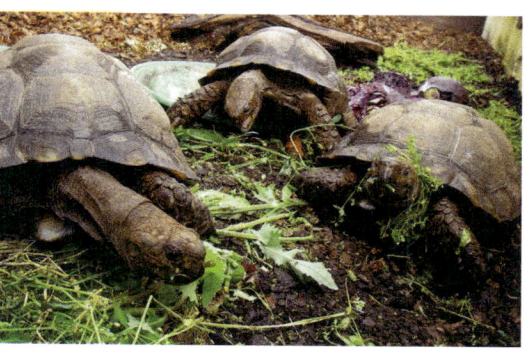

Fig. 5.5. Burmese Brown *(Manouria emys)* tortoises feeding (Eleanor Lien-Hua Tirtasana Chubb).

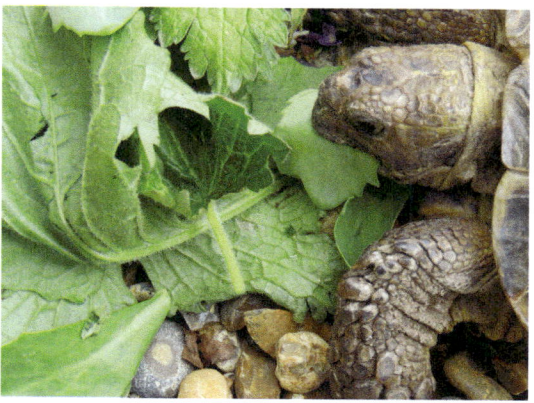

Fig. 5.6. Horsfield's tortoise (*Agrionemys horsfieldii*) feeding.

important to observe your tortoise frequently during the day. You will become familiar with normal feeding behaviours so that any change will be noticed and can be acted upon quickly.

Omnivorous tortoises will need feeding less frequently, perhaps three to four times per week. This is because the food will include much richer animal material, as well as plants. This makes it even easier to overfeed omnivores. Again, they should eat everything offered with enthusiasm and finish within

Tortoise Diets

63

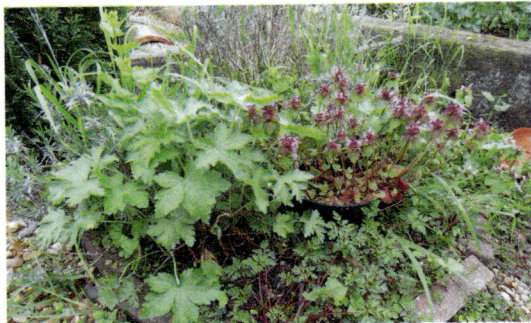

Fig. 5.7. Some natural planting allows grazing and foraging for Mediterranean tortoises.

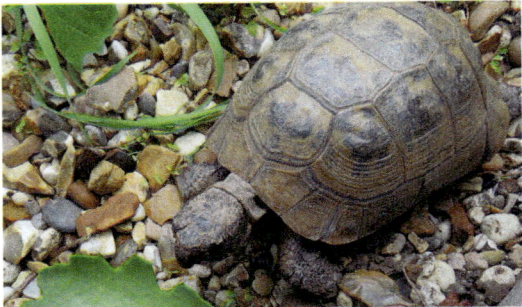

Fig. 5.8. Tortoise having taken a bite out of a leaf, showing the shape cut out which matches the beak.

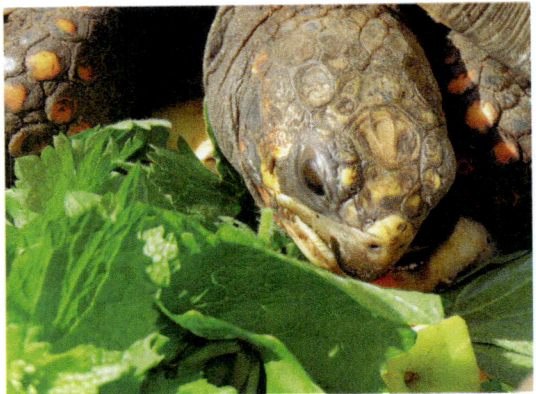

Fig. 5.9. For omnivores such as Red-footed tortoises, it is important not to load the diet with too much fruit and mushrooms, or with the animal protein provided, as at least 80% of the diet should be green leaves from weeds and growing plants.

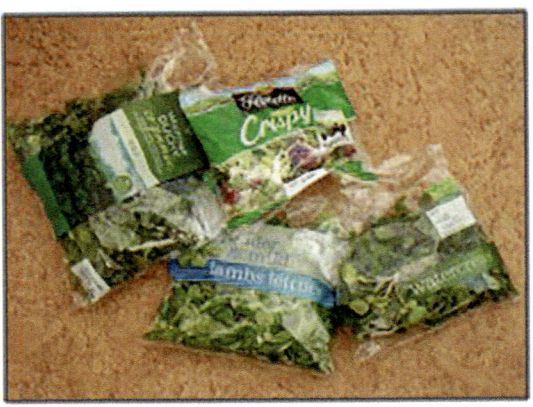

Fig. 5.10. Some shop-bought foods, which should be used to the minimum but are the best of a bad bunch, given that wild plants and growing plants from the garden or greenhouse are always better choices.

about 20 minutes. The bulk of the meal should be weeds, succulents and flowering plants, with about a quarter comprising fruit and a small amount of animal protein, as shown in Fig. 5.9.

What shouldn't I feed my tortoise?

In captivity tortoises can be capricious in their eating habits. They may easily become 'addicted' to one favourite type of food or may suddenly decide not to eat something they were previously perfectly happy with. Favourite foods are not always the best foods for tortoises to eat. I love chocolate but if my diet consisted solely of chocolate, it would not be very good for me!

Peas and green beans have been fed as favoured foods in the past, and most tortoises will tuck into these with gusto. However, these legumes are high in protein and contain phytic acid, which impairs the uptake of calcium and other minerals, making them a poor food choice. Chard, spinach and kale, along with sweet (bell) peppers (and some berries), contain oxalic acid, which is also not recommended as it also inhibits calcium uptake. In years gone by tortoises were commonly fed cat and dog food as part of their diet. Both of these are very harmful as they contain high levels of protein and fat – even more so in the case of cat food. These high-protein, high-fat animal protein food sources should never be fed to herbivores. They are also a poor choice for omnivores because of the high fat content (Highfield, 1996).

People have told me that their tortoise has eaten 'nothing but cucumber' for over 50 years. In reality, this is unlikely to be the case. The tortoise may well have been grazing on garden plants without the owner noticing. The point is well made, however, that some tortoises can be very fussy when offered food in captivity.

I once looked after Edith, a large, aged female Spur-thighed tortoise *Testudo graeca whitei*, who had become very unwell. This was due to a long-term poor diet and overlong hibernations/brumations. She had eaten only lettuce and tomato for at least 30 years. When offered any other items she refused to eat them. I had to hand-feed her for 2 years, gradually introducing more appropriate food items, such as those described in the sections below. Eventually she started to feed herself and accepted a wider variety of foodstuffs. Tortoises often take a very long time to show the effects of poor husbandry and can take an equally long time to start to recover.

In the past during the early years of tortoise keeping, cat or dog food, along with bread and milk, were advised as suitable food items. Before there was anything like the understanding we now have of their dietary needs, some veterinary advice was to tube-feed tortoises with high-energy, liquid foods. One owner brought a very young tortoise to me, so ill as to be near death. She had been feeding it milk 'as it was a baby' and she thought 'that's what babies eat'.

I once came across owners who used to give their male Hermann's tortoise a weekly 'treat' consisting of a plate of the family's Sunday roast, including meat, vegetables, roast potatoes and of course gravy. During the Ninja turtle phase of the 1980s it was not unusual for owners to be feeding turtles, terrapins and tortoises on pizza. Tortoises will eat these types of food with apparent relish, but they are not good for them. They are a long way from natural food items.

The owner of a female Hermann's tortoise, Tina, in the UK, once asked me how to prevent any spread of bird flu into her aviary of captive birds. Apparently, she was being visited by a lot of wild birds all coming into her garden to steal Tina's ham sandwich, given to her daily for breakfast. My suggestion that this was not a suitable part of her diet was met with incredulity, as it was felt that she should not be deprived of her favourite food.

All the food items mentioned above are totally unsuitable for tortoises and will cause great harm to them.

Tortoises do not need foods high in calories – largely because they are ectotherms, and so do not need to burn food internally in order to generate their own body heat. Any salad or vegetable foods bought in shops and stores for our tortoises will usually be too high in calories. If we feed this sort of diet, we are feeding our tortoises the equivalent of fast-food diets (Jepson, 2010). We all know that convenience or fast food can be very appealing. The smell and taste might be good, but nutritionally this type of food is very poor, being low in fibre and high in fat. This makes fast food a poor choice for us on a regular basis. For the same reasons shop-bought food for tortoises is not good for their health. The foods we can buy are also much too low in calcium, an essential mineral for normal bone growth and development. Figure 5.10 shows some of the least bad options of bought foods available throughout the year.

Food choices for tortoises in captivity should be guided by the rule:

- low protein, low fat, high fibre, high vitamin and mineral (calcium).

Bean sprouts, pea shoots, spinach, chard, cabbage, kale and broccoli are all a definite 'NO'. Better choices include lamb's lettuce, watercress, Romaine lettuce, rocket or pak-choi, but all in small amounts and limited as much as possible.

Levels of toxins such as oxalates should also be considered, because they inhibit calcium uptake (Rendle, 2019). Watercress and coriander, for example, have very low oxalates, while spinach is high in oxalates and should be avoided. Another consideration is foods that have high levels of goitrogens, which can cause hypothyroidism, such as brassicas (cabbage, kale, broccoli) and should largely be avoided (Rendle, 2019). The other major consideration is the ratio of calcium to phosphorus in the food (see below), as foods with a high proportion of calcium and a low proportion of phosphorus should be chosen for food (Highfield, 1996, 2000; Highfield and Highfield, 2009).

What should I be feeding my tortoises on?

The diet of any species contains two types of nutrients: macronutrients and micronutrients.

1. Macronutrients – large organic food molecules which make up the bulk of the diet. These consist of:

- Proteins – used to make up the body structure; essential for growth.
- Carbohydrates – used to provide energy; these are the main source of any calories needed to generate energy.

- Fats and oils – also used to provide energy and calories, and to make some body structures and chemicals such as hormones.

2. **Micronutrients** – found in minute amounts but essential for normal bodily functions. These include:

- Vitamins – organic substances made by plants and animals and essential for the maintenance of good health and metabolism.
- Minerals – inorganic elements absorbed by plants and animals and also essential for the maintenance of good health and metabolism.

Additionally, the diet must provide:

- Fibre – which allows peristalsis (movement of food) through gut and helps maintain gut bacteria (the normal gut flora required for digestion).
- Water – which is essential for metabolic processes to take place, for the removal of toxic wastes and for temperature regulation.

In tortoises the low demand for calories, combined with a very large bony structure (the shell), means that in general the diet should be:

- Low in fats, oils and proteins
- High in vitamins and minerals (in particular calcium)
- High in fibre

These are your guiding principles for all decisions regarding food and diet. This includes omnivores (they will eat more protein) and herbivores.

Essentially, we should be providing a plant-based diet for our captive tortoises. Some species – the tropical tortoises, which are omnivores – will need the addition of a small amount of higher-protein foods (including animal protein) but the bulk of the diet should remain as plant material. As much of that as possible should be naturally growing, or planted to grow, in our gardens to try to provide variety and the most nutritionally beneficial foods (Highfield, 1996; 2000).

Is it best to feed my tortoise on a natural diet?

Yes, as stated, the best diet is the one that is most similar to the diet available to tortoises in the original environment. The closer the diet we provide is to that which the tortoise has evolved and adapted to eat over millions of years, the healthier the tortoise will be. The development and adaptation of their body structures, their physiology and behaviour are all based on, and adapted to, that natural diet.

It is a challenge for us to get that completely right in captivity, as set out in Table 5.1.

Do all tortoises eat the same things all the time?

Tortoise demands for nutrients will change with the seasons (particularly in the times leading up to hibernation/brumation, and emergence from it, if the tortoise is a species that does hibernate). Nutrient demands will be affected by gender and activity levels, including preparation for mating, mating itself and egg-laying in females. Table 5.2 indicates other things that affect the amounts and types of food required.

What sort of foods are best for herbivorous tortoises?

Mediterranean species and Horsfield's tortoises need a complete diet of mixed weeds and flowering plants. This is as close to their natural diet as possible. King (2020) provided a very useful list of edible plants in the UK, which is useful across Europe.

Some readily available examples of edible plants in Europe include: grasses, dandelions, vetches, sowthistle, herbs, hawkbit, plantain, deadnettle, cat's ears, trefoils, nipplewort, mallow, garlic mustard. Names of many of these plants are provided in Table 5.3.

Grazing species such as Sulcatas (*Centrochelys sulcata*) and Leopard tortoises (*Centrochelys pardalis*) need around 70% mixed grasses and hays, plus around 30% flowering plants, succulents and weeds (Kabigumila, 2001).

Table 5.4 lists suitable plants for tortoise enclosures. Information about suitable weeds and flowering plants for tortoises can be found on TheTortoiseTable App at www.thetortoisetable.org.uk.

Natural habitats encourage a tortoise to eat well. It is a good idea to grow 'tortoise-friendly' weeds and flowering plants in your garden if you can, so that you can be sure they have not been sprayed with chemicals which could injure your tortoise. Your tortoise will enjoy walking around and finding his own healthy diet (Fig. 5.13). There should be grass available for grazing species, as shown in Fig. 5.15.

Are some plants poisonous to tortoises?

There are poisonous plants that are toxic to tortoises. These should not be planted in enclosures,

Table 5.1. Macronutrients and micronutrients.

- What tortoises eat varies from species to species. A tortoise's diet should be based on what types of food it is likely to eat in its natural environment.
- In general, the bulk of the tortoise diet should be plant materials, which provide the necessary carbohydrates, fats, oils and proteins, as well as acting as a source of fibre.
- Some tortoises (particularly tropical tortoises) will require their diets to be supplemented by a small amount of higher-protein foods, including animal material.

Macronutrients and fibre:	• Plant material tends to be low in protein and high in fibre. Animal material has a higher protein content and often is lower in fibre. Getting the proportions of each type of macronutrient right is the big challenge when feeding captive tortoises. • Generally, the plant material offered should be naturally grown wild plants/weeds, with some cultivated flowering and succulent plants. • Commercially produced plant foods, such as those you might buy in the store, shop or supermarket, have too much protein and fats/oils with too little fibre. They are also often grown using many chemicals such as fertilizers and pesticides. The long-term effects of these are largely unknown within long-lived species such as tortoises. • The hard stems and leafy materials found in naturally growing plants are the best source of fibre, as they contain a high percentage of this undigestible material, which is essential for gut health and digestion. • Without enough fibre, the tortoise can become constipated. The free movement of food through the gut is essential for effective digestion to take place throughout the length of the gut. The fibre is also needed to provide a suitable environment for the normal gut flora and fauna, including helpful bacteria, which are vital in the digestive processes.	
Micronutrients: Vitamins required	Vitamin A (retinol)	Required for normal skin and tissue linings. This fat-soluble vitamin is needed on a regular basis as a supplement, as tortoises do not have good fat reserves.
	Vitamins B1 (thiamine), B2 (riboflavin), B3 (niacin), B6 (pantothenic acid), B7 (biotin), B12 (folate and folic acid)	The water-soluble B vitamin complex provides essential components for many metabolic pathways, including normal blood, muscle and nerve function, digestion, growth and development.
	Vitamin C (ascorbic acid)	Water-soluble and essential for skin and bone development. It is also important for normal function of the immune system and is an antioxidant.
	Vitamin D3 (cholecalciferol)	Fat-soluble and required for the uptake of calcium. Sunlight on the surface of the skin allows the tortoise to make vitamin D3 (see Chapter 4 on artificial light and heat). If there is insufficient sunlight, supplementation is needed to ensure the body has enough to take up calcium, particularly in young animals whose shells and bones are actively growing.
	Vitamin E (tocopherols and tocotrienols)	Fat-soluble and required as an antioxidant and for immune system function.
Micro-nutrients: Minerals required (the list is not exhaustive)	Calcium	For normal bone growth and development; for normal blood clotting and for muscle function.
	Phosphorus	Often found with calcium in food and is also essential for bone growth and development. The ratio of calcium to phosphorus needs to be high so that there is always much more calcium available.
	Sodium	For normal body fluids, muscle and nerve function.
	Potassium	For normal body fluids, muscle and nerve function
	Iron	Needed for the production of red blood cells.
	Iodine	For thyroxine production. This hormone has an influence on almost all metabolic processes.
	Manganese	Needed for effective digestion.

Continued

Table 5.1. Continued.

	Selenium	For immune system function.
	Magnesium	Essential in metabolism especially of sugar and for the function of some hormones.
	Copper	For normal growth and development and for the production of red and white blood cells.
	Cobalt	For normal growth and development and for the production of red and white blood cells

---

Box 5.1. Relationship between vitamins and minerals

(See also Chapter 7 on common illnesses and diseases)

The essential micronutrients are in balance with each other and the proportion of each relative to the others is also key to a balanced diet.

The ratio of calcium to phosphorus is one such example. The proportion of calcium compared with phosphorus in the diet should be higher, giving a ratio of at least 2:1. As an example, Nutrobal® (a Vetark® product), a calcium supplement to be added to food, has a 46:1 ratio of calcium to phosphorus. This means that for every one part of phosphorus, there are 46 parts calcium. This is very high, as the supplement is designed to add high levels of calcium to the diet. Both calcium and phosphorus are essential in the diet and are involved in normal bone formation. Generally, however, the higher the phosphorus levels in foods, the lower the calcium levels and it is only wild-grown plants and weeds that have the ideal higher levels of calcium needed for healthy bone formation. Examples of useful nutritional supplements are shown in Fig. 5.11.

In addition, in order to take up adequate calcium from the diet, vitamin D3 is required (see Chapter 4 on artificial light and heat). The relationship between these vitamins and minerals forms the basis for many metabolic processes – an excess or deficiency in one of them will upset the natural homeostasis necessary for growth and repair of bones.

There are many examples where deficiency in one nutrient will lead to poor uptake of another. The nutrients may be supplied in the diet but not available to the tortoise, due to disease.

---

or given as supplementary feed. Tortoises generally do not eat toxic plants, but the risk is always there, particularly if they are hungry. These plants are best avoided in any location near the enclosures, as well as the enclosures themselves.

Toxic plants are listed in Table 5.5 but the list is not exhaustive. If in doubt, check a reliable source such as TheTortoiseTable App or www.thetortoisetable.org.uk

What do I feed my tortoises at times of the year when weeds and flowering plants are not growing?

In colder climates (particularly during the winter months), growing suitable food plants or collecting them can be difficult as they are in short supply; many of the plants shown in Fig. 5.16 will die back over the winter. It is difficult to find enough weeds, or to grow enough natural food, although greenhouses, cold-frames and trays indoors can be used. Plants can also be grown in tortoise enclosures indoors.

In situations where indoor plant-growing is not possible, buying foods such as salad leaves can provide a short-term solution. Suitable examples are Romaine and red leaf (Lollo rosso) lettuces, or lamb's lettuce.

These foods must have the addition of food supplements (Fig. 5.11), to increase the available calcium in the diet. Lumps of chalk and eggshells can be used to provide additional calcium in enclosures, as shown in Fig. 5.14 above and, for juveniles, in Fig. 5.18 below.

Additional fibre should also be provided through addition of soaked tortoise cobs, or pressed food, which is made up of dried grasses and hays. These become a sort of mash when soaked and can be mixed in with the leaves provided in the diet. Examples include Pre-Alpen cobs (Fig. 5.19) and Arcadia® freshly pressed tortoise food. Any available safe weeds should continue to be included to this dietary mix.

In the UK and Europe this could include the following weeds (which remain available over much of the winter), also described in Table 5.3: plantain (*Plantago lanceolata*), hardy geranium (*Geranium* spp.), campanula (*Asterales campanula*), hosta (*Hosta* spp.), deadnettle (*Lamium* spp.), sedum or

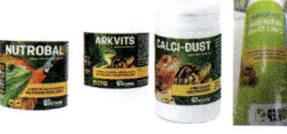
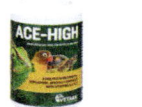
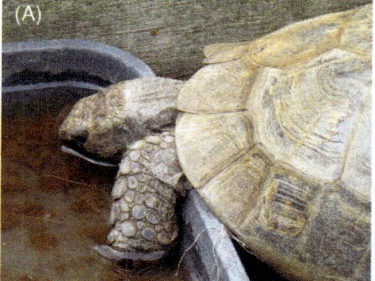
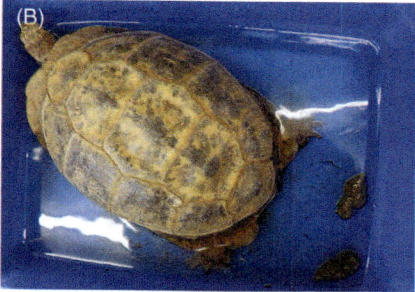

Fig. 5.11. Example of vitamin and mineral supplements.

Fig. 5.12 (A) Tortoise drinking. This large tortoise can lean over the edge of the water tray but ideally this should be sunk into the ground so that it is level with the substrate for easy access. (B) Tortoise placed in a bath for drinking purposes and to excrete wastes.

Box 5.2. Sources of water (Fig. 5.12)

The following are uses of water for tortoises:

- Provision of correct humidity levels
- Water to drink
- Water to bathe in
- Water to aid shedding of skin
- Excretion of toxic wastes from proteins in the diet

Adult tortoises get much of the water they require from their food. In the wild they often live in arid places where water is in short supply, especially in summer.

One of the most supportive things we can do for tortoises in captivity is to provide regular access to fresh water (Fig. 5.12). Any health problems will be made much worse if the tortoise is also dehydrated. Offering fresh water at all times is an easy way to help your tortoise avoid illnesses related to dehydration.

Dehydration-induced illnesses include reduced kidney or liver function, together with the development of bladder stones or reproductive issues.

---

ice plant (*Sedum* spp.), buddleia (*Lamiales buddleja*), bristly ox-tongue (*Pieris echioides*, *Helminthotheca echioides*) and ivy-leaved toadflax (*Cymbalaria muralis*). Clover (*Trifolium* spp.) is a very popular legume with tortoises but it is high in nitrogen, and therefore high in protein, so should be given only occasionally as a treat.

Commercially available diets are also available and can be useful at this time of year. These can be used to supplement the diet of non-hibernating, grass-eating species, increasing fibre when naturally growing weeds are not readily available (Fig. 5.19).

How do I grow suitable plants for tortoise food, out of season in a northern climate?

This can be achieved in a number of ways.

- Grow weeds/wild plants from seed in a greenhouse, heated sheds, or in trays indoors on windowsills (e.g. dandelions and plantains, as shown in Fig. 5.17A).
- Grow edible plants in a greenhouse (e.g. Opuntia cactus – prickly pear, coleus, spider plants as shown in Fig. 5.17B).

What sort of foods are best for omnivorous tortoises?

Tropical species such as Red-footed (*Geochelone carbonaria*), Yellow-footed (*Geochelone denticulata*) and Burmese Brown (*Manouria emys*) tortoises need around 75–80% weeds, flowering plants and leafy greens, plus 15–20% fruit and mushrooms, with 5% (or less) of animal protein (Fig. 5.20). The animal protein could include snails, slugs, insects, woodlice, maggots, caterpillars, pinkies, chicken.

Can I just go out and collect plants from the wild and feed them to my tortoise?

If you cannot supply enough weeds and other plants from your garden alone, you might need to collect some from the wild. However, please bear the following in mind.

- Do not collect from any areas where the plants may have been sprayed with pesticides or herbicides, or where they are exposed to a high level of

Table 5.2. Factors affecting amounts and types of food required.

Factor	Effects
Species	Diet varies according to the species of tortoise, and the type of food it is likely to eat in its natural environment.
Age	Young animals require more calcium for healthy growth. They also need proportionately more food than an adult as they are gaining weight as body structure, rather than simply maintaining body weight.
Size	Larger individuals and species need more food.
Season	In the tropics, seasons are largely constant, with little annual change; in temperate regions the type of food availability will vary from season to season so the nutritional value of food and its water content changes throughout the year.
Breeding status	Female tortoises need additional calcium in their diet for the normal formation of eggs.
Temperature	As ectotherms, the external temperature largely determines metabolic rate. The higher the temperature, the more active the tortoise will be and so the greater the need for food.
Humidity	Levels of humidity can alter levels of activity and therefore can impact nutrient needs.
Daylength	Longer days mean greater activity.
Quality and quantity of light	Natural sunlight is the best source of light, as it provides all the necessary wavelengths for normal activity and growth. Artificial light sources may limit some natural metabolic processes because they do not necessarily provide adequate amounts of the entire natural spectrum. For example, insufficient ultraviolet B (UVB) levels will reduce the ability to make vitamin D3 in the skin, which in turn reduces the ability to take up calcium. This is covered in more detail in Chapter 4 on artificial light and heat.

Table 5.3. Available growing food plants readily eaten by captive tortoises, from 'Wild Flowers and Plants Safe for Tortoises to Eat' (source: The Tortoise Table www.thetortoisetable.org.uk). See Appendix 3 for images of common food plants.

Common name	Latin name	Aromatic (providing scent/smell within the environment)
The list is not exhaustive but identifies commonly available plants which tortoises like to eat. Feed freely, or sparingly within a varied diet of as many safe plant types as are available.		
Alexanders (horse parsley, smyrnium)	*Smyrnium olusatrum, S. perfoliatum*	
Archangel	*Angelica sylvestris*	
Bristly oxtongue (bristly ox-tongue, bristly ox Tongue)	*Picris echioides; Helminthotheca echioides*	
Buddleia (butterfly tree)	*Lamiales buddleja*	✓
Cactus	*Opuntia* spp.	
Campanula (bell flower, trailing bell flower)	*Asterales campanula*	✓
Cat's ear (cat's ears, cats ears, catsear)	*Hypochaeris radicata*	
Chicory	*Cichorium intybus*	
Corn salad (lamb's lettuce, lambs lettuce)	*Valerianella* spp., esp. *Valerianella locusta*	
Cranesbill, hardy geranium	*Geranium* spp.	✓
Creeping thistle (field thistle, prickly thistle, Canada thistle)	*Cirsium arvense*	
Dandelion	*Taraxacum officinale*	
Deadnettle (white dead nettle, red or purple deadnettle, spotted deadnettle)	*Lamium purpureum; Lamium maculatum*	
Evening primrose	*Oenethera* spp.	✓
Forget-me-not (forget me not)	*Myosotis* spp.	
Garlic mustard	*Alliaria* spp.	✓
Goat's beard (goats beard, salsify, Jack-go-to-bed-at-noon)	*Tragopogon* spp.	
Goose grass, cleavers	*Galium* spp.	
Hawkbit	*Leodontodon* spp.	

Table 5.3 Continued.

Hawk's beard	*Crepis* spp.	
Herb Robert, geranium	*Geranium robertianum*	✓
Hibiscus	*Hibiscus* spp.	
Lavender	*Lavendula* spp.	✓
Lilac	*Syringa* spp.	✓
Mallow, tree mallow, lavatera	*Lavatera* spp., *Malva terrestris*	
Marigold	*Calendula* spp.	
Marjoram	*Origanum majorana*	✓
Mint	*Mentha* spp.	✓
Mulberry tree	*Morus* spp.	
Nipplewort	*Lapsana communis*	
Oregano	*Origanum vulgare*	✓
Pansey/viola	*Viola* spp.	✓
Broadleaf plantain (broad-leaved plantain, greater plantain, common plantain, hoary plantain, rat-tail plantain, rat's tail plantain)	*Plantago major*; *Plantago media*	
Ribwort plantain (narrowleaf plantain, narrow leaf plantain, English plantain)	*Plantago lanceolata*	
Rose (leaves and petals)	*Rosa* spp.	√
Sedum, ice plant	*Sedum* spp.	
Snapdragon	*Antirrhinum*	
Sowthistle, blue sowthistle (common blue sowthistle, alpine blue-sow-thistle)	*Sonchus oleraceus* and spp., *Cicerbita* spp. inc. *C. macrophylla, C. alpina, C. plumieri*	
Speedwell	*Veronica* spp.	
Thyme	*Thymus* spp.	√

exhaust fumes. These chemicals are likely to be toxic to your tortoise.
- Do not disturb wildlife within the area where you are collecting.
- Also be aware that some countries have legislation which prohibits the collection of some or all native wild plant species. If collection is permitted, do not take the whole plant. It is better to take some leaves so that the plant can regrow, rather than pulling up everything, including the roots. In addition, if there is an area where there are groups of one plant species, try not to collect all the plants of any given species.
- In Europe, The Habitats Directive (1992) *The Natura 2000 Network* also includes Special Protection Areas (SPAs) classified under the Habitats and Birds Directive. Following the findings of a review in 2016, the European Commission launched a new Action Plan 'to rapidly improve the practical implementation of the Habitats and Birds Directives. The Action Plan also aims to accelerate progress towards the EU goal of halting and reversing the loss of biodiversity and ecosystem services. Collectively these sites are often referred to as 'Natura 2000 sites' and are now the largest coordinated network of protected areas anywhere in the world' – The Habitats Directive (europa.eu). Plants must not be taken from these areas.
- In the UK it is against the law to pick any part of a plant that is on the protected species list of the 1981 Wildlife and Countryside Act (Wildlife and Countryside Act 1981, available at legislation.gov.uk) Similar general protection is given to all plants in Northern Ireland, under the Wildlife (Northern Ireland) Order, 1985 The Wildlife (Northern Ireland) Order 1985 (legislation.gov.uk)
- The Canadian wildlife Act was amended in 1994 About the Canada Wildlife Act - Canada.ca to include all land species of flora and fauna.
- The US Endangered Species Act of 1973 Endangered Species Act | U.S. Fish & Wildlife Service (fws.gov) also provides federal protection to plant species.
- You should only pick cultivated plants in the following places if you have been given specific permission:
  - Authority/District/council-owned parks, verges, roadsides and roundabouts
  - Community gardens
  - Neighbours' gardens

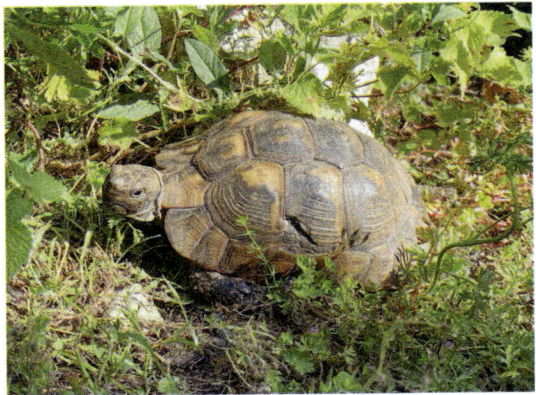

Fig. 5.13. Tortoise in a well-planted environment with a range of shrubs, herbs and flowering plants.

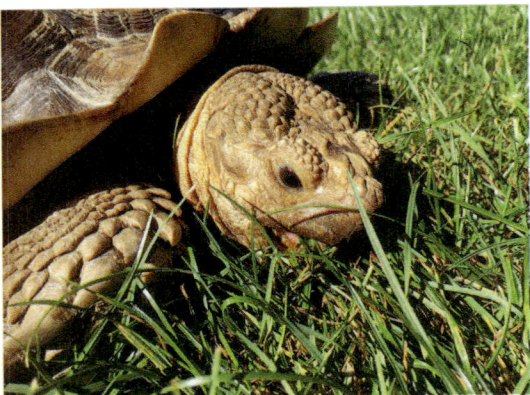

Fig. 5.15. Grazing Sulcata.

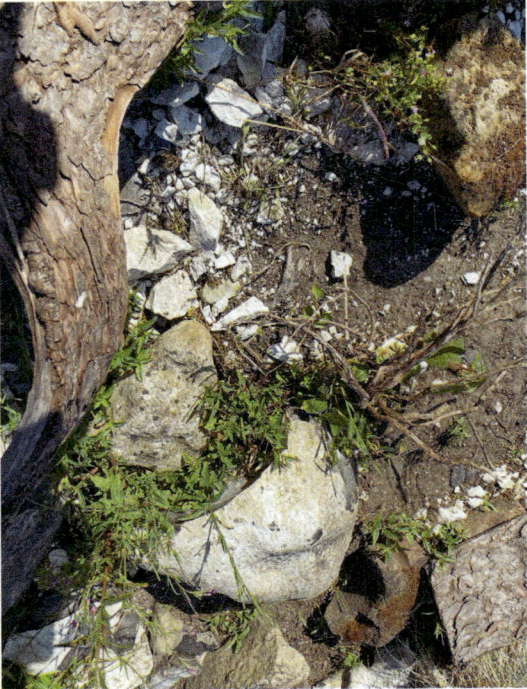

Fig. 5.14. Provision of calcium in enclosures to ensure access to this essential mineral.

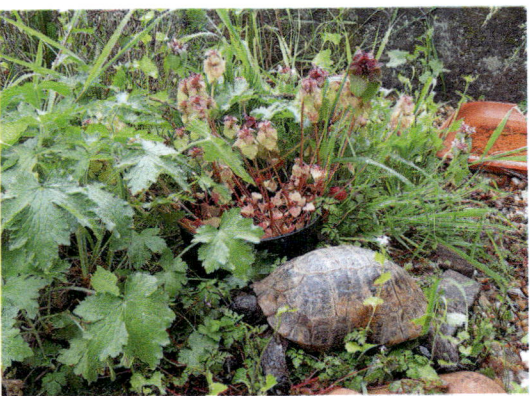

Fig. 5.16. Tortoise in a well-planted enclosure in the UK which includes pink deadnettle, hardy geranium, sowthistle, garlic mustard, herb Robert and plantain.

How can I change the diet of a tortoise that has been poorly fed over a long period of time?

It can take a long time for a tortoise to unlearn bad habits, or to come to accept a better diet. Sometimes the tortoise might need to be hand-fed initially to make the food as easy to pick up as possible. (Note that hand-feeding tortoises as a general principle is not a good idea as they can become addicted to that as well and refuse to eat on their own.)

Positioning the food in the corner of the enclosure may also help, so that there is minimal movement of the food, and the tortoise gets a piece of food every time they take a bite. This is particularly useful if the tortoise is blind or has neurological damage. When there is a poor appetite, the tortoise can be very easily put off and is soon discouraged if the food cannot be easily gathered into the mouth.

The following tips might prove helpful.

- Introduce the new food slowly and in small quantities.
- Cut the new food up into very small pieces and add it slowly to the tortoise's existing diet, increasing the volume bit by bit.
- Try moistening the new and the old food and mixing them together. It is almost impossible for the tortoise to separate pieces that are stuck together, and at least some of the new diet will be ingested.
- Liquidizing the food mixture of old and new so that there is only one type of food is sometimes needed. This makes the food mixture into a pulp which is very easily taken in, or used in hand-feeding where the tortoise needs some encouragement initially. Mashing the food into a pulp makes it even more difficult for the tortoise to pick out and reject new types of food.
- The smell of a cucumber or ice plant (sedum) is often enough to tempt even the most stubborn of tortoises. Juices from a cucumber smeared over the new food or the thinnest of slithers mixed in can encourage many tortoises to eat the new food.
- For arid and semi-arid species, you can try finely chopping dried grasses and moistening the mixture with warm water to release the sweet smell before mixing it with the new food.
- Once you have offered the food, move away so that the tortoise cannot see you.
- Once a pattern is established, start to decrease the amount of food from the old diet, and increase the amount from the new diet, until there is no unsuitable food left. This can take some time, but if you proceed slowly and are consistent then there is no reason why it should not work.

Table 5.4. Suitable types of shrubs and flowering plants for grazing, cover and shade (TheTortoiseTable App 2024).

Plants chosen for their added value to wildlife and because they can be food items.
Some are hardy, others may require over-wintering in a greenhouse in colder climates.

Astilbe	Bears breeches (Acanthus)	Bergamot (Monarda)	Blue sowthistle (Cicerbita)
Bristly oxtongue (Picris)	Harebell (Campanula)	Cat's ear (Hypochaeris)	Chameleon plant (Houttuynia)
Butterfly bush (Buddleia)	China doll (Radermarchera)	Clarkia	Coleus
Cone flower (Echinacea)	Tickseed (Coreopsis)	Couch grass (Elymus)	Cranesbill (Geranium – hardy)
Creeping thistle/ Spear thistle (Cirsium)	Firecracker flower (Crossandra)	False heather (Cuphea)	Deadnettle, pink/ white/ spotted (Lamium)
Twinspur (Diascia)	Saxifrage (Echeveria)	Wych Elm (Ulmus)	Evening primrose (Oenothera)
Fescue grass (Festuca)	Field madder (Sherardia)	Flowering currant (Ribes)	Forget-me-not (Myosotis)
Elephant grass (Pennisetum)	Globe thistle (echinops)	Gloxinia (Gesneiaceae)	Goats beard (Tragopogon)
Ground elder (Aegopodium)	Hawk's beard (Crepis)	Hawkbit (Leontodon)	Haworthia
Heartleaf iceplant (Aptenia)	Hebe	Hedge woundwort (Stachys)	Hibiscus
Hollyhock (Alcea)	House Leek (Sempervivum)	Ice-plant/ Sedum (Crassulacea)	Oat grass/ cat grass (Avena)
Jacaranda	Kidney weed (Dichondra)	Knapweed (Centaurea)	Lady's purse (Calceolariaceae)
Lamb's lettuce (Valerianella)	Lavatera	Lilac (Syringa)	Lipstick plant (Aeschynanthus)
Maize/corn (Zea)	Mallow (Malva)	Marigold (Calendula)	Marjoram (Origanum)
Mazus	Mexican petunia (Ruellia)	Michaelmas daisy (Aster)	Millet (Panicum)
Mimulus	Mind-your-own-business (Soleirolia)	Mint (Mentha)	Mother of pearl plant (Graptopetalum)
Mulberry tree/ bush (Morus)	Navelwort (Umbilicus)	Nemesia	Nipplewort (Lapsana)
Prickly pear (Opuntia cactus)	Oregano (Origanum)	Pampas grass (Cortaderia)	Pansy/ violet (Viola)
Peperomia	Plantain (Plantago) broadleaf and narrowleaf	Polka dot plant (Hypoestes)	Prayer plant (Maranta)
Purple loosestrife (Lythrum)	Red valerian (Centranthus)	Chia (Salvia)	Scotch thistle (Onopordum)
Sea holly (Eryngium)	Sedge (Carex)	Sow thistle (Sonchus)	Spider plant (Chlorophytum)
Spiraea	Teasel (Dipsaceae)	Thyme (Thymus)	Timothy grass (Phleum)
Wall lettuce (Mycelis)	Wheat (Triticum)	Yellow archangel (Lamium)	Zinnia

Table 5.5. Plants to be avoided in enclosures or as food items (TheTortoiseTable App 2024).

PLEASE CHECK FOR TOXICITY IF THE PLANT IS NOT LISTED HERE. THE LIST IS NOT EXHAUSTIVE.

Some of these species are extremely toxic and can kill tortoises very quickly. Many contain a group of plant chemicals called alkaloids as the toxin.

Aconitine, for example, causes paralysis of the nervous system, lowers pulse rate and stops the heart from beating.

Colchicine in crocuses has similar effects to arsenic, causing serious damage to the stomach and bowel, often leading to death.

Solanine, a glycoalkaloid found in the leaves and stems of the nightshade family, including potatoes, aubergines, tomatoes, can be fatal if the plant has high enough levels within.

Persin, the fungal toxin in avocado, also causes gastric damage, vomiting and diarrhoea, potentially leading to death.

Aconite (Aconitum)	Allium	Alstroemeria	Anemone
Aquilegia	Arnica	Arum lily/Lords and ladies	Ash
Avocado	Baneberry (Actaea)	Bird's foot trefoil (Lotus)	Blackthorn (Prunus)
Borage/heliotrope (Boraginales)	Broccoli/cabbage/cauliflower/ kohlrabi (Brassica)	Broom (Cystisus)	Bryony (Bryonia)
Camassia	Castor oil plant (Ricinus)	Cedar (Cedrus)	Celery (Apium)
Coltsfoot (Tussilago)	Comfrey (Symphytum)	Chrysanthemum	Cotoneaster
Cow parsley (Anthriscus)	Crocus species	Cyclamen	Dock (Rumex)
Elder (Sambucus)	Eucalyptus	Euonymus	Euphorbia species Poinsettia/spurge
Fat-hen/Goosefoot/ good King Henry (Chenopodium)	Feverfew (Tanacetum)	Flamingo flower (Anthurium)	Flax/linseed (Linum)
Foxglove (Digitalis)	Frangipani (Gentianales)	French marigold (Tagetes)	Giant cane (Arundo)
Gladiolus	Grape hyacinth (Muscari)	Greater celandine (Chelidonium)	Gound ivy (Glechoma)
Groundsel (Senecio)	Hellebore (Helleborus)	Hemlock (Conium)	Hogweed (Heracleum)
Holly (Ilex)	Horse chestnut (Aesculus)	Hyacinth/bluebell (Hyacinthoides)	Hydrangea
Iris species	Ivy species (Hedera)	Japanese/Wood anemone	Juniper (Juniperus)
Kerria	Laburnum	Lantana	Laurel (Prunus)
Leopard's bane (Doronicum)	Ragwort (Ligularia species)	Lily (Lilium)	Lily of the valley (Convallaria)
Lobelia	Lupin (Lupinus)	Lychnis (Silene)	Mimosa (Acacia)
Mistletoe (Viscum)	Montbretia (Crocosmia)	Mullein (Verbascum)	Daffodil (Narcissus species)
Nerine	Nightshade, Garden/ Deadly; Jerusalem cherry Tobacco plant; Wolfberry (Solanacaea species)	Oak (Quercus)	Oleander (Nerium)
Onion/chives/leek/garlic (Allium)	Passionflower (Passiflora)	Pea (Pisum)	Peace lily (Spathiphyllum)
Peony/Tree peony (Paeonia)	Philodendron	Photinia	Pieris
Pine (Pinus)	Plumbago/Statis	Pokeweed (Phytolacca)	Poppy (Papaver species)
Potato (Solanum)	Primrose/cowslip/primula species	Ragwort/Silver dust (Senecio)	Ranunculaceae species: Clematis/buttercup/ columbine/delphinium
Red maple/Sycamore (Acer)	Rhododendron/Azalea species	Rhubarb (Rheum)	Ribes: red/white/black (currants)
Santolina	Snowdrop (Galanthus)	St John's Wort (Hypericum)	Sweet chestnut (Castanea)
Toad lily (Tricyrtis)	Toadflax/Yellow toadflax (Linaria)	Toadstools and mushrooms (apart from edible varieties in shops) can be very toxic	Tulip (Tulipa)
Viburnum	Wallflower (Erysimum)	Walnut tree (Juglans)	Wild carrot (Daucus)
Wisteria	Wood sorrel (Oxalis)	Yew (Taxus)	

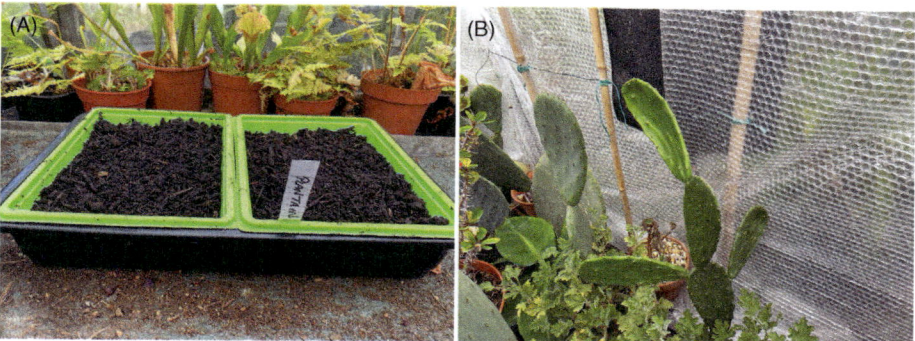

Fig. 5.17. Indoor growing of tortoise food plants. (A) Under-lights trays of plantain. (B) Opuntia cactus in the greenhouse.

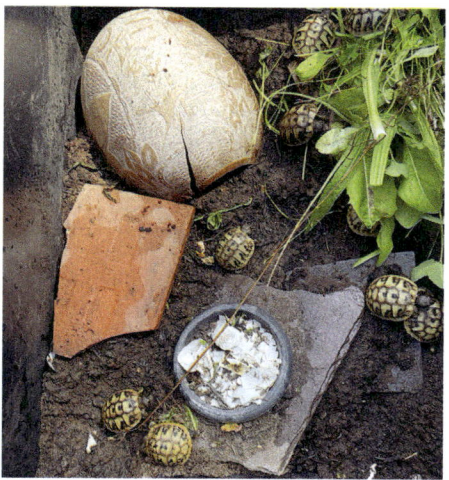

Fig. 5.18. Additional calcium provided to juveniles as egg-shells and calcium grit or chalk lumps.

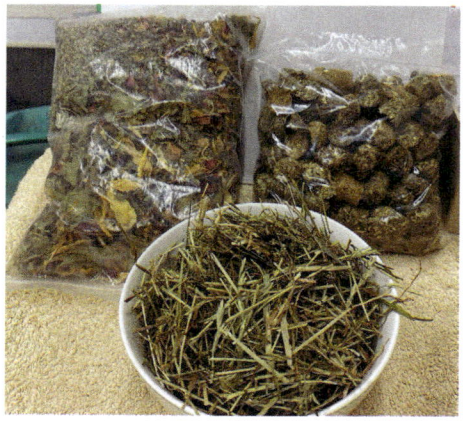

Fig. 5.19. Commercial diets: dried flowers, Pre-Alpen cobs® and Readigrass®.

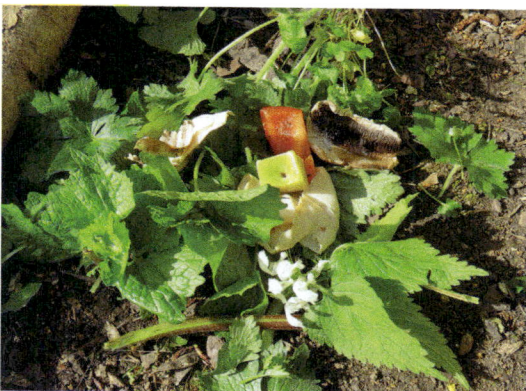

Fig. 5.20. Varied, leafy plant-based diet for omnivores, with added fruit and mushrooms.

Table 5.6. Commercial diets, pellets and cobs, which can increase the fibre content and variety of plant species supplied over the winter.

Type	Commercial products
Pellets	Pro Rep Tortoise food®
	Pre-Alpen cobs®
	Lucky Reptile Herb Cobs®
	Mazuri Tortoise Diet Pellets®
Flower mixes	Pro Rep Tortoise Flower Mix®
	Pro Rep Juvenile Tortoise Botanical Mix®
	Zoo Med Tortoise Flower Food Topper®
Grass and hay products	Readigrass® for Horses Friendship Estates
	Arcadia Freshly Pressed Tortoise Food®
	Zoo Med Grassland Tortoise Food®
	Timothy hay

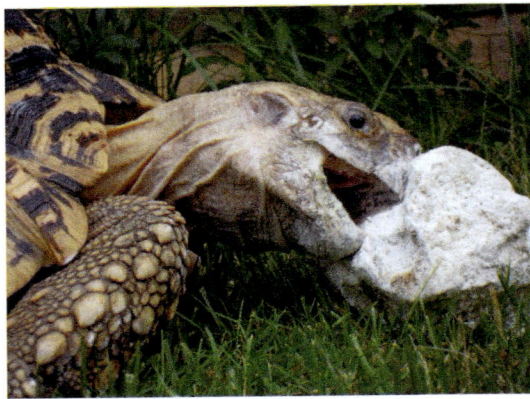

Fig. 5.21. Enclosure with supply of chalk lumps, here being readily eaten by a Leopard tortoise (Eleanor Lien-Hua Tirtasana Chubb).

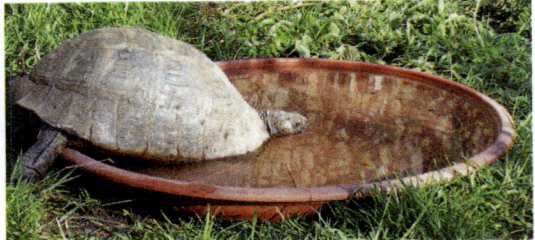

Fig. 5.22. Tortoises should have free access to water in shallow trays sunken into the substrate (Eleanor Lien-Hua Tirtasana Chubb).

Should I add nutritional supplements to my tortoise's food?

In captivity a tortoise's diet will never be exactly the same as that found in the wild. Because of this a nutritional supplement of vitamins and minerals, given three to four times a week for adults, is recommended. This ensures that there is no shortage of essential vitamins and minerals in the diet. Calcium and other mineral and vitamin supplements should be offered to ensure that there is no shortage of these essential micronutrients.

Suitable supplements include those shown in Table 5.7 and Fig. 5.11. These should always be used according to the manufacturer's instructions and over-supplementation should be avoided.

Note that cuttlefish has been used as a rich calcium source in the past, but due to over-fishing in some regions, for conservation and biodiversity reasons, alternatives such as calcium or chalk lumps or grit have been used here.

Why is the calcium:phosphorus ratio important?

Calcium and phosphorus are often found together in food items. They are both involved in normal bone growth and development.

The calcium:phosphorus (Ca:P) ratio should always be in favour of calcium for tortoises. Growing tortoises need calcium for their shells, as this provides support which is essential for normal bone development. Without calcium they can experience calcium-related deficiencies such as pyramiding of their shells, poor bone strength in their limbs and a resultant flattened body appearance, particularly towards the tail. This flattening reduces the space required for normal-sized organs to fit inside the shell. This can be particularly harmful for the lungs and can cause breathing difficulties (see Chapter 7 on common illnesses and diseases).

Due to the large shell and high calcium requirements, the ratio of calcium to phosphate should be at least 2:1, which means two parts calcium to every one part phosphorus (Rendle, 2019). A ratio of 3:1 calcium:phosphorus would be even better. This is especially true when feeding juveniles or egg-laying females, where the demand for calcium is highest. Additional sources of calcium, such as lumps of chalk, grit and granules, should be available in enclosures (Fig. 5.21). Calcium powder in the soil of outdoor enclosures can be taken up by growing food plants, which is a more effective and natural way of providing high calcium in the diet.

In many shop- or store-bought plants (such as the lettuces previously referred to) the ratio of calcium to phosphorus is much lower than in weeds and other naturally occurring plants. This makes the addition of calcium supplements even more important when using such foods as part of the diet.

Is there any danger of giving too much supplement?

Supplements should be used according to the manufacturer's guidance to avoid risk of overdose. It should be noted that with oral vitamin D3 supplements, there is no limiting pathway or buffering system preventing the absorption of vitamin D3 from the gut (Baines *et al.*, 2016). It is therefore possible to overdose this vitamin through supplementation, in a way that is not possible when the vitamin is manufactured by the skin in the presence of sunlight (see Chapter 4 on artificial light and heat).

Table 5.7. Suitable nutritional supplements.

Product	Manufacturer	Contents	Form
Arkvits®	Vetark	Mix of Nutrobal and Ace-High	Powder to sprinkle on food
Nutrobal®	Vetark	High calcium levels, vitamin D3	Powder to sprinkle on food
Calcidust®	Vetark	Calcium	Calcium powder to dust food
Zolcal-F Feed®	Vetark	Calcium, vitamin D3	Liquid for oral supplementation in drinking water or on food for quick uptake
Zolcal-D® Supplement	Vetark	Calcium and vitamin D3	Liquid for oral supplementation in drinking water or on food for quick uptake where deficiencies have been identified
Ace-High®	Vetark	Vitamins A, B1, B2, B6, B12, C, D3, E, Calcium, phosphorus, Na, Fe, K, Co, I, Mn, Se, Mg, Cu	Multivitamin and mineral powder supplement
Botanical Calcidust®	ProRep	Calcium carbonate, magnesium carbonate, bee pollen, cactus flower, dandelion, plantain, chickweed, nettle leaf, milk thistle, rose petal, marigold flower, Echinacea, hibiscus flower, mulberry leaf, prickly pear	Powder to sprinkle on food, made more palatable by the addition of pollen
Calcidust®	ProRep	Calcium carbonate	Powder to sprinkle on food
Tortoise calcium blocks®	ProRep	Calcium carbonate	Blocks of solid calcium to gnaw on, also wears down the beak

Water provision

Although not a nutrient, water is (as we all know) essential for life. Although many tortoises are adapted to live in arid conditions and have mechanisms to retain available water, in captivity free access to water is best practice. As this book emphasizes throughout, we cannot completely recreate the natural environment. The additional stresses of being in captivity mean that we should offer as much support as possible to our tortoises. Allowing the tortoise to bathe and drink as needed (Fig. 5.22) is one easy way to provide support and to prevent any health problems due to dehydration (see Chapter 7 on common illnesses and diseases).

Conclusion

As can be seen, the key to feeding a healthy diet for your tortoise lies in providing as wide a variety of appropriate food types as possible. While all tortoise diets should be largely based on weeds, flowering plants and succulents, different types of tortoises will require these items in different proportions, while some might need additional items. For some tortoises, such as Mediterranean and Horsfield's tortoises, weeds, flowering plants and succulents should make up 100% of the diet.

For others like the large grazers, Leopard tortoises (*Centrochelys pardalis*) and Sulcatas (*Centrochelys sulcata*), for example, the diet should consist of mainly grasses with one-quarter to one-half flowering and succulent plants.

For the omnivores, such as Red-footed (*Geochelone carbonaria*) and Yellow-footed (*Geochelone denticulata*) tortoises or Hingebacks (*Kinixys* spp.), around three-quarters of the diet should be weeds, flowering plants and succulents, with the remaining quarter being fruits and mushrooms, together with a small percentage of animal protein.

For all tortoises, fresh water should always be freely available and accessible, while vitamin and mineral supplementation at least three times per week is also recommended.

Providing a good diet, suited to the needs of the individual species, is the cornerstone to ensuring that your tortoise remains fit and healthy throughout its long life. A poor diet can have a dramatic impact on the well-being of tortoises – particularly juveniles, which are very susceptible to damage from growth deformities such as pyramiding and lumpy shells, collapsed or soft shells, or weakened and thin bones on the limbs. We have improved our knowledge in this area considerably in recent years. Foods that were commonly fed are now known to be completely unsuitable and harmful. If we stick to the principle of trying to emulate the natural diet, we have the best opportunity to get things right.

References and Further Reading

Baines, F.M., Chattell, J., Dale, J., Garrick, D., Gill, I., Goetz, M., Skelton, T. and Swatman, M. (2016) How much UV-B does my reptile need? The UV-Tool, a guide to the selection of UV lighting for reptiles and amphibians in captivity. *Journal of Zoo and Aquarium Research* 4(1), 42–63.

Celse, J., Catard, A., Caron, S., Ballouard, J.-M., Gagno, S., Jardé, N., Cheylan, M., Astruc, G., Croquet, V., Bosc, M. and Petenian, F. (2014) Management guide of populations and habitats of the Hermann's tortoise. *LIFE*, 8.

Highfield, A.C. (1996) *Practical Encyclopaedia of Keeping and Breeding Tortoises and Freshwater Turtles*. Carapace Press, London.

Highfield, A.C. (2000) *The Tortoise Trust Tortoise and Turtle Feeding Manual*. Carapace Press, London.

Highfield, A.C. and Highfield, N. (2009) *Keeping a Pet Tortoise*. Interpet, Dorking, UK.

Jepson, L. (2010) *Mediterranean Tortoises*. Kingdom Books, Interpet, Dorking, UK.

Kabigumila, J. (2001) Sighting frequency and food habits of the Leopard tortoise *Geochelone pardalis* in Northern Tanzania. East African Wildlife Society. *African Journal of Ecology* 39, 276–285.

King, L. (2020) *Edible Plants for Tortoises in the UK*, 4th edn. Available from: books@tlady.clara.co.uk

Lumbis, R. and White, C. (2022) Ch 5 Nutritional welfare. In: Rendle, M. and Hinde-Magarity, J. (eds) *BSAVA Manual of Practical Veterinary Welfare*. BSAVA, Quedgeley, UK, pp. 124–146.

McArthur, S., Wilkinson, R. and Meyer, J. (2004) *Medicine and Surgery of Tortoises and Turtles*. Blackwell, Oxford, UK.

Milton, S.J. (1992) Plants eaten and dispersed by adult leopard tortoises *Geochelone pardalis* in the southern Karoo. *African Journal of Zoology*, 27(2).

Moskovits, D.K. and Bjorndda, K.A, (1990) Diet and food preferences of the tortoises *Geochelone carbonaria* and *G. denticulata* in northwestern Brazil. *Herpetologica* 46(2), 207–218.

Rendle, M. (2019) Ch 4 Nutrition. In: Girling, S.J. and Raiti, P. (eds) *BSAVA Manual of Reptiles*, 3rd edn. BSAVA, Quedgeley, UK, pp. 49–70.

Rouag, R., Ferrah, C., Luiselli, L., Tiar, G., Benyacoub, S., Ziane, N. and El Mouden, E.L. (2008) Food choice of an Algerian population of the spur-thighed tortoise, *Testudo graeca*. *African Journal of Herpetology* 57(2), 103–113.

The Tortoise Table App: available from www.thetortoisetable.org.uk

Vetter, H. (2006) *Chelonian Library 2. Hermann's Tortoise. Testudo hermanni, T. boettgeri and T. hercegovinensis*. Chimaira, Frankfurt, 325 pp

Wegehaupt, W. (2009a) *Mediterranean Tortoises, Where and how they live in the wild*. Kressbronn, Germany.

Wegehaupt, W. (2009b) *Naturalistic Keeping and Breeding of Hermann's Tortoises*. Kressbronn, Germany.

Wegehaupt, W. (2021) *Feeder Plants for Mediterranean Tortoises*. Kressbronn, Germany.

6 Health Checks – Indicators of Good Health

Abstract
This chapter looks at checks that can be carried out regularly by tortoise keepers to ensure their tortoises are in good health, and how to look for signs of the tortoise being unwell. The main indicators of well-being are behavioural. Is the tortoise behaving normally? To answer this the keeper needs to know what 'normal' behaviour is for their tortoise. The need for observation of the tortoise on a regular basis is highlighted. Levels of activity, types of daily behaviour and diet-related behaviours are discussed. The tortoise's appetite is a good indicator of how well they are feeling. When unwell, a failure to feed is a clear sign of health problems. This chapter links to Chapters 7, 8 and 12 in this book.

There are also physical signs and symptoms of disease to look for as indicators of the tortoise becoming unwell. These physical changes include waste products becoming abnormal, or changes to the physical appearance of the tortoise. Measurements of weight and length can be taken as a way of keeping regular records of change as the tortoise grows and develops. These records can also show sudden changes in weight in adult tortoises, which can be useful in monitoring health.

Some first aid techniques are discussed, but only briefly, as this is covered in Chapter 7 on common illnesses and diseases. The need to seek veterinary advice, as necessary, to ensure that any health issues are treated promptly is highlighted. It is very important that we avoid compromising the tortoise's welfare through lack of attention to behaviour. Observations of the physical and mental state of the tortoise are essential for monitoring good health. Veterinary advice should be sought for any health issues or disease identified through health checks.

Top 10 health checks are described along with general maintenance through nail and beak trimming if necessary. All the suggestions in this chapter focus on maintaining health and welfare through a suitable captive environment, easy-to-carry-out checks and keeping good records.

How do we check if our tortoise is healthy?

The first check should be to ensure that environmental conditions are suitable for the species of tortoise being kept. If the environment is not right the health can never be optimal. There should be regular checks of temperatures, lighting sources and cleanliness of a suitable substrate. Provision of a suitable-size enclosure, appropriate humidity levels, planting to create microclimates, opportunities for basking, hides and shelters (as described in Chapter 3 on the captive environment) are essential in maintaining health. Keeping enclosures clean, providing fresh water (see also Chapter 19 on health and safety) and checking daily that your tortoise is behaving 'normally', are a key part of health checks.

There are some simple regular checks on health that we should carry out on a daily, weekly and monthly basis.

Daily

Check for any signs of injury or damage by observation without causing the tortoise stress. Check eating habits and any waste products. Check that there are no changes in behaviour. Is the tortoise in the usual places? Is the tortoise moving around as usual?

Weekly

Check that the tortoise is drinking normally by placing it in a warm bath, even when water is freely available in the enclosure. This will give an added opportunity to observe waste products and to check for cleanliness or build-up of dirt or faeces, especially around the tail. Visually check for any obvious injuries, or any changes to the head, limbs, tail or shell.

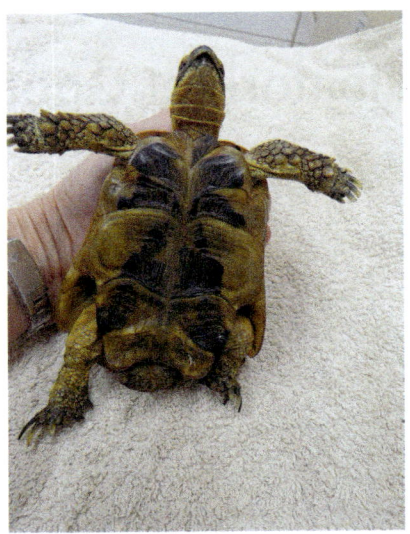

Fig. 6.1. Physical examination of underside of plastron.

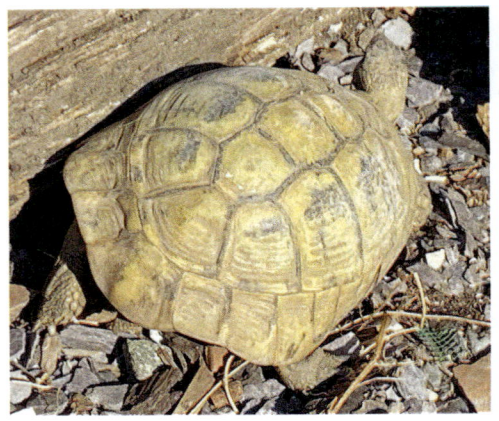

Fig. 6.3. Hermann's tortoise (*Testudo hermanni*) basking.

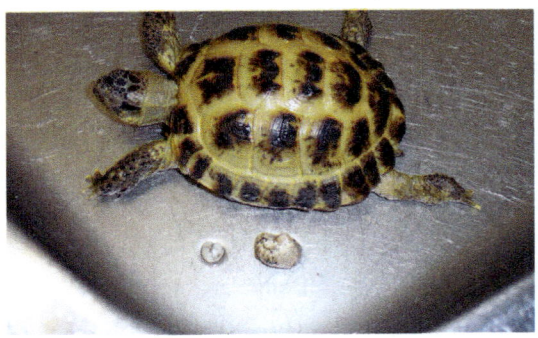

Fig. 6.2. Male Horsfield's tortoise with bladder stones that passed out of the cloaca.

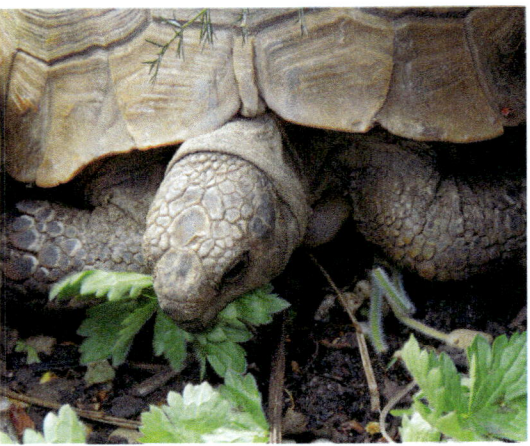

Fig. 6.4. Spur-thighed tortoise (*Testudo graeca*) eating.

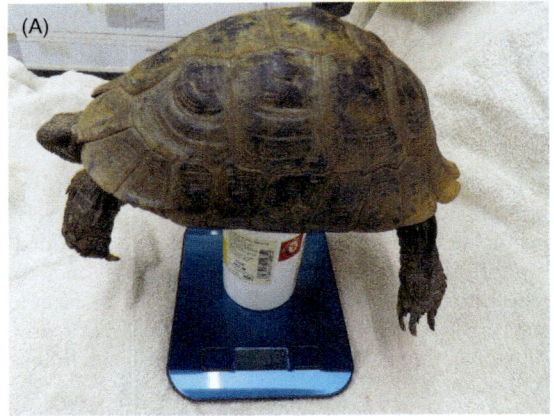

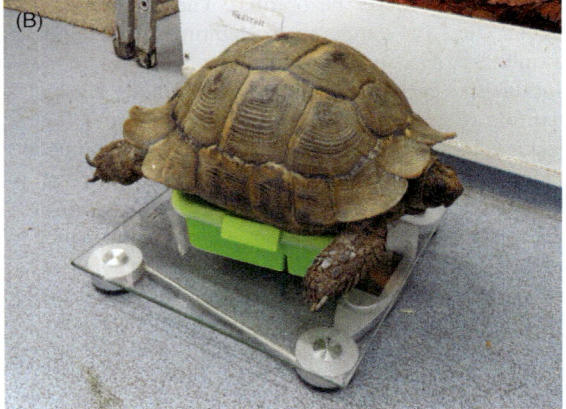

Fig. 6.5. Weighing (A) smaller tortoises and (B) larger tortoise while reducing stress by not placing onto their backs is preferable.

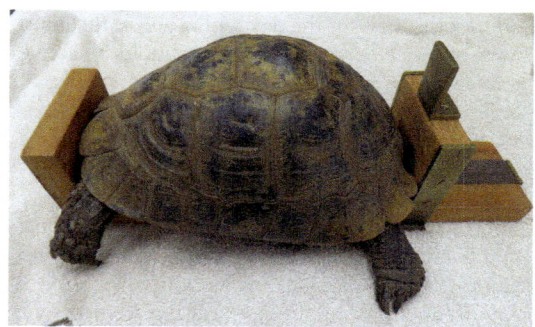

Fig. 6.6. Measuring SCL of tortoises (in millimetres) using a ruler set into wood with a solid fixed end and a movable end. This can also be done using a hardcover book at each end with a ruler under the tortoise.

Monthly

Carry out the full checks described below to check for injury, lumps, swellings, length of beak and nails, inside of the mouth. Check the head and limbs for any changes, and examine the skin and shell closely. Weigh and measure your tortoise as set out below, to keep a record of any sudden changes. Growth should be slow and steady in juveniles, although some of the larger species will grow much faster (e.g. Sulcatas).

Record keeping – what do I need to know?

Keeping good records is the best way to see changes over time. Looking at the physical appearance of the tortoise, measuring weight and length and noting any signs and symptoms are straightforward ways to check health. Monitoring waste products is also essential, to ensure that bodily functions are taking place as they should. Health check forms (Ebenhack, 2012; Chitty and Raftery, 2013; Raftery, 2019) to collect background information can be completed on your PC, tablet, laptop or phone, using a number of different apps. Choose the option that gives you the greatest flexibility and accessibility. Example tortoise health records are shown in Appendix 1, p. 271.

As you will see below in the list of Top 10 health checks, behaviour is number one. Is the tortoise behaving normally? To answer this, you as the keeper need to know what 'normal' behaviour is for your tortoise (Deane and Valentine, 2022; McBride and Hinde-Megarity, 2022). The need for observation of the tortoise on a regular basis is key to spotting any changes. Levels of activity are important (McArthur *et al.*, 2004; Chitty and Raftery, 2013). Is the tortoise getting slower or moving less? When looking at the types of daily behaviour seen, is the tortoise basking or hiding more than usual? Is the tortoise agitated or calm? Is the tortoise refusing to move or holding its body parts in unusual positions? Is the tortoise trying to escape the enclosure repeatedly, or showing discomfort when passing urine or faeces?

Feeding and drinking are very important behaviours in indicating how well the tortoise feels (see Chapters 8 and 9 on behaviour and emotions).

I once looked after a juvenile male Horsfield's tortoise who was having difficulty passing urine and faeces. Having tried to bathe him repeatedly in lukewarm water without success, he was taken to a veterinarian, who X-rayed him. On the X-ray there were a number of stones (some large in comparison with the size of the tortoise, which was only 70 mm in length) in the lower part of the bladder trying to pass out. Several had started to pass into the cloaca. It was felt that if we could support the tortoise to pass these with lubricants in the cloaca, this would be preferable to removing them surgically.

We continued bathing and encouraging the tortoise to drink and after 2 days the tortoise started to produce a collection of small stones and pieces of gravel into the water. Then a much larger stone was felt to be in the cloaca and the tortoise was straining to pass it. I have never seen a tortoise look so distressed as he tried to squeeze the stone out. I helped him by applying some pressure behind the stone, like pushing a pea along a tube. The relief on his face as the stone passed out of the vent was amazing to see, as it was very large (as shown in Fig. 6.2). Given that tortoises do not have the capacity to show facial expressions (see Chapter 9 on emotional states), this animal conveyed his high levels of distress through bulging eyes and rapid head and limb movements. This is an extreme example but indicates the need to observe tortoises while they carry out all their daily activities.

Reproductive behaviours can also give good indications of physical health. The tortoise is unlikely to try to breed if feeling unwell, or if there are bodily systems or organs that are not functioning as well as they should. Engagement with other tortoises, or avoidance, may also signal problems. All of these behavioural signs may indicate changes in health, as reported by Warwick *et al.* (2013).

These checks and signs only work, of course, if the tortoise is being kept in suitable environmental conditions. As discussed in Chapter 3 on the captive environment, and in the chapters on different species of tortoises (Chapters 13–17), a tortoise cannot maintain good health if its basic needs are not being met. If the environment is not optimal in terms of temperature, lighting, substrate, humidity, diet and water availability, the tortoise will never be completely healthy. As discussed in Chapter 7 on common illnesses and diseases, without suitable environmental conditions the tortoise may be surviving but not thriving.

Any identified potential health issues or disease should be acted upon immediately and veterinary advice sought as necessary. A review of husbandry and environmental conditions should also be carried out. Any environmental causes of identified health problems should be addressed to prevent a recurrence of the problem.

Top 10 Checks for a Healthy Tortoise

The Top 10 checks include: (1) Behaviour; (2) Length/weight ratio; (3) Feeding; (4) Drinking; (5) Urates; (6) Faeces; (7) Mouth and beak; (8) Nose, eyes, ears; (9) Lumps, bumps, swellings; and (10) Skin/nails/shell damage.

1. Behaviour

Look for any changes in behaviour (see Chapters 8 and 9 on behaviour and emotional states). Note that for normal behaviour to be shown, temperature ranges must be correct, i.e. the preferred optimal temperature zone (POTZ) must be provided for any species that you keep. A temperature gradient (defined by the POTZ) is required during the day, and similarly during the night. Suitable humidity levels should also be provided.

Normal behaviours include basking to increase body temperature, walking, feeding, resting and hiding, together with making use of retreats for shelter from the sun or rain. Temperature regulation continues throughout the day and is one of the main drivers of movement. The tortoise should be active and lively when warm.

Your tortoise should actively explore its environment, climbing over obstacles, for example, within its enclosure. Other exploratory behaviours include sniffing and looking at the surroundings. The tortoise should also be seeking out natural foraging and grazing, to find suitable food items, which will vary according to the tortoise's species and the natural food sources.

Any reduction in activity and movement, or changes in normal behaviours, should be an early warning of potential health issues developing. Failure to feed or to produce normal wastes (see below) should be seen as potentially very serious and appropriate veterinary advice should be sought.

2. Length/weight ratio, or weight over time

To obtain the length/weight ratio you need to measure the straight carapace length (SLC) in millimetres (mm) and weigh the tortoise in grams (g) (Figs 6.5–6.7).

Length can be compared with weight by using the Jackson ratio (Jackson, 1980). (Note that the Jackson ratio can only be used with Spur-thighed and Hermann's tortoises. It is not suitable for use with Horsfield's or Marginated tortoises, or any species other than Spur-thighed and Hermann's tortoises. The Jackson ratio is based on comparing weight and length using a coefficient calculated as 0.191 for these two species. As reported in Rendle (2019) the Jackson ratio is based on:

$$\text{Weight}(g) = c \times \text{SCL}(cm)^3$$

where c is the coefficient and = 0.191.

Table 6.1. Examples of POTZ and relative humidity values (from Scheelings, 2019; Varga, 2019).

Tortoise species	Preferred optimal temperature zone (POTZ) (°C)	Relative humidity (RH) (%)
Spur-thighed *Testudo graeca*	20–28	30–50
Hermann's *Testudo hermanni*	20–28	30–50
Leopard *Geochelone pardalis*	25–35	40–75
Sulcata *Geochelone sulcata*	25–35	40–75
Red-footed *Geochelone carbonaria*	21–27	50–60
Bell's Hingeback *Kinixys belliana*	24–28	50–80

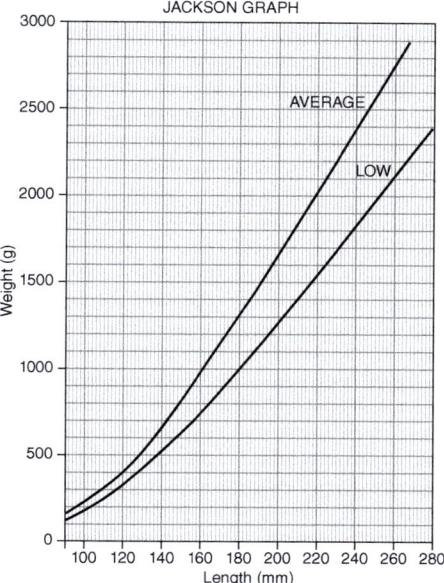

Fig. 6.7. The ratio between weight and length, as an indication of body condition, can be identified through the Jackson ratio for Spur-thighed and Hermann's tortoises only. This ratio has been used from the early days of tortoise keeping, when these were the main species in captivity. This ratio should not be used for any other species (Jackson, 1980).

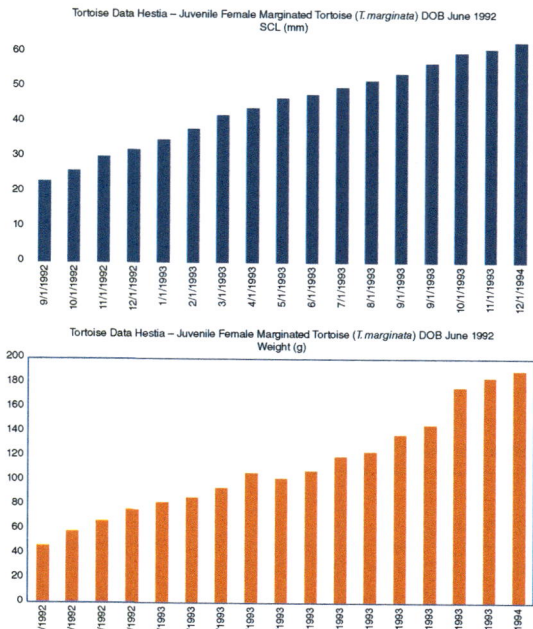

Fig. 6.8. Monthly records of juvenile growth by weight and length in female Marginated tortoise (*Testudo margianta*) Hestia, 1992–1994.

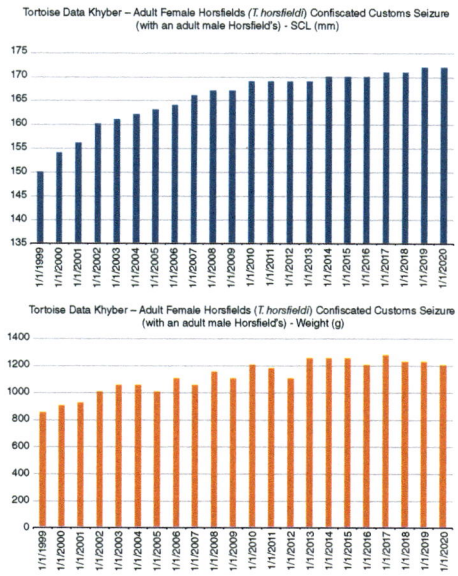

Fig. 6.9. Annually logged records of adult female weight in Horsfield's tortoise (*Testudo horsfieldi*) Khyber, 1999–2020.

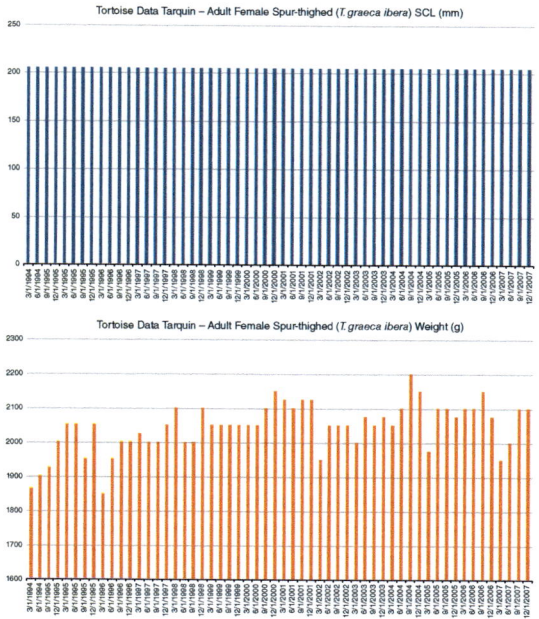

Fig. 6.10. Quarterly records of adult female weight in Spur-thighed tortoise (*Testudo graeca ibera*) Tarquin, 1994–2007.

> **Box 6.1.** Calculation of the bone density ratio (see also Chapter 12 on hibernation)
> I have used the bone density ratio as an indicator of body condition for a number of years. As this is not species-specific, it is less accurate than a ratio where a coefficient has been calculated (such as Jackson's ratio). It gives a general indication of condition and whether the tortoise is very heavy or very light in weight compared with length. For many species, however, we simply do not have accurate data on growth rates or body condition.
> The mathematical calculation to compare length with weight is shown in the formula below, where:
>
> L = straight carapace length in centimetres (cm), not millimetres (so convert millimetres to centimetres by dividing by 10; for example: 1 mm = 0.1 cm; 25 mm = 2.5 cm; 10 mm = 1 cm; 100 mm = 10 cm)
> W = weight in grams
> Bone ratio (N) = Weight (g) / (Length (cm))^3
> Bone density ratio (N) formula:
> N = W(g) ÷ L(cm)^3

Table 6.2. Bone ratio results and meaning.

Tortoise size	Bone density ratio results (based on similar figures as the Jackson's ratio coefficient of 0.191)
Healthy tortoise less than 15 cm length	Healthy tortoise Bone value (N) is 0.22–0.25
Healthy tortoise greater than 15 cm length	Healthy tortoise Bone value (N) is 0.20–0.23
If N ≥ 0.25 (greater than or equal to 0.25)	Tortoise is obese
If N ≤ 0.17 (less than or equal to 0.17)	Tortoise is underweight

Raftery (2019, p. 94) reported a calculation for body condition in tortoises based on the SCL (L), the maximum carapace width (at its widest point) (W) and the maximum height from the bottom of the plastron to the top of the carapace (H). This has been calculated for the Californian Desert tortoise (*Gopherus agassizii*) by Mader and Stoutenberg (1998) as:

$$\text{Predicted body weight}(g) = 0.588(L \times W \times H) + 388$$

There is a great deal of further work needed in this field to identify coefficients for other tortoise species based on their shape and dimensions.

The bone density ratio also compares the SCL to the weight. It is not species-specific and for most tortoise species we do not have a specific coefficient with which to work. We do not have data on what a 'normal' weight is for a given length, neither do we have data on what that comparison suggests in terms of body condition.

The relationship, or ratio, between length and weight is often used to assess the tortoise's health prior to hibernation. This assessment has been a primary use of the Jackson ratio as an indicator of whether the tortoise is a good weight to sustain itself during the hibernation period when it will not be feeding (see Chapter 12 on hibernation). You may be guided, having calculated one of these ratios, whether your tortoise is of suitable weight to hibernate.

Note that tropical tortoises cannot be hibernated at all (see Chapters 3, 14, 15 and 17). Young tortoises can be hibernated for short periods of time (see Chapter 12 on hibernation). Tortoises that are unwell, or have recently been unwell, should not be hibernated. If in any doubt, seek specialist veterinary advice before hibernating your tortoise.

Health can also be monitored by weighing your tortoise every month (see Figs 6.8–6.11). This could be part of your regular health checks, and will help to identify sudden weight changes, or trends of weight loss or gain. Weight gain may indicate egg production in females. Gradual weight loss may be an early indicator of a number of health issues, or of disease (McArthur *et al.*, 2004; McArthur, 2012; Chitty and Raftery, 2013).

Regular weighing is also effective when checking growth rate in hatchlings and juveniles. Young tortoises should grow steadily and not too quickly. Very rapid growth is one of the causes of distorted growth, lumpy pyramided shells and leg deformities. These are often seen in cases of metabolic bone disease (see Chapter 7 on common illnesses and diseases).

In adults, weight should remain fairly constant over time. In a 2–3 kg tortoise, for example, weight changes of 200 g over a month would not be considered abnormal. Weight can show a pattern of fluctuation over the months. A tortoise of that size can lose 200 g simply when passing urine, or the tortoise can drink a similar weight of water whilst submerged in a bath.

3. Feeding

All healthy tortoises will overeat given the chance, particularly hatchlings. Tortoises that are not eating are generally not well, unless they are preparing for hibernation (see Chapter 12 on hibernation). Tortoises should take a range of food items offered, rather than being picky and selecting only a few favoured foods. Herbivorous tortoises should be foraging and browsing for available food plants in their enclosures.

If additional food is given, the tortoise should feed readily with a good appetite. The same is true of omnivorous tortoises when given plant and animal protein. Any reduction in appetite, or complete failure to feed, is an indication of the tortoise being extremely unwell.

4. Drinking

Healthy adult tortoises in the wild, eating a natural diet, can only drink when water is available (Fig. 6.12). They will seek out water in the environment, taking plants early in the morning when there is dew on the leaves. They will also take droplets of water from each other's shells and from stones where dew forms. In captivity they should have freely accessible water available to them at all times (see Chapter 3 on the captive environment). This is a simple but essential husbandry requirement to ensure that no additional stress or disease is caused by lack of available water in captivity.

Offering a bath once a week, in addition to the freely available water, gives the keeper the opportunity to observe the tortoise drinking and any waste products being passed. The tortoise will dip its head into the water and hold it under the surface as it draws in water, which can be seen as pulse-like movements along the neck.

Hatchlings and juveniles need access to water, and a suitably humid environment to allow normal growth. Sick or recuperating tortoises need greater access to warm water, as hydration is most important in staying healthy and well. They should be bathed daily. Bathing before and after hibernation is also essential (see Chapter 12 on hibernation) to allow full hydration and a full bladder before, and rehydration after, the hibernation.

Bathing involves the tortoise sitting in a shallow bath of tepid/lukewarm water in order to drink. The water should be around 30–35°C. Offering water in a small bowl is not usually helpful to the tortoise, which must be able to sit in the water in order to take in water. Water may also be absorbed through the cloaca into the bladder.

Bathing is not primarily for washing or cleaning purposes, but any mud, dirt or faeces can be removed for good hygiene once the tortoise has had a drink (Fig. 6.13). A soft brush can be used to gently clean off any dirt or faeces on the shell or legs, or trapped around the tail. This should be done after the tortoise has had a drink. This is another opportunity to check for damage or abnormalities as described below.

5. Urates

These are the toxic wastes produced by the kidneys from protein metabolism (as with our urine). Uric acid is the main waste product formed, but it is virtually insoluble. It is therefore converted to more soluble salts called urates (Figs 6.14 and 6.15). These nitrogen-containing wastes must be removed from the body before they build up and become toxic. In herbivorous terrestrial tortoises the urates, when passed, should be white and milky. Any change in these wastes should be acted upon. If the urates become solid or gritty, dehydration may be the cause. Bathe the tortoise more often and ensure that fresh water is readily available. If the urates become yellow, or even green, there may be infection. Failure to produce any urates may also be an indicator of significant disease of the bladder or kidneys, or a more general systemic bodily problem. In all these cases veterinary advice should be sought.

6. Faeces

These should be very dark green/black, fibrous, solid but soft. Faeces are often produced in the bath, (or in the car during a journey). In herbivores, the faeces should not smell unpleasant. They should not be runny, nor be pale or red in colour. Runniness might indicate diarrhoea or poor digestion of food. If the food is undigested having passed through the gut, the individual food items will still be identifiable – flower parts, stems

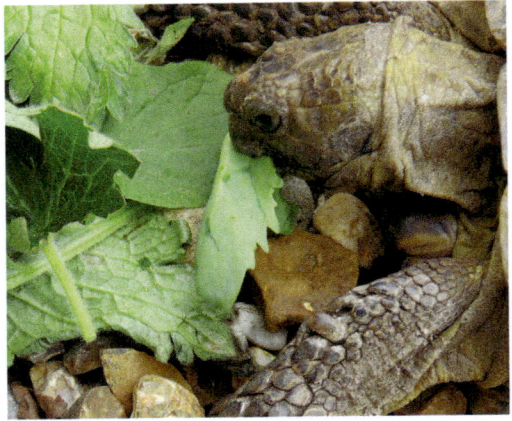

Fig. 6.11. Herbivorous Horsfield's tortoise (*Testudo horsfieldi*) feeding with good appetite on a variety of weeds.

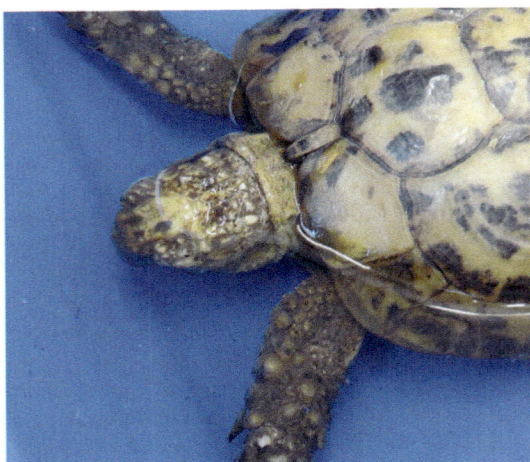

Fig. 6.12. Tortoise drinking with head submerged in bath.

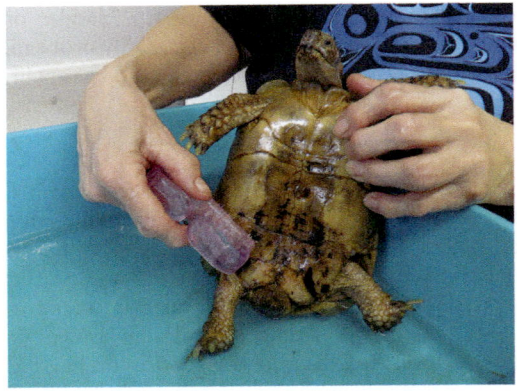

Fig. 6.13. Tortoise being cleaned with a soft brush.

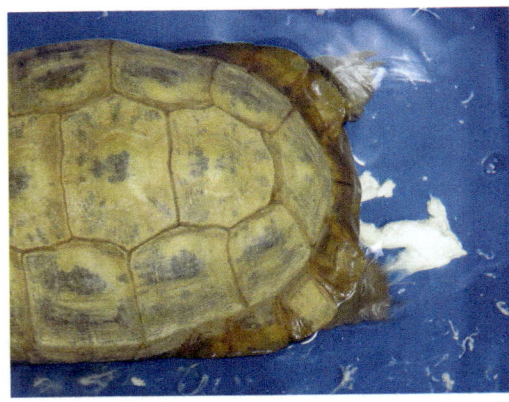

Fig. 6.14. Tortoise producing normal urates, which are white, soft and creamy in consistency.

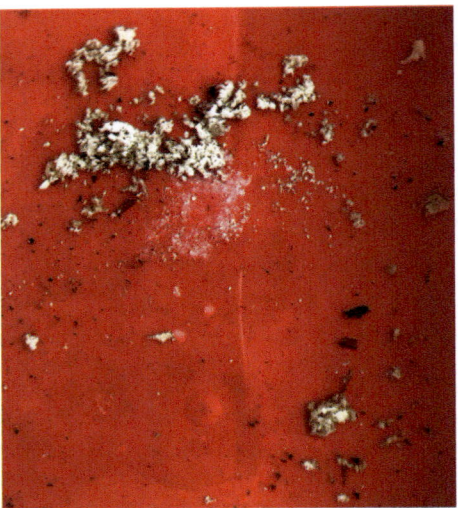

Fig. 6.15. Tortoise producing gritty wastes, which are darker, sometimes yellow, with hard crystals or granules.

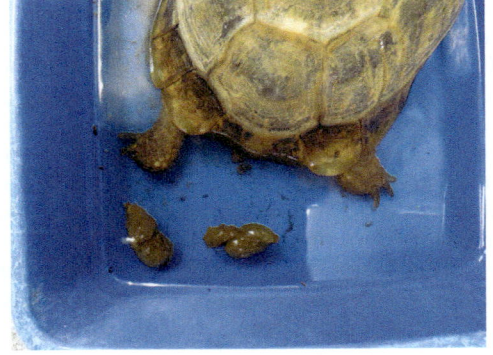

Fig. 6.16. Tortoise producing normal faeces.

and leaves. This sort of loose, or smelly, form of faeces should be seen as a sign of potential disease and may require veterinary treatment (see Chapter 7 on common illnesses and diseases). Tortoises that have been fed on unsuitable food items will often have faeces that smell unpleasant. The smell is because the tortoise has been unable to properly digest some of the foods eaten. Usually this will be a strong smell, sometimes acidic and rancid. Again, if this persists veterinary advice should be sought.

Tortoises can be infected with *Salmonella*, *Campylobacter* and *E. coli* (see Chapter 7 on common illnesses and diseases), any of which can cause runny faeces. These pathogens are potentially a risk to humans.

A high level of worm eggs may cause the faeces to become runny, and the worms themselves may be seen if there is a high infestation. The faeces should be tested for the species of worm present and the number of eggs (worm count) by sending to a laboratory (e.g. reptile parasite and worm count testing by Wormcount Vet Lab).

Some years ago, a veterinary student conducted a study with my Mediterranean tortoises and, from faeces samples, found two types of nematode worm eggs: ascarids (roundworms) and oxyurids (pinworms). None of the tortoises showed symptoms of infestation. Following treatment with two doses of oxfendazole, interestingly 80% of the male tortoises with a worm burden responded to the treatment, whereas only 37% of the females were cleared of eggs. This would be an interesting further study to identify any relevant differential factors between the genders, such as: eating patterns; volume of food eaten (as females are larger); whether the doses of treatment were less accurate in smaller animals; or some physiological difference related to reproductive hormones was at play.

Treatment to reduce the egg numbers should be carried out. Drugs such as oxfendazole (products: Parafend® and Panacur®) can be tubed into the tortoise's gut to reduce worm and egg numbers. This should be done with a soft silicone tube passed into the tortoise's stomach to minimize potential damage to the delicate membranes lining the gut. Consult your veterinary professional for advice (see Chapter 7 on common illnesses and diseases).

7. Mouth and beak

Mouths and beaks should be checked monthly for any signs of redness or infection. Check that the mouth and tongue colour is a healthy pink. Any redness may be a sign of infection and veterinary advice should be sought.

Stomatitis, or mouth rot, can be seen as cheesy yellow or white patches in the mouth. There may be red spots on the tongue. This is a serious condition caused by infection or damage and should be treated by a veterinarian immediately. It is common after hibernation in tortoises that were not well before or during hibernation. It is often a sign of a poor functioning immune system.

It is important to become familiar with the normal appearance of your tortoise's mouth by regular examination (Figs 6.18–6.20). This involves opening the mouth and looking inside. To do this, support the tortoise on a firm surface such as a worktop or table with a towel for the tortoise to gain some purchase with the nails and feet. The tortoise may be reluctant to allow you to hold its head – unsurprisingly, as this is an unusual thing to happen and would normally mean the tortoise is being attacked by a predator.

Place the tortoise flat onto the towel you have prepared and allow the tortoise to rest there. Putting an object such as a book or small cardboard box about 5 cm high under the front legs, so that the front of the body is elevated, will encourage the tortoise to put the front legs and head out. Once the head is out you can quickly hold it between thumb and first finger. Tortoises are very strong and will resist this, which is stressful for them. Hold the head with one hand and gently open the mouth with the forefinger of your other hand. Once you have looked inside, release the head and allow the tortoise to return to the enclosure. Once a month for the sake of good health is reasonable, but this sort of handling should be kept to a minimum as it is stressful for tortoises. Try to ensure that the back legs remain on the surface, as this reduces stress (Williams, 2017; Williams and Beck, 2021).

There will be a variation in colour depending upon the species and the corresponding external skin colour. Some tortoises have very yellow skin and scales, for example, and so the inside of their mouths may also be yellowish. You should be aware of this and know what is normal for your tortoise. Only if you know what is normal will you know if there has been change. For example, some foods (e.g. dandelions) can stain the tongue and mouth a dark brown colour, which may look like a disease. You need to be aware of these effects.

The beak can become overgrown easily, if the diet is too rich in protein and not enough opportu-

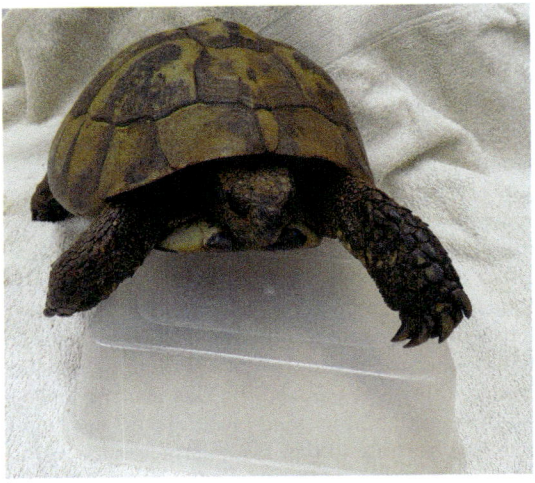

Fig. 6.17. Tortoise with front raised on a small box to encourage the head to be extended.

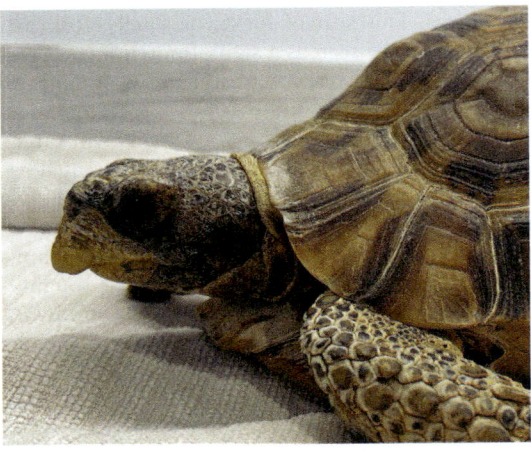

Fig. 6.19. Overgrown beak.

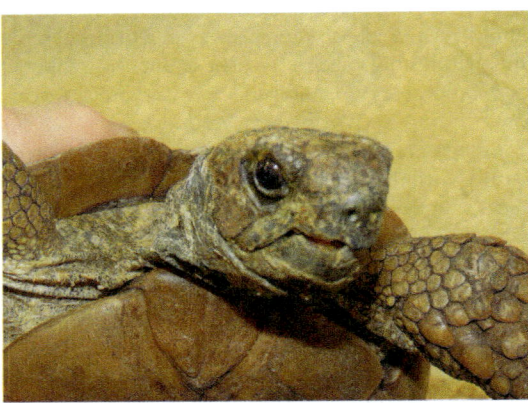

Fig. 6.20. Deformed beak – this has occurred due a very old injury, which now needs managing with regular trimming so that the tortoise can eat.

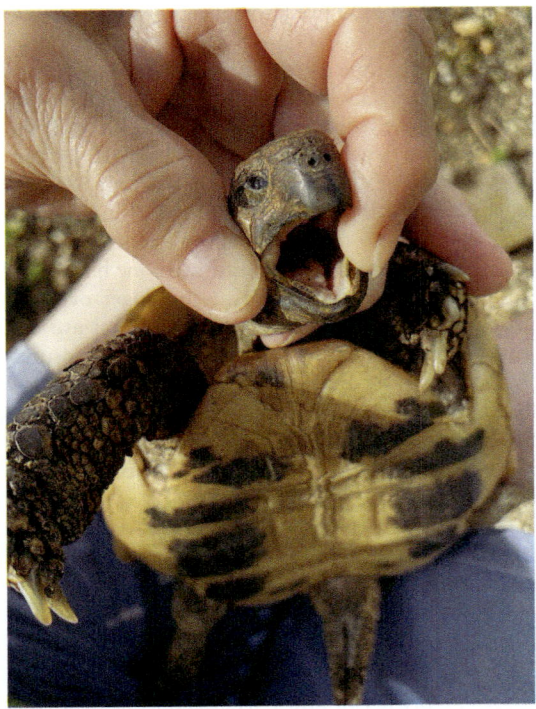

Fig. 6.18. Tortoise's mouth being opened and examined, with back legs on surface.

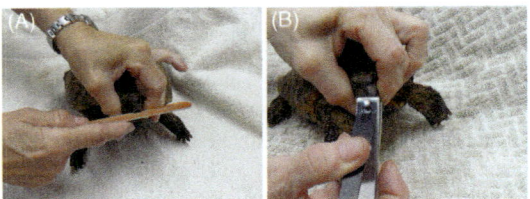

Fig. 6.21. Beak trimming using (A) an emery board and (B) nail clippers. The emery board may take a little longer but there is less possibility of damaging the tortoise. The nail clippers shown have a narrow opening, which restricts the possibility of cutting too much away.

nities are provided for wearing down on hard stems and rough fibrous plant material. The overgrowth can easily be trimmed using clippers. It is important

to try to prevent this excess growth with improved diet, but where this does happen, trimming of the upper beak to a straight line is needed to ensure that the tortoise can eat properly. This can also be done with a small sanding device such as a Dremel or an emery board/nail file.

If in any doubt about your ability to carry out these health checks and maintenance, seek veterinary advice – this is always preferable to causing the tortoise (or yourself) any damage.

8. Nose/eyes/ears

The appearance of the face and the sense organs should be checked regularly for any damage (Figs 6.22 and 6.23). Tortoises can damage their faces while feeding, or through trauma from objects in the environment, despite the tough scales in place for protection. Infection within the head may also manifest itself through changes in the scales of the head (see also section 9). Changes in the scales of the head may indicate disease (Fig. 6.24) (see Chapter 7 on common illnesses and diseases).

The nares, or nasal openings, should be open and clear. Sometimes a tortoise will have a slight difference in shape between the two openings, or one may be larger than the other. You will be aware of this from regular observations of your tortoise. It is also possible for food items to get stuck in the openings and passages. Pieces of grass or seeds are not uncommon and can usually be removed with a cotton bud or similar soft item. Any discharge from the nares is cause for concern, as it may indicate infection. Any tortoise with such a discharge should be referred to a vet (see Chapter 7 on common illnesses and disease) as runny nose syndrome, or rhinitis, also called testudine intranuclear coccidiosis (TINC), is common in some species (McArthur et al., 2004; McArthur, 2012).

The eyes should be clear, bright and open. As tortoise age their eyes may become opaque as, like most animals, they can develop cataracts. Cloudiness may also be caused by the deposition of cholesterol. Any swelling of the eyelids can indicate a disease such as vitamin A deficiency, or more general problems. Any tortoise when feeling unwell may close its eyes, as it will feel too unwell to open them. There may be a localized problem with the eye or eyes, or an underlying problem, perhaps related to poor immune function (see Chapter 7 on common illnesses and disease). Eyes that are closed for much of the time indicate significant illness and should be referred for veterinary advice as a matter of urgency.

Ears can be a site of abscesses, which may remain undetected for years. The ear is a large, slightly concave scale, behind the eye, with no external ear structure. The scale or membrane is a common site for infections leading to swelling or bleeding. These infections require veterinary treatment for the removal of abscesses or infection (see Chapter 7 on common illnesses and diseases).

9. Lumps/bumps/swellings

In addition to checking the face, the rest of the body should be checked for any hard lumps (Figs 6.25 and 6.26). These are often signs of abscesses and infection. Unlike in humans, the infected material, or pus, inside is solid and cheesy and it cannot normally be dispersed with antibiotics or other drugs. Abscesses are usually surgically removed and therefore veterinary treatment is required (see Chapter 7 on common illnesses and diseases). There may be swellings or lumps on an individual limb, which may indicate a localized infection, or there may be more generalized swelling in both hind limbs, or even in all four limbs. Such swelling may be due to fluid build-up (oedema). Oedema may indicate more generalized problems and be due to poor liver or kidney function, or indeed to any number of health issues, such as poor circulation or problems with the reproductive system. Veterinary advice should be sought. Swelling may also be due to infection or gout, both of which require veterinary treatment (see Chapter 7 on common illnesses and diseases).

10. Skin/nails/shell damage

Any skin injuries or wounds should be referred to a vet. Keep the site of wounds clean with disinfectant products such as Tamodine Wound (Vetark®). This has anti-fungal and antibacterial properties. F10® products can also be used as a disinfectant, both within the environment and for skin conditions, as can Hibiscrub® (Molnlycke). Small wounds can be treated with first aid and good hygiene for cleanliness. If they persist, spread or become worse, veterinary advice should be sought.

Shell damage can also be treated with iodine products, although if severe, bleeding, or wet, it should be referred to a vet for treatment such as antibiotics, as there may be underlying infection.

Nails can become overgrown in the same way that we can see in beaks (Figs 6.29 and 6.30). If the substrate in the enclosure is varied and contains soil, rocks and stones, normal walking should wear the nails to a suitable length. However, diet or the environment can prevent this normal wear from happening

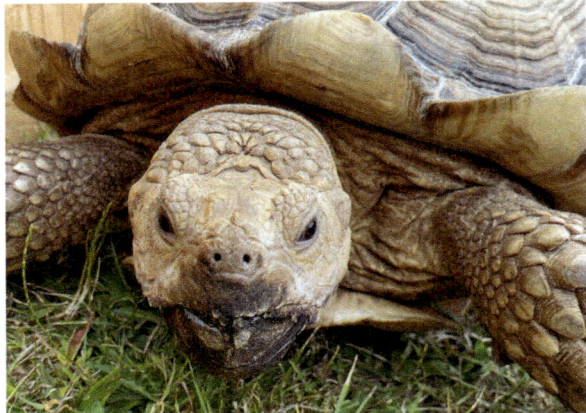

Fig. 6.22. Tortoise face showing normal nares (or nostrils) and eyes.

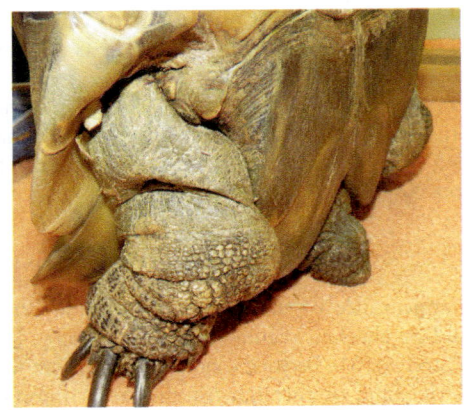

Fig. 6.25. Leg swellings due to fluid retention or infection.

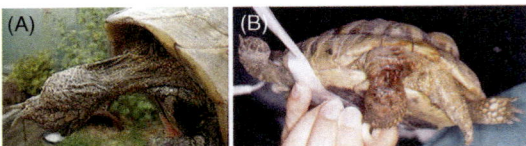

Fig. 6.26. (A) Leg abscess (Eleanor Lien-Hua Tirtasana Chubb). (B) Leg abscess being removed (William Lewis).

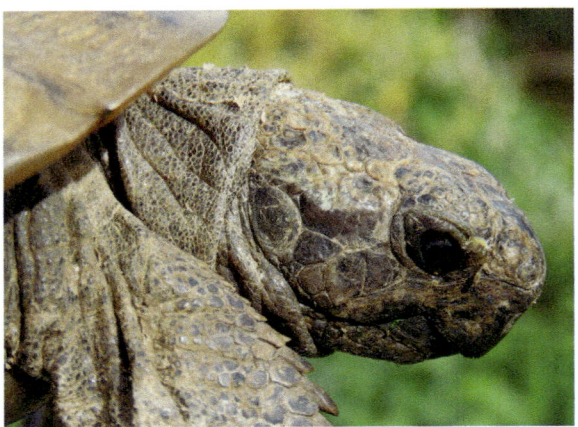

Fig. 6.23. Tortoise face showing normal eye and ear.

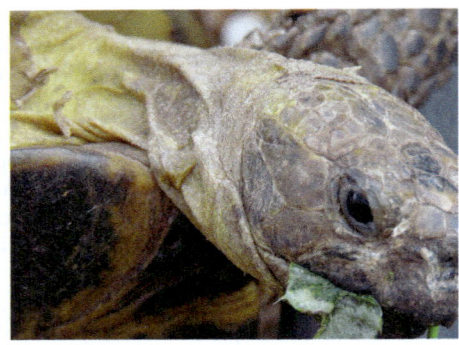

Fig. 6.27. Skin problems such as excess sloughing may indicate underlying health issues.

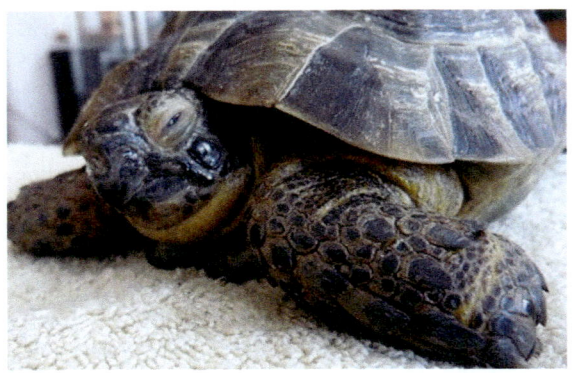

Fig. 6.24. Abnormal eye largely closed (Eleanor Lien-Hua Tirtasana Chubb).

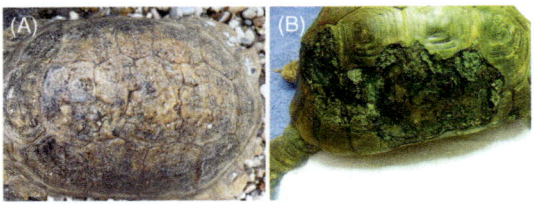

Fig. 6.28. (A) Shell damage due to fire. (B) Shell damage in females due to excess ramming or butting by males (Eleanor Lien-Hua Tirtasana Chubb).

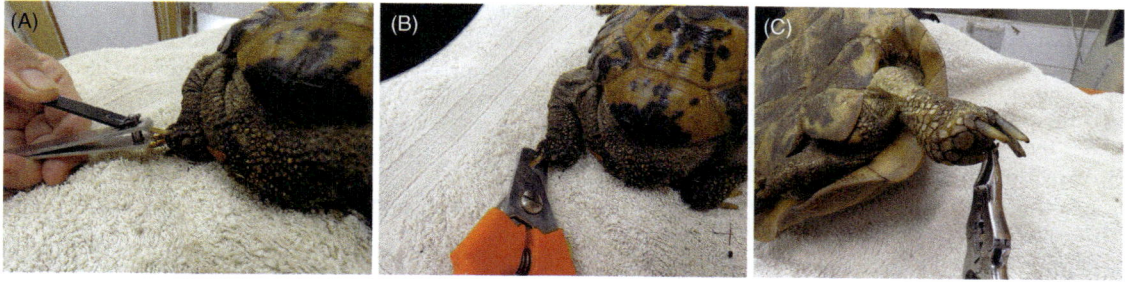

Fig. 6.29. (A) Nails being trimmed with small narrow nail clippers. (B) The clippers are sprung for strong nails. (C) The clippers have narrow pointed ends to fit between small gaps in nails but care should be taken with the pointed ends. If in any doubt, seek veterinary advice on nail clipping.

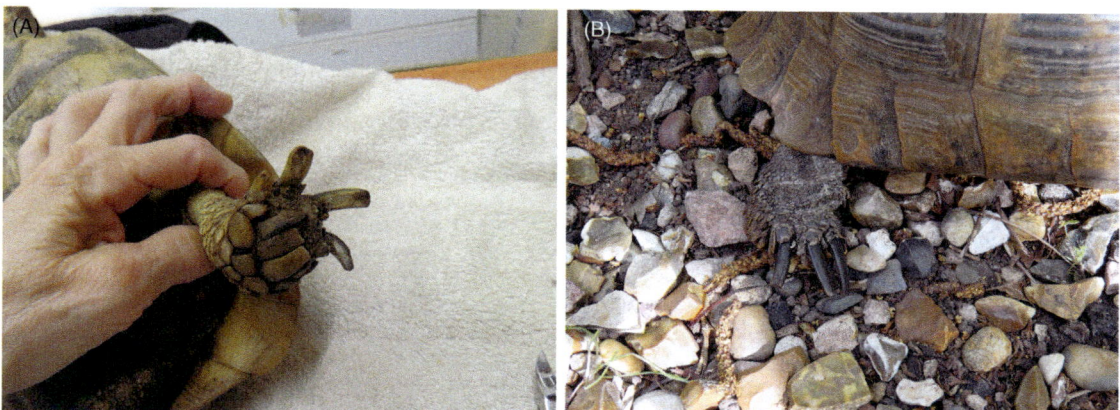

Fig. 6.30. (A) Pale nails and (B) dark nails. The latter are much more difficult to trim without damage to the living part of the nail, as the blood supply cannot easily be seen.

and nails can become long. They can also grow into the skin of the foot if left for a long period. The tortoise should be placed flat onto a work surface or table on a towel you have prepared. Examine one foot and leg at a time allowing the tortoise to keep the other limbs in contact with the surface. In the same way that the tortoise will withdraw their head for protection, limbs will also be withdrawn. Again, the tortoise will resist you holding a limb and may be very strong when trying to pull it into the shell space. Try to keep these handling and checking activities to a monthly event, to reduce stress but maintain a good handle on the health and well-being of your tortoise.

Note that if the nail is cut too short and the blood supply is damaged, the nail will bleed. This is painful and to be avoided. Pale-coloured nails show where this blood supply is as the 'quick' but with dark nails this is hard to see (Fig. 6.30).

How do I make best use of my health checks?

During your daily and weekly health checks, and your thorough monthly check and measure/weigh-in, you will get to know your tortoise better. Physical handling to ensure that there are no significant changes can be carried out with the minimum of stress. Regular checks and observations will allow you to become familiar with your tortoise's behaviour (Warwick *et al.*, 2013). This will allow you to spot any changes quickly, so that you can act to rectify the situation, seeking veterinary advice when needed. Keep a record of what you observe using a simple recording form.

If you are attempting to breed from your tortoise(s) this will be particularly important, as you will see if females are likely to be carrying eggs and will be able to observe courtship and mating behaviours (see Chapter 11 on breeding).

When carrying out your Top 10 health checks, ask yourself these questions:

- In general, is the tortoise bright and alert?
- Is the tortoise behaving normally?
- Are the eyes clear, dark and bright?
- Are the nares (nostrils) clean and dry?
- Are the nails or beak overgrown? If they are overgrown, then ask the vet to show you how to trim them, so that you can do this regularly if needed. Ensure that there are stones and rocks available in the tortoise's enclosure to help stop them overgrowing in future.
- Is the shell clean and free from damage?
- Is the tail area clean and free from faecal matter?
- Is the tortoise eating normally?
- Is the tortoise passing faeces regularly and, if so, is the poo solid like a little log and very fibrous (if soft or runny, then diet may need reviewing; or there may be a worm problem)?
- Has the tortoise received an annual check of faeces for worm eggs? Samples can be taken and sent to laboratories for a worm count which will identify if worm eggs are present and which species. If the results show high worm egg counts, treatment should be carried out with an antihelminth drug such as oxfendazole. Consult your veterinary practitioner for advice.
- Is the tortoise passing urine regularly and is it clear? If there are urates, they should be runny like egg whites, soft and milky.

Conclusion

This short list of regular health checks can be vital in maintaining good health and welfare. Spotting changes early is the key to keeping your tortoise healthy. Observing, checking and measuring, when combined together, can provide an early-warning system of developing health problems.

This time is very well spent for you and your tortoise. The sooner you spot any problems, the sooner you can get help and advice and the sooner they can be rectified. This saves on veterinary bills, which is good for you and good for the tortoise. The longer a condition goes unnoticed and undetected, the more likely it is that the solutions will take longer and cost more. The quicker any changes are acted upon, the healthier the tortoise will remain.

Tortoises have very specific requirements to remain healthy in captivity, as this book sets out. The suitability of some species as pets is questionable given these requirements. While in our care we have to do our best to maintain the tortoises in optimum condition. These simple health checks are a very good way of doing this.

References and Further Reading

Chitty, J. and Raftery, A. (2013) *Essentials of Tortoise Medicine and Surgery*. Wiley Blackwell, Chichester, UK.

Deane, K. and Valentine, A. (2022) Ch 2 Assessment and recording methods tool kit. In: Rendle, M. and Hinde-Megarity, J. (eds) *BSAVA Manual of Practical Veterinary Welfare*. BSAVA, Quedgeley, UK, pp. 18–70.

Ebenhack, A. (2012) *Health Care and Rehabilitation of Turtles and Tortoises*. Turtle and Tortoise Preservation group. Living Art Publishing.

Jackson, O.F. (1980) Weight and Measurement data in tortoises and their relationship to health. *Journal of Small Animal Practice* 20, 269

McArthur, S. (2012) Chelonian Medicine: Improving Standards for Captive Chelonia in the UK. In: *Proceedings of Tortoise Welfare UK Conference* 17 November 2012

McArthur, S., Wilkinson, R. and Meyer, J. (2004) *Medicine and Surgery of Tortoises and Turtles*. Blackwell, Oxford, UK.

Mader, D.R. and Stoutenberg, G. (1998) Assessing the body weight of the Californian Desert tortoise (*Gopherus agassizii*) using morphometric analysis. In: *Proceedings of the Association of Reptilian and Amphibian Veterinarians Annual Conference* pp. 103–104

McBride, A. and Hinde-Megarity, J. (2022) Ch 3 Animal behaviour. In: Rendle, M. and Hinde-Megarity, J. (eds) *BSAVA Manual of Practical Veterinary Welfare*. BSAVA, Quedgeley, UK, pp. 71–103.

Raftery, A. (2019) Ch. 6 Clinical examination. In: Girling, S.J. and Raiti, P. (eds) *BSAVA Manual of Reptiles*, 3rd edn. BSAVA, Quedgeley, UK, pp. 89–100.

Rendle, M. (2019) Ch. 4 Nutrition. In: Girling, S.J. and Raiti, P. (eds) *BSAVA Manual of Reptiles*, 3rd edn. BSAVA, Quedgeley, UK, pp. 49–69.

Scheelings, T.F. (2019) Ch. 1 Anatomy and physiology. In: Girling, S.J. and Raiti, P. (eds) *BSAVA Manual of Reptiles*, 3rd edn. BSAVA, Quedgeley, UK, pp. 1–25.

Varga, M. (2019) Ch. 3 Captive maintenance. In: Girling, S.J. and Raiti, P. (eds) *BSAVA Manual of Reptiles*, 3rd edn. BSAVA, Quedgeley, UK, pp. 36–48.

Warwick, C., Arena, P., Lindley, S., Jessop, M. and Steedman, C. (2013) Assessing reptile welfare using behavioural criteria. *In Practice* 35, 123–131.

Williams, J. (2017) Stress in Chelonia (tortoises, terrapins and turtles). *The Veterinary Nurse* 8(5).

Williams, J. and Beck, D. (2021) Stress, anxiety, fear and frustration in different reptile species: How to reduce these negative emotional states during veterinary procedures. *Veterinary Nursing Journal* 36(7), 213–216.

7 Common Illnesses and Diseases in Tortoises

Abstract

This chapter describes some of the more common conditions seen in pet tortoises. It highlights signs and symptoms that should be looked out for, when carrying out regular checks on the health of captive tortoises. Disease due to inadequate husbandry is discussed along with infectious disease. Measures to reduce disease transmission where several tortoises are kept in one household are identified. First aid for tortoises is addressed, so too is the prevention of disease (see also Chapter 6 on health checks). Support and recuperation of tortoises following veterinary treatment is also described.

The value of keeping accurate records of health, observations and physical measurements is described. This information can then be provided to any veterinary practitioner whose advice you may seek in the case of an unwell tortoise. Wherever possible you should consult a veterinarian who has experience and training in exotics, in particular tortoises.

This chapter is no substitute for veterinary treatment. If you are concerned about your tortoise, you should seek advice from a qualified professional at the earliest opportunity.

What if something goes wrong?

This chapter is designed to help you recognize illness and disease more quickly, enabling you to get veterinary help for your tortoise as soon as possible. Many health problems of tortoises in captivity are caused by poor husbandry. Husbandry issues are highlighted, with suggestions for improvements that will allow you to better meet your tortoise's needs.

The more accurate your own records and observations, the more useful this information will be to any veterinary practitioner whose advice you seek (Deane and Valentine, 2022). Veterinarians who see small animals may, in some cases, also have experience and additional qualifications in exotic veterinary medicine (Ebenhack, 2012). As reptile and tortoise veterinary treatment is considered to be a specialist area of expertise, it is always advisable to seek out an experienced and qualified specialist veterinarian.

This chapter highlights signs and symptoms to look out for, as part of your regular checks on your tortoise's health. Diseases due to infection are also discussed, along with measures to reduce transmission, where several tortoises are kept in one household. First aid for tortoises is addressed, as is the prevention of disease.

How do I know something is wrong?

Chapter 6 on health checks should be read before this chapter. Chapter 6 details the simple checks that can be made to assess the health of your tortoise on a regular basis. The better the husbandry and the more the captive environment mimics the natural environment, the more likely it is that a tortoise will stay healthy and well. Tortoises will always need support in captivity. Once we remove choices in terms of access to a natural environment, inevitably we interfere with a tortoise's ability to regulate its bodily needs. This applies to tortoises kept as pets in areas that are in their natural habitat, as much as it does to those kept in colder, more northerly climes. The degree of support required might be greater in the latter case, but the principles of providing a range of environmental options, so that the tortoise can achieve homeostasis, apply equally.

Homeostasis may be defined as the self-regulation of all biological systems to maintain stability. The physiology of the body of any animal is in a dynamic equilibrium, which is impacted by many factors (as described here). To achieve homeostasis, tortoises need to be able reach their preferred body temperature. Tortoises need access to heat and sunlight (and, at times, artificial light, which mimics the sun), water, suitable humidity levels, appropriate

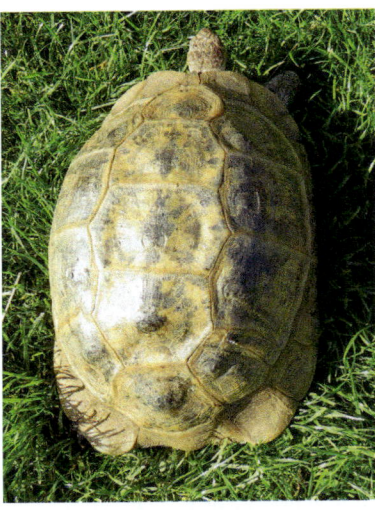

Fig. 7.1. Tilly, one example of a 'survivor', is a very large female Spur-thighed tortoise (*Testudo graeca whitei*) who weighs 3800 g and measures 298 mm (12 inches) in length.

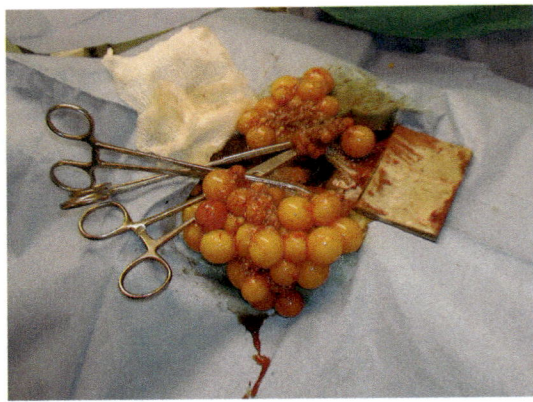

Fig. 7.2. Incomplete egg production as seen in follicular stasis, where many small eggs without shells remain in the reproductive tract and often have to be surgically removed by spaying the tortoise (William Lewis).

space and environmental enrichment together with a suitable diet for their species.

Once taken from the natural environment, or having been born into a captive environment, all of these factors may be distorted by the facilities we provide. If we fail to provide what is required, there will be a negative impact on the tortoise's metabolism and health.

Healthy tortoises can cope with less-than-optimal conditions, as described below. However, a tortoise that is weakened by disease, or is recovering from trauma or illness, needs to be kept under optimum environmental conditions to give the best possible opportunity for recovery.

This is one reason why a tortoise that is recuperating from illness or injury would never be a candidate for hibernation/brumation. The additional pressures of hibernation (which by definition takes place in less-than-optimal conditions) will significantly limit the opportunities for repair and regeneration of tissues and bodily functions.

Physiological compensation

In many cases tortoises cope remarkably well with the reduction in normal daylight hours and light intensity, low temperatures, excessively long hibernations/brumations and a poor diet, often experienced in captivity. They may do so for many years. I have seen tortoises that have been hibernated/brumated regularly for 5–6 months of the year, repeatedly for over 50 years, who are still moving around, feeding and surviving.

Figure 7.1 shows Tilly, a very large Algerian Spur-thighed tortoise, *T. graeca whitei*, whose owner had never provided any additional heat or light sources. Tilly had been a 'garden tortoise' in the UK for approximately 45 years, going to sleep for hibernation/brumation in October and, depending on the severity of the winter, not waking until March or even April. She had been fed exclusively on lettuce, cucumber and tomatoes. Having the freedom of the whole garden, however, had meant that she had also eaten weeds such as dandelions and plantains. Most of her diet was not suitable for good health and, over time, she had become unwell.

Initially Tilly had coped with her environment by becoming inactive. The low temperatures for much of the year prevented her normal levels of movement and feeding. She showed what we might describe as physiological compensation, whereby her body adapted to poor diet and low temperatures (Matthew Rendle, personal communication). Her reproductive system did not function as it should have, leading to a condition called follicular stasis or pre-ovulatory ova stasis (McArthur *et al.*, 2004; Chitty and Raftery, 2013). This means that her body tried to produce eggs as normal, but the captive environment, including the lack of a male to stimulate egg production, prevented complete egg formation. The retained eggs (or follicles) sat in the body cavity, taking up space, potentially impacting lung capacity, interfering with liver function and eventually causing infection. Figure 7.2 shows part of the surgical procedure to remove retained eggs. A large number and the yellow yolk sacs can be seen very clearly.

Tilly was surviving, but not thriving. She was not healthy or well. This was largely unnoticed by her owner. Her body was hanging onto life in every possible way, trying to compensate for the conditions. Over the years, excessively long hibernation/brumation periods (see Chapter 12 on hibernation) weakened her, making her sluggish and slow to recover when she emerged from hibernation/brumation each year. She was not feeding as well as she had been. As this was all happening very slowly and gradually over 40 or more years, no sudden changes were observable.

She had put on weight as the follicles built up, but this was assumed to be a healthy sign rather than a worrying one. Eventually her body could no longer physiologically compensate, and she stopped eating and walking altogether, and simply sat with eyes closed. It was only at this point that her owner sought veterinary help and advice. By then the only possible solution to prolong Tilly's life and improve her health was to remove the follicles. This involves traumatic and extensive surgery, with a long recovery period, or expensive medical implants. Long-acting gonadotropin-releasing hormone (GnRH) agonists (e.g. Deslorelin) may be given as an implant such as Suprelorin®F (Virbac) to reduce the numbers of follicles being produced (Johnson, 2013; Bardi et al., 2021). In some situations, both surgery and implants may be used.

Without being kept warm and given antibiotics, Tilly would not have survived after the surgery. This is another reason that, more frequently, veterinarians are now using Suprelorin®F implants alongside an improved environment, rather than waiting until the tortoise is fit enough for surgery. This approach is being used with good success using long-acting GnRH agonists.

Reluctantly Tilly's owner had to give her up, as he was unable to provide the specialist care she needed. Tilly is now in a sanctuary where her needs are better met.

This is a very sad but all too common scenario that I have encountered many times over the past 30 years. Tilly's owner became very distressed when he realized that he had not provided Tilly with adequate care. This was not intentional – he was following advice that may have been current 40 years ago. He had failed to appreciate that, as we have learnt more about the conditions under which these animals should be kept, the advice has changed considerably. It was difficult for him to give up a much-valued companion to whom he was very attached. Tilly was associated with his late wife; their children had grown up with her in the garden and now his grandchildren were also very fond of her. The high levels of attachment people feel towards their tortoise because it 'has always been there' may be surprising, but these emotions are clearly strongly felt by many tortoise keepers. My unpublished MSc research data (Southampton, 2011) identified a high level of attachment by owners, similar to that seen in dog owners. In part this is due to the longevity of the tortoise, and the idea that it had 'always been there and always will be'.

Illness and disease

The types of illness and disease seen in tortoises depends on many factors, as shown in Table 7.1.

Table 7.1. Factors causing different types of illnesses and diseases in tortoises.

Factor	Comments
Species of tortoise	Some species are more susceptible to certain types of disease and particular disease-causing organisms
Age of tortoise	Young tortoises can tolerate less environmental disruption. Their much smaller body size and mass makes them more susceptible to external effects such as dehydration, while degenerative diseases are a natural part of the ageing process and so more likely to be seen in aged animals
Gender of tortoise	Male and female tortoises can become ill because of: the nature of their reproductive biology; whether they live alone; the proximity of other tortoises; the amount of available space; and opportunities for normal reproductive behaviour
History of the tortoise	How long the tortoise has been in captivity; whether wild-caught or captive-bred; whether recently subjected to transportation either within the country or from overseas; whether the tortoise has been in contact with other tortoises
Husbandry provided	Health may be affected by: the suitability of diet; temperatures available during the daily cycle; lighting sources; humidity levels; conditions provided and duration of hibernation; hygiene quality of enclosures; and whether the tortoise has been kept as a solitary animal or in a group

The types of illnesses and diseases commonly seen in tortoise are described below under the following categories:

1. Endoparasites causing disease
   (A) Microparasites – viruses, bacteria, protozoa
   (B) Macroparasites – worms
2. Ectoparasites causing disease – ticks, fleas, fungi
3. Shell and skin disease
4. Diet-related disease
5. Liver disease
6. Kidney and urinary disease
7. Diseases due to hibernation duration
8. Injury and damage by predators, other tortoises, or the environment
9. Drowning
10. Tumours
11. Eye diseases
12. Reproductive diseases
13. Prolapses

Appendix 2 shows an example record for observations to monitor tortoise health, weight, length, signs, symptoms, treatments, preventative therapy.

1. Endoparasites causing disease

(A) Microparasites – viruses, bacteria, protozoa

Diseases caught from other tortoises caused by microparasites

Tortoises can be infected by a number of organisms which cause disease (pathogens). Some of these are newly emerging, having been identified only relatively recently (Kolesnik *et al.*, 2017). Some are transmissible to humans, as described in Chapter 19 on health and safety.

Testing for pathogens is now more readily available than in the past. Tests for *Mycoplasma* (Jacobson *et al.*, 2014) bacteria and herpes viruses can be carried out by taking a swab from the mouth and nasal passages, for example. These can then be posted to laboratories for identification of organisms.

These infections are mainly caused by parasitic viruses and bacteria. They are all obligate parasites which complete their life cycles within the host's cells. There are also single-celled organisms (protozoa) that reproduce using spores, which can cause disease. One example of these is coccidia, which cause a range of diseases affecting respiratory, digestive and many other body systems.

Upper respiratory tract disease (URTD)/ runny nose syndrome (RNS) or rhinitis

The bacterial mycoplasma infections (*Mycoplasma agassizii*) linked to upper respiratory tract disease (URTD), or runny nose syndrome (RNS), as it is also known, infect the nasal passages and cause a cold-like discharge, or runny nose. This infectious disease is very easily passed from one tortoise to another. Spur-thighed tortoises, in particular, are susceptible to this disease. There is a danger of spreading disease when mixing tortoise species for this reason. Some species are more resilient and can act as a reservoir or source of infection to other species. For example, the more delicate North African subspecies of *Testudo graeca*, such as *T. g. graeca* and *T. g. nabeulensis*, can contract URTD from the Turkish subspecies, *Testudo graeca Ibera*, very easily.

This discharge is seen as a clear fluid initially, coming from one or both nares (nostrils) due to irritation of the nasal passages, in the same way that we get a runny nose if we have a cold or flu virus (Fig. 7.3). This sign can sometimes be caused by a foreign body (such as a seed or piece of plant material) stuck in the nasal passage. If this is the case the discharge will be seen as coming from only one nostril. Subsequent removal of the object will cause the discharge to stop. In many cases, however, the discharge is more likely to be a sign of infection such as that caused by *Mycoplasma*.

This is a common ailment of Spur-thighed tortoises, and one that can recur. Environmental factors may impact the disease. For example, I had six *Testudo graeca graeca* show a runny nose on the same day in a particular year. This was possibly due to additional environmental conditions (such as high humidity levels), contributing to an existing underlying infection. Often the symptoms stop, and tortoises recover without treatment. Even if this is the case the tortoise will still need additional support (such as extra bathing) to ensure that it does not get dehydrated by the fluid loss.

In other cases, the discharge may become thicker, cloudy and turn yellow in colour, all of which suggest that the infection is progressing and becoming more serious. Veterinary treatment should definitely be sought at this point, if it has not been already.

The nasal discharge can be removed by 'milking' it away from the nasal passages. Upward pressure from a thumb placed under the tortoise's chin can be used to push the discharge out of the front of the nares from where it can be wiped away. This will allow the tortoise to breathe more easily, as tortoises cannot sneeze or clear their nasal passages unaided. This is, however, only a temporary and short-term first-aid measure.

Testing for the infectious organism is advisable. This will allow the specific pathogen causing the infection to be identified and so ensure that any treatment offered is the best one to deal with this pathogen. Such testing is much more readily available today and it allows treatment to be more effective as it rapidly targets the offending organism (Marschang, 2011; Marschang and Hyndman, 2023). Testing services are available through veterinary practices and also directly by posting samples to a laboratory (e.g. Laboklin, based in the UK).

Stomatitis inflammation and infection in the mouth and pharyngeal cavity

This condition is often associated with an underlying condition, or poor immune function, which allows opportunistic viruses or bacteria to infect the mouth. It is frequently seen post-hibernation/brumation in animals that have been hibernated/brumated for over-long periods (see section on hibernation below).

The tortoise's mouth may look red, ulcerated or have necrotic (dead tissue) plaques (seen as yellow deposits) on the sides or roof of the mouth, or on the tongue. All of these are painful and likely to cause the tortoise to stop feeding.

Treatment of stomatitis involves addressing any underlying conditions and providing optimal

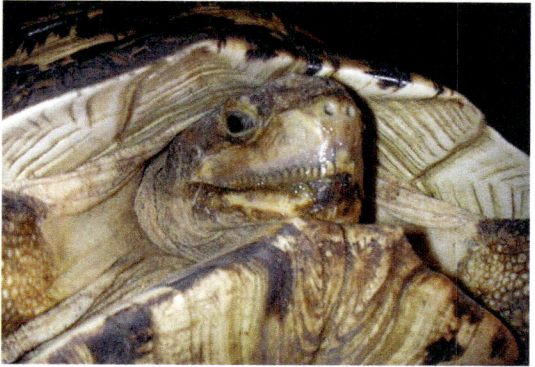

Fig. 7.3. Leopard tortoise with nasal discharge, a typical symptom of URTD. Discharge can also be seen from the mouth and eyes (Eleanor Lien-Hua Tirtasana Chubb).

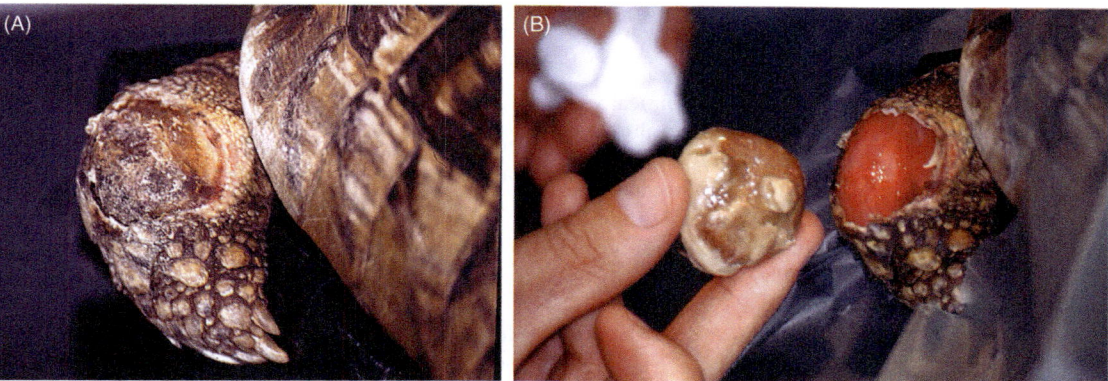

Fig. 7.4. (A) Leg with abscess estimated to have been present for 5 years. (B) Abscess removed and size of hole left behind (William Lewis).

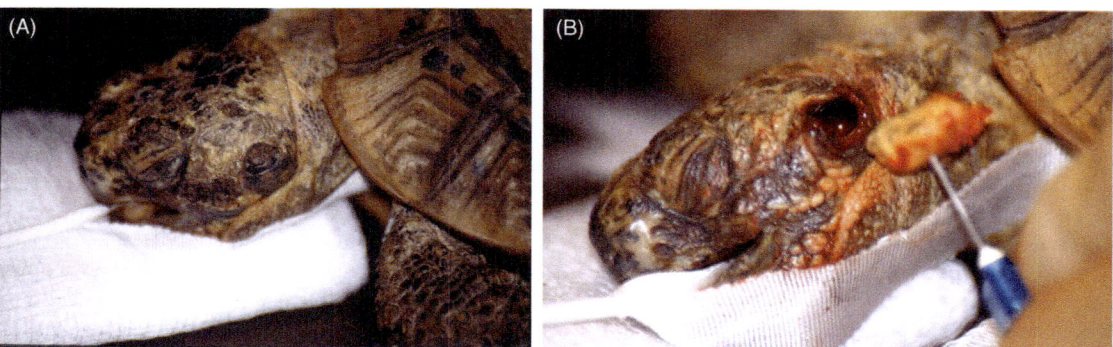

Fig. 7.5. Ear (aural) abscess. (A) Before treatment. (B) Removal showing abscess (William Lewis).

Common Illnesses and Diseases

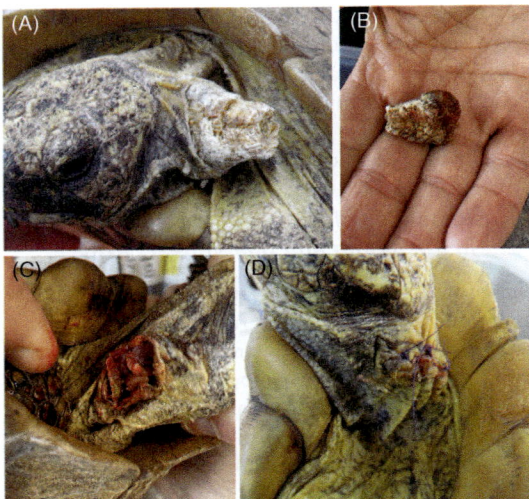

Fig. 7.6. (A) Skin abscess on the side of the neck that had been present for at least 3 years; the angles show that this was so large as to be preventing normal withdrawal of the head (Sian Bewick). (B) The abscess removed. (C) The wound left behind. (D) The wound stitched closed.

environmental conditions. Antibiotic, antiviral and antifungal treatments may be given systemically (spread through the whole body by giving orally or by injection) and treatment of the actual damaged tissues and plaques in the mouth may be needed.

Upper respiratory tract disease may cause infection in the mouth. Hypovitaminosis A may also be a cause. Infections can be caused by herpes viruses. Where the infection is caused by bacteria such as *Pseudomonas*, this is more likely to be a secondary infection with an underlying suppressed immune system.

Flagellates or ciliates

These single-celled protozoans are common in tortoises and a normal part of the gut flora and fauna. However, if their numbers increase to very high levels (usually because the tortoise is already unwell), the tortoise may show signs of gut irritation and inflammation, such as diarrhoea. Treatment may then be needed, for example with metronidazole, under veterinary supervision. A fresh faecal sample (otherwise the organisms quickly die off) can be used to identify different species of flagellate, many of which belong to the Trichomonas order. Paramecium-type organisms such as *Balantidium coli* would be one example from the ciliates.

Abscesses

Abscesses may be formed over very long periods of time in the soft tissues of the limbs, tail or head. They are not caught from other tortoises generally but are often caused by bacteria.

The abscess will be a hard mass of infected tissue and may have remained undetected for a long time, as shown in the leg abscess in Fig. 7.4A and B.

One site where abscesses are often found is the ear. Tortoises have no outer ear, but the eardrum is seen as a scale on the surface of the head. The cavity behind is quite large and can be the site of infection.

Abscesses may develop slowly over many months or years as shown in Fig. 7.4, the ear abcess in Fig. 7.5A and B. They often remain unnoticed until they are very large and protrude from the side of the head or limb. Abscess development may be associated with low levels of immunity, or chronic stress resulting from environmental conditions, or the presence of other tortoises. Stomatitis in the mouth may allow infection to ascend up the Eustachian tube into the ear.

Treatment involves surgery to remove the abscess. It is important to ensure that all the infected pus is removed. Unlike pus in humans, in tortoises the infected material is hard. Because of this it cannot easily be dispersed through the use of antibiotics (if it is due to a bacterial infection) and can only be removed by surgery, as shown in Fig. 7.6A–D. Lancing, as can be achieved for humans, cat or dogs, is not successful in reptiles.

General effects of microparasites

Herpes viruses in tortoises can be a very serious form of infection. Some herpes viruses cause only a minor illness, but other forms of herpes have recorded 100% death rates (Kolesnik *et al.*, 2017). Viral disease can infect many organs in tortoises, causing lesions, swelling, respiratory and liver damage. Herpes viruses have been associated with URTD and stomatitis (Marschang and Chitty, 2019).

Herpes viruses causing high fatality rates is a relatively newly reported phenomenon in tortoises. However, it is becoming more common in tortoises that have been in close contact with large numbers of others. Tortoises kept in high concentrations in pens used for 'farming' or 'ranching' as a method of large-scale captive breeding in their home countries, for example, are very susceptible to infectious diseases (see Chapter 20 on tortoise keeping in the past, present and future).

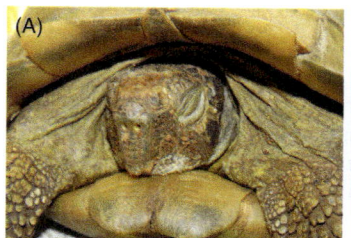 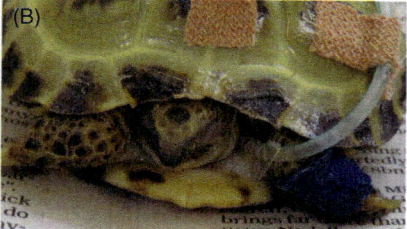 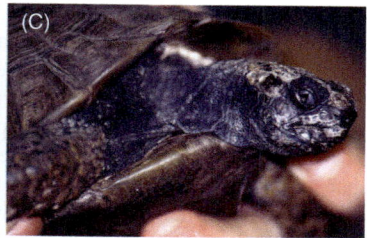

Fig. 7.7. (A–C) Very unwell tortoises, whose survival is at risk. The tortoise in (C) is very near death (William Lewis).

Horsfield's tortoises are very common in the pet trade currently, and many more of the hatchlings and juveniles being sold are becoming ill due to these infections. Where keepers have other tortoises (of whatever species), there is a high risk of the disease being passed to previously healthy animals. Herpes viruses, in all species, are a 'for life' infection which can often lie dormant in nervous tissue, but are still present. Recovered animals show intermittent infections and shedding (recurrence or recrudescence), especially when stressed, meaning that the virus may re-emerge to cause disease.

Strict quarantine must therefore be followed when introducing new tortoises. The suggested quarantine time is at least 3 months (6 months is best practice) (Highfield, 1996), with testing for *Mycoplasma* and herpes viruses before introduction. Testing does not always show up the herpes virus, which is always present in an infected animal. Even polymerase chain reaction (PCR) tests, which recognize the genetic material from pathogens, will only pick up the virus if the individual is shedding. Therefore, a negative PCR test result does not mean an animal is clear of infection, just that it is not shedding the virus at that time (Kolesnik *et al.*, 2017).

Infections of intranuclear coccidiosis (TINC) have also been reported in tortoises relatively recently (Hofmannova *et al.*, 2019). The systemic disease caused by these intracellular protozoa (single-celled organisms) was first seen in Radiated tortoises (*Astrochelys radiata*). Symptoms include lethargy, anorexia, swelling, dehydration, weakness and weight loss. These generalized symptoms are due to the presence of the TINC organisms in many of the body's organs and systems – respiratory, digestive, urinary, reproductive and endocrine systems. This results in the tortoise becoming very ill indeed, with many dying despite receiving veterinary treatment.

Many of these bacterial, viral and protozoal diseases require prompt veterinary treatment if the tortoise is to have any chance of survival.

Generalized signs

Generalized signs that may have a number of causes include:

- Lethargy – general failure to move and feed
- Tortoise subdued or depressed
- Eyes closed and/or swollen
- Anorexia – failure to feed (see below re hibernation)
- Hiding in shelter continuously
- Failure to bask to gain heat

In all these instances the tortoise will be feeling very ill; examples are shown in Fig. 7.7. Some of the specific signs, such as swollen or closed eyes, may not always be recognized as a generalized symptom. The tortoise may be diagnosed as lacking in vitamin A, for example. If the underlying cause of disease is not identified correctly, appropriate treatment cannot be given. Often there is underlying infection or very poor husbandry or hygiene practices at play. These create the circumstances that mean that the tortoise may be (just about) surviving but not thriving.

It must be noted that tortoises can also carry a number of diseases that cause no symptoms but that are transmissible to humans (see Chapter 19 on health and safety).

(B) Macroparasites – worms

Parasitic diseases transmitted from other tortoises and their waste products in the environment

These are diseases caused by much larger parasites, such as worms, ticks, mites (especially in imported species) and fleas. These are termed macroparasites as they are often big enough to be seen with the naked eye.

Worms – intestinal parasites

Most worms seen in tortoises are nematodes or roundworms. Tapeworms and trematodes (flukes) are

Common Illnesses and Diseases

not common in terrestrial tortoises, although may possibly be present in recently wild-caught tortoises.

Roundworms come from different sub-groups such as ascarids, oxyurids (also known as pinworms) or spirurids – all different groups of parasitic worms that live in tortoise intestines. These worms reproduce using eggs, which are secreted in the faeces of the tortoise. They can live in the environment for a long period of time, in the soil for example, but are also small enough to be blown around and transferred to a neighbour's garden.

Tortoises do naturally carry a small worm load, as do many wild animals. In the wild the worms are not found in high numbers, as the tortoise will defecate and then walk away. This means that the chances of tortoises getting reinfected is low, as they rarely come into contact with faeces – their own or that of other tortoises. In captivity, however, in smaller enclosures, the situation is very different. It is much more likely that the tortoise is able to ingest faeces (and therefore worm eggs) if the enclosure is small, or overcrowded, and the hygiene is poor.

There are some worm species where the eggs in fresh faeces are not infective but have to remain in the faeces for some time before they are at the infective stage. This means that old faeces are also a problem. Lack of cleaning to remove faeces, and therefore reduce the number of the eggs in the environment, represents a significant health issue (Eatwell and Hedley, 2019).

Nematodes can be debilitating if found in high concentrations. The visceral larval migration (movement of the larvae through the body) before ending up in the intestines can cause liver or respiratory disease, when large numbers of larvae are present.

They can increase in numbers if the tortoise already has poor immunity levels. They can cause gut blockages if present in very high numbers or cause severe damage to the intestine. Both can be fatal.

An example of high levels of endoparasites in captive tortoises comes from Ellerd *et al.* (2022). In the USA, 87.5% of tortoises sampled at a trade show tested positive for endoparasites. Oxyurids were found to be very prevalent across this study (14 out of 16 tortoises).

In the past, routine annual worming of tortoises was commonplace. However, the drugs used to kill these parasites have a potential toxicity to tortoises, and therefore are not used without risk. Some tortoises will have been wormed when there was no reason to do so as they had no worms or eggs present in the faeces.

A more modern approach is to test first for the presence of worms, usually via worm egg counts of faeces samples. The faeces sample has a special flotation fluid added, which allows the eggs to float to the surface, before being checked microscopically for the numbers and types of worm eggs or larvae seen. Worming treatment is only given if sufficient numbers are present in a faecal float (Eatwell and Hedley, 2019).

Anti-helminth drugs, including benzimidazoles (fenbendazole, oxfendazole) and emodepsid (Panacur® Profender®), can be given to tortoises as a worming treatment, which should be carried out under veterinary supervision. Some anti-parasitic drugs, such as ivermectin, are known to be fatal to tortoises, even though they can be safely used to treat other species. These treatments are accessible and frequently sold in pet shops.

Treatment for endoparasites, or the use of antibiotics, may well damage normal gut flora and fauna, causing the tortoise to be unable to digest food properly. This may mean restocking of the gut with useful bacteria, for example with fresh faeces from healthy animals. Probiotics that promote the growth of healthy gut flora, such as Reptoboost®, may also assist in this regard.

2. Ectoparasites causing disease – ticks, mites, biting flies and fleas

Ticks, mites, biting flies and fleas are rare in tortoises in captivity in many countries, unless the animal is recently wild-caught.

If these are present, they are generally easily seen on the skin or shell surface (Fig. 7.8). They can be removed chemically with permethrin or F10 preparations.

Flies can lay eggs in open wounds in any country, and the eggs will develop into maggots if undetected. The maggots will eventually hatch but, while developing, they may cause significant damage to soft tissues. Flushing with chlorhexidine and physical removal of maggots may be effective in treatment. All of the treatments listed here require veterinary supervision.

When maggots are internal in the body cavity, removal can be very difficult and of course would be done by a qualified veterinary practitioner.

3. Shell and skin disease

Tortoises slough their skin, as all reptiles do. This normal shedding of the skin takes place throughout the year.

Vitamin A excess or deficiency can cause inflammation and excess shedding. Any patches of redness, or

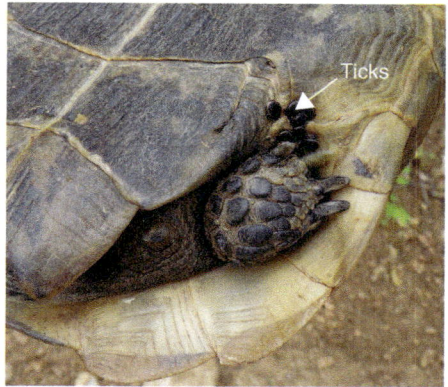

Fig. 7.8. Large number of ticks on a wild Spur-thighed tortoise (*Testudo graeca ibera*) in Thessaloniki, Greece. The animal was injured, possibly from a road traffic trauma, and looked unwell.

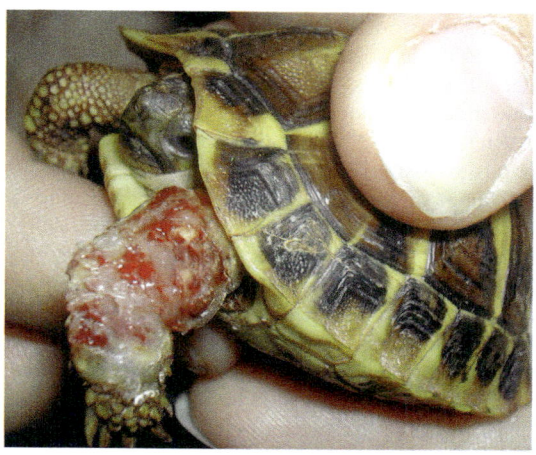

Fig. 7.9. Infected skin on the front leg of a very young tortoise, due to fungal infection (William Lewis).

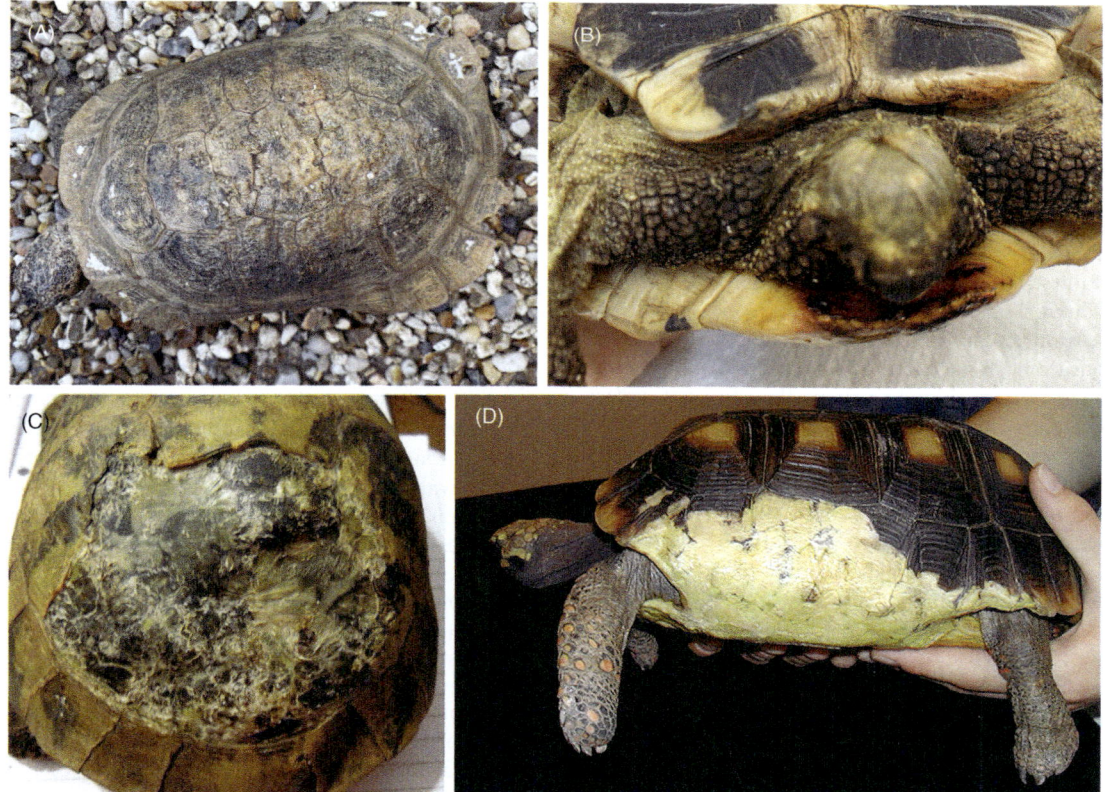

Fig. 7.10. (A) Shell damage on the carapace due to fire, now repaired, plus there are three holes previously drilled into this tortoise's shell where repeated attempts have been made to attach a string to tether the tortoise. (B) Shell damage under the tail, which is bleeding. (C) Much of the carapace is damaged due to infection (Eleanor Lien-Hua Tirtasana Chubb). (D) Shell damage repaired (William Lewis).

Common Illnesses and Diseases

obvious wear on the feet or limbs, may indicate that the tortoise has been kept on a very hard substrate that is causing excessive loss of skin. This husbandry issue should be addressed alongside any treatment.

Veterinary investigation is required if skin shedding is excessive or if there are signs of infection. If the skin or shell is physically damaged, opportunistic infections of bacteria or fungi may result (Fig. 7.9).

The shell is made of bony plates (also known as scutes and shields) covered with a very thin layer of keratin. It is therefore well supplied with blood and any significant damage to the underlying bone will lead to bruising and bleeding, which can be seen at the surface (see predation below).

Where the shell has previously been damaged, patches of dead bone may be seen as new growth occurs, which will eventually be lost as the new bone grows to replace it and will then be covered with keratin (Fig. 7.10A–D).

Where there are lesions (holes or wounds) from no obvious cause such as injury, infection from bacteria or fungi should be considered. Where the shell is damaged so that underlying tissues can be seen there is great opportunity for infection to reach the internal tissues and organs (Fig. 7.11). Veterinary advice should be sought immediately. Figure 7.12 shows stages of treatment post-spay where the shell flap became infected and was lost, leaving a very large hole which had to be treated and protected until new shell growth covered the gap. As mentioned above, flystrike leading to maggot infestation is a major hazard in these cases.

Pinkness of the plastron, where blood is close to the surface, can indicate internal infection such as septicaemia, or infection of the bone under the keratin. This may cause blood or tissue fluid to pool under the keratin shield. However, if the area turns pale again when pressed, this is less likely to be the case. Marginated tortoises, as an example, have very pale areas on their shells that allow sight of pink or red areas very easily. This may be identified as septicaemia when in fact it is due to normal blood flow near the surface when the tortoise is warm (Fig. 7.13).

Softness of the shell is not normal in terrestrial tortoises. The shell should be hard and completely solid. Growth occurs between the keratin shields or plates, and should be seen as a thin white line (Fig. 7.14).

If growth is taking place very rapidly, this line may widen and become yellow in colour; it may feel softer than the surrounding shell. This is indicative of overfeeding (see diet, below), leading to very fast growth and shell deformities (Fig. 7.15).

Where the shell is very misshapen, flattened or deformed, the likely cause is dietary (see below).

4. Diet-related disease

(See also Chapter 5 on diet).

It is very easy to overfeed tortoises or to feed them the wrong types of food. The closer we can get to their naturally available diet, the more likely it is that their dietary needs will be met. This means giving food items, on a daily basis and on a monthly and annual cycle, that are based on what is available in the natural habitat at that time.

Overfeeding

Overfeeding is a common problem in tortoises, as they are biologically adapted to seek food and eat what they find – all of it! They do not know when they will find food again. For herbivorous tortoises in the wild this means walking (often long distances) to find suitable plants that they can reach.

Walking keeps tortoises physically fit and uses up calories. This means that they can largely eat everything they can find in the wild without becoming overweight or obese. For omnivorous tortoises the same principles apply, but they may need to feed less frequently as their diet is higher in protein and fats.

The demand for calories in tortoises is low, when compared with a mammal such as a cat or dog. This is because they do not need to generate heat energy to keep warm. Because tortoises are ectotherms, they are unable to do this and must gain heat energy from the sun or other artificial external sources.

It is very easy to overfeed tortoises in captivity for three reasons:

1. They often exercise less than animals in the wild as their space is restricted, so there is less opportunity to walk any real distance.
2. Tortoise keepers often feed their tortoises daily. This means that much more food is provided than the tortoise actually needs, or would be able to find in the wild.
3. In captivity the food given is often of a higher nutritional level than 'scrub grasses' in the wild.

Tortoises in captivity are often overweight. Nutritional excesses can lead to fatty liver syndrome and obesity, particularly when the diet is high in fats. High protein levels can lead to dehydration and gout in adults and to metabolic bone disease (see young tortoises, below). High nitrate levels (linked to protein levels) can lead to hypothyroidism or iodine deficiency.

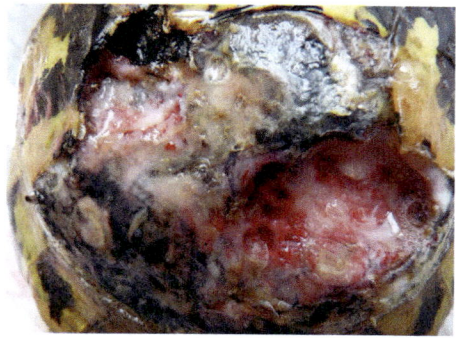

Fig. 7.11. Tortoise with extensive shell damage in which the underlying tissue can be seen as the shell has been entirely lost due to infection (Eleanor Lien-Hua Tirtasana Chubb).

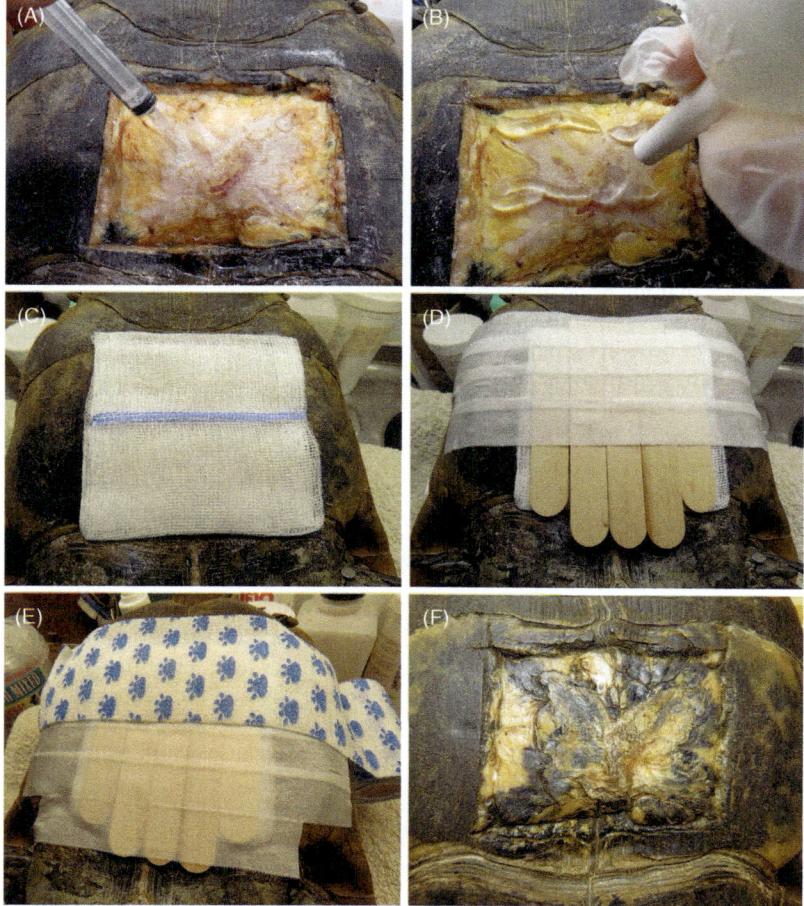

Fig. 7.12. Infection in the shell flap following a tortoise spay meant that the flap was lost and had to re-grow. This sequence shows how the internal organs of the body were protected from infection and physical damage, as the shell healed. This large section of shell completely healed over, which took around 10 months. The dressing was replaced twice weekly. (A) The area was washed with sterile saline; (B) completely covered in Intrasite gel (Smith & Nephew®); and (C) covered in sterile gauze. (D, E) Jumbo-size wooden lolly sticks were taped into position. (F) The almost healed shell.

Common Illnesses and Diseases

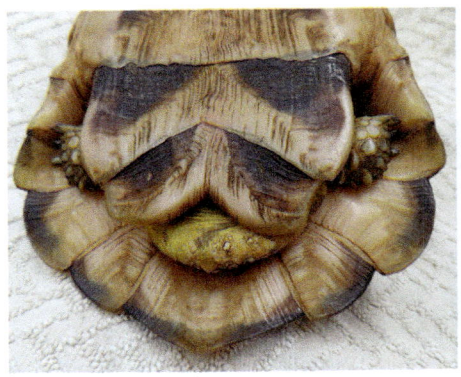 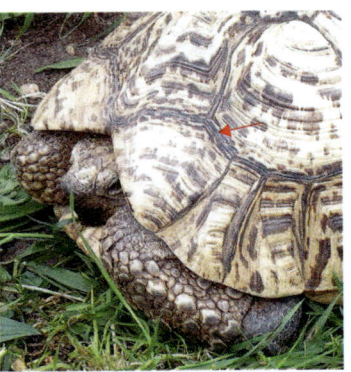 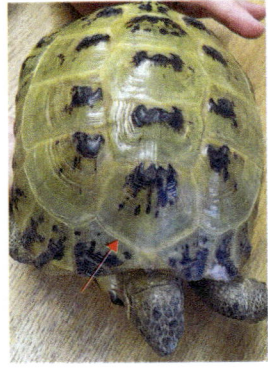

Fig. 7.13. Shell pinkness on Marginated tortoise (*Testudo marginata*).

Fig. 7.14. Normal white growth line (red arrow).

Fig. 7.15. Wide yellow growth line (red arrow) (Eleanor Lien-Hua Tirtasana Chubb).

Excess or deficiency of vitamins, minerals or other nutrients can also potentially cause disease.

Inappropriate feeding – imbalance in dietary nutrients

Diet for captive tortoises may be more limited in variety than the foodstuffs that might be found by a tortoise in the wild. It might also include inappropriate items, such as animal protein being given to herbivorous tortoises. High-protein plant material such as peas, beans or sweetcorn can also have harmful effects on herbivorous tortoises. These tortoises should be eating a high fibre and calcium diet with very low protein levels.

Tortoises can very easily become addicted to one or two food items, which will limit the dietary range even more and thus exacerbate the effects of an imbalance. I once looked after an elderly female Spur-thighed tortoise who had lived on cucumber for over 50 years, having refused all other food items offered by her owner. In reality, she had been eating weeds in the garden during the summer months, but her owner did not think that these counted as anything nutritious. In fact, these weeds were what was keeping the tortoise going, as cucumber has virtually no nutritional value and consists largely of water.

As stated, high levels of fibre and calcium are needed for both herbivorous and omnivorous tortoises alongside low protein and fat content. Herbivorous tortoises do not eat any high-protein foods. Feeding fatty sources of animal protein can be damaging for omnivorous tortoises. Nor should omnivores be given too much meat as a proportion of the diet. In omnivorous tortoises the proportion of animal protein, fruit and mushrooms should be around 5–10% of the total.

It should also be noted that there is a difference between invertebrate protein and mammal, bird or fish (vertebrate) protein in the diet. The quality and nutrient composition of invertebrates such as insects, given as part of the diet of omnivores, is less predictable than that of vertebrates, including the protein content and profile (Capitan, 2022). This could impact the likelihood of some diseases developing, such as gout, due to the variability of the diet fed to the invertebrates themselves (Martin Lawton, personal communication).

Vitamin and mineral deficiencies and excesses

It is possible for tortoises to become ill if they take in too much or too little of essential vitamins and minerals. These essential micronutrients are in equilibrium and the proportion of each, relative to the others, is also key to a balanced diet.

The ratio of calcium to phosphorus is one such example. The proportion of calcium compared with phosphorus in the diet should be higher, so that there is a ratio of at least 2:1 calcium to phosphorus in the diet (Highfield, 1996). Both calcium and phosphorus are essential in the diet as they are involved in normal bone formation, together with good muscle and nervous function. Generally, however, the higher the phosphorus levels in foods, the lower are the calcium levels. It is only wild-grown plants and weeds that have the ideal (higher) levels of calcium needed for healthy bone formation (see young tortoises, below).

In order to take up adequate calcium from the diet, vitamin D3 is also required (see Chapter 4 on artificial light and heat). The relationship between these vitamins and minerals forms the basis of many metabolic processes – an excess or deficiency in any one of them will upset the natural homeostasis of others, or interfere with the uptake of nutrients.

A balanced and varied diet can only be achieved if the foodstuffs that are available are as varied as possible. This balanced and varied diet is vital if good health is to be maintained and disease prevented.

Gout effects

I have seen elderly female tortoises unable to eat and clearly in distress from gout, which is caused by a build-up of uric acid – in this case in the joints of the jaw (Fig. 7.16). This is a very serious condition and results in high levels of pain. I have seen the leg joints affected in other cases. Euthanasia may be the most humane option.

Dietary disease in young tortoises

Hatchlings and young tortoises are much more susceptible to the effects of overfeeding or an inadequate diet. This often leads to poor growth, resulting in deformities of the limbs, tail, jaws and shell (Fig. 7.17). Depending on the extent of deformity, the internal organs may also be affected adversely.

Metabolic bone disease

One of the very common consequences of dietary imbalance and/or overfeeding is metabolic bone disease. This is caused by one or more of the following:

- Deficiency of calcium in the diet.
- Excess of phosphorus in the diet.
- High protein levels in the diet.
- Overfeeding leading to very rapid growth.
- Inadequate provision of correct UVB (see Chapter 4 on artificial light and heat.
- Inadequate dietary vitamin D3.
- Low environmental temperatures preventing normal digestion.
- High environmental temperatures leading to increased metabolism and growth but an inability to absorb sufficient calcium and lay it down into bone.

The causes above may lead to different types of disease and a range of consequences to the body's size, shape and proportion (Fig. 7.18). Very commonly, nutritional secondary hyperparathyroidism is the identified cause of metabolic bone disease. This refers to increased parathyroid hormone (PTH) levels, which reduce calcium levels in the blood. The parathyroid glands regulate calcium and phosphorus levels in the blood through PTH (Rendle and Calvert, 2019). The condition leads to kidney damage, which then exacerbates the calcium metabolism problem, leading to renal secondary hyperparathyroidism (Johnson, 2019). This is the result of long-term kidney disease.

The plastron and the carapace of the shell can both become deformed. This is often seen initially as shell pyramiding where the carapace becomes lumpy rather than smoothly domed. The dome of the carapace may become flattened, as the developing muscles pull the shell downwards when it lacks the solidity and strength to resist as it normally would. This type of deformation is particularly common in the pelvic region, as the stronger muscles there are able to pull the carapace down even further. Such 'pancake' or flattening effects lead to reduced space in the body cavity (Fig. 7.18).

This will have consequences for organ development and function. Lung capacity may be limited. Liver function may be negatively impacted. The capacity to reproduce, carry and, particularly, to pass eggs in females will be much reduced (see reproduction, below). Hibernation/brumation of animals with severe deformities should be approached with extreme caution, and if it is to be attempted it should be kept short. This allows the tortoise to experience a natural cycle, but without the stress of an extended dormancy.

A maximum 4–6 weeks of hibernation/brumation in tortoises with metabolic bone disease would be recommended. In some cases, the deformities are so severe, and the lung capacity so limited, that it may be safer not to hibernate at all.

The shell may be too small for the tortoise's body, leaving parts exposed that would normally be protected by the shell. Or the pressure of the deformed shell on certain parts of the body such as the head or tail, or on eggs, may lead to deformed growth or production. This is also likely to impact negatively on the tortoise's ability to walk.

The shell may become soft, with fluid leaking between the scutes or shields of the shell. This extreme situation, linked to very high uric acid levels, is likely to be fatal for the tortoise.

Table 7.2. Effects of nutritional deficiencies and excesses.

Nutrient	Excess	Deficiency
Calcium	Hypercalcaemia would not normally be seen unless extensive treatment for metabolic bone disease (see young tortoises, below) had been given. Hypercalcaemia can lead to renal failure, calcification of soft tissues and ultimately death.	Hypocalcaemia would lead to metabolic bone disease as it is linked to high phosphorus levels. Prolonged hypocalcaemia (from calcium or vitamin D deficiency) may result in hyperparathyroidism (see young tortoises, below).
Phosphorus	Hyperphosphataemia would not normally be seen in a healthy tortoise. If, however, there is kidney disease, the uptake of phosphorus from the blood may be impaired. Phosphate retention may result from nutritional secondary hyperparathyroidism.	Hypophosphataemia is unlikely as there is always more phosphorus available in the diet than is needed.
Vitamin A	Hypervitaminosis A causes excess skin sloughing and can cause pain and lameness.	Hypovitaminosis A may result in swollen eyelids, swelling of the legs (oedema), kidney and liver damage. A lack of Vitamin A in the diet may result in a reduced immune system response leading to increased susceptibility to infection. This may be a contributing factor in development of stomatitis in the mouth.
Vitamin D	Hypervitaminosis D3 – high levels of D3 are not usually seen even where supplements are given. However, when LED lights are used to replace fluorescent UVB sources, the full range of UVB wavelengths may be lacking. This may lead to overproduction of vitamin D3 (see Chapter 4 on artificial light and heat). As yet these effects have not been studied, but have been associated with hypercalcinosis. Calcification of soft tissues may be seen.	Hypovitaminosis D may lead to poor calcium uptake with the consequent effects of low calcium on bone development. Low blood calcium levels can result in egg-laying problems (dystocia) and neurological and muscular problems. Calcification of soft tissues may be seen, but is more likely with hypervitaminosis D.
Protein	Gout can be the result of a long-term high-protein diet. This is a very painful condition where the joints become swollen, and movement is limited due to a build-up of uric acid. Visceral gout may lead to liver and kidney damage or failure.	Protein demand is low in tortoises, making a deficiency unlikely.

The lifespan of many of these animals is severely shortened. Many of them do not reach adulthood. Those who do so will often have limited, pain-filled lives, unable to function normally (Fig. 7.17A–C).

The limb bones may be weakened as available calcium is insufficient to meet the combined demands of growth in both the shell and the bones. The limb bones may be thin, soft and lacking strength. This means that movement may be impaired, or even impossible. The tortoise may not be able to hold its own body weight up in order to walk normally (Fig. 7.18). This is a particular problem for the larger, heavier species such as Leopard and Sulcata tortoises.

The jaw may be over- or under-shot, deformed and soft. This may interfere with normal feeding, as the beak usually cuts piece of food for the tortoise to ingest. This may mean a lifetime of beak care through burring (using a sanding tool such as a Dremel), or clipping with hand-clippers, to reduce the overgrowth and allow normal feeding.

The tail may be shortened, or an abnormal shape (Fig. 7.19). The tortoise may be unable to retract it into the shell. Left exposed, the deformed tail may scrape along the ground and can become worn and damaged. This can lead to skin damage and abscesses, which often need surgical shell treatments.

Once such deformities have occurred, it is unlikely that they can be corrected. Improved diet and in particular giving sufficient calcium and vitamin D3 can prevent further damage but the tortoise will always be deformed.

Vomiting or regurgitation

Tortoises do not normally vomit but can regurgitate food. The most likely causes of regurgitation would be ingestion of a foreign body, infection in the gut or large numbers of parasitic worms. Veterinary attention should be sought for a tortoise who regularly regurgitates food, as it is a sign that something potentially serious is wrong.

One case of this that I observed involved a large male Radiated tortoise called Brian, who had been captive-bred in the UK. The tortoise was well supplied with calcium and the husbandry was effective. The shell growth appeared to be largely normal but had been more rapid than would have been the case in the wild. The shell was hard and domed, but quite thickened at the front of the plastron where the head extends out. This meant the opening for the head was smaller than would normally be the case (Fig. 7.20).

One day Brian had eaten some large pieces of pepper. One of these had apparently damaged his oesophagus as it moved from his mouth down his throat and into the stomach. The bruising and inflammation that resulted led to several episodes of what looked like vomiting, but was probably regurgitation, as he tried to eat again. This behaviour was very distressing to observe, as the tortoise was clearly in great difficulty and discomfort.

Veterinary treatment involved reducing the inflammation and giving pain relief. Subsequent feeding was restricted to smaller food items, and the episode was not repeated.

5. Liver disease

Liver disease is often the result of poor diet (see reproductive disease, below).

Fatty liver (hepatic lipidosis) is common particularly in older captive tortoises (Fig. 7.21). There is an over-representative number of female tortoises treated for this due to a physiological lipidosis association with follicle development. This is largely due to poor diet. The main causes are a diet high in fats and carbohydrates or where high-protein foods have been given to herbivorous tortoises. Fatty liver is often associated too with generally poor husbandry, including keeping the tortoise at temperatures that are too low or hibernating/brumating the animal for excessively long periods.

The liver processes digested foods and stores fat for use during hibernation/brumation and egg production. Damage to the liver from excess fat may lead to the follicles not proceeding through the oviduct normally, where more fat and albumin are added in the shell-gland part of the process (see female reproduction, below). When the liver is diseased the effects are very general, because it is a very large organ involved in many aspects of metabolism.

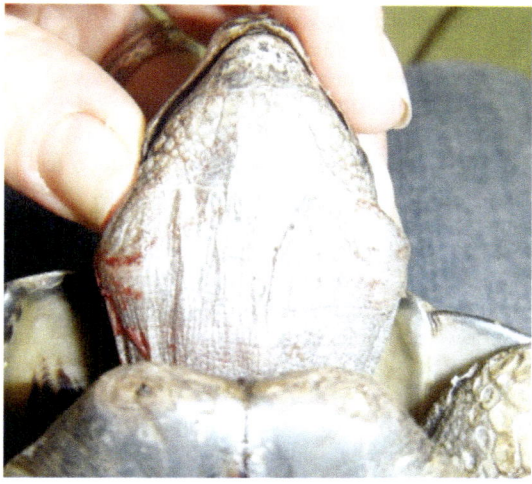

Fig. 7.16. Swelling due to gout may be seen in joints of the jaw (Eleanor Lien-Hua Tirtasana Chubb).

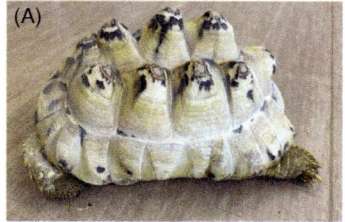 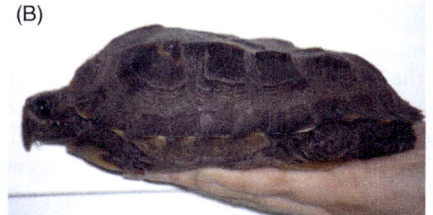 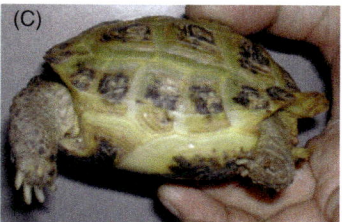

Fig. 7.17. Deformed tortoises due to metabolic bone disease. (A) Severe pyramiding in Leopard tortoise. (B) Shell collapse (William Lewis). (C) Soft shell (William Lewis).

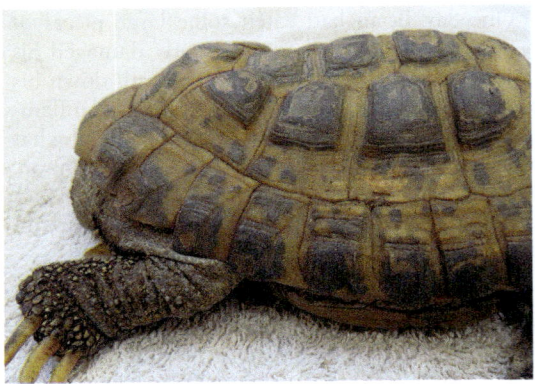

Fig. 7.18. Flattened body cavity as the shell is pulled down by pelvic muscles.

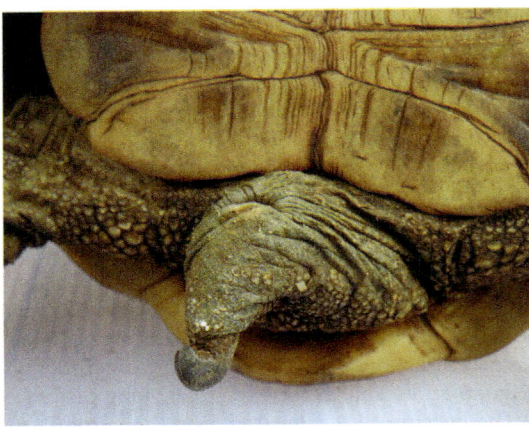

Fig. 7.19. Deformed tail in male Hermanns tortoise leading to damage.

The impact is seen throughout the entire body. One common sign in the later stages of liver disease is a failure to feed, or anorexia. Part of the pathogenesis (the way in which the disease develops) is that the storage of fat in the liver cells (hepatocytes) is excessive. These cells can no longer function properly. Thus, there are fewer liver cells functioning normally in the liver. This can reduce efficiency of food digestion and the many detoxification processes that the liver carries out. The effect is that the tortoise will suffer toxicity due to the liver dysfunction.

In ageing tortoises, a general reduction in activity, greater lethargy and reduced feeding may all have underlying causes related to poor liver function. That said, a healthy normal tortoise, like most animals with a liver, will show a good power of regeneration of a damaged liver.

The liver can be stimulated to function more efficiently using anabolic steroids, which can alter metabolism to boost the reduction of fat in the liver cells. These can also increase appetite in non-feeding tortoises. Hydration with plenty of warm baths is also essential in these situations, together with a reduction in fat content in the diet (Brown *et al.*, 2019).

6. Kidney and urinary disease

The kidneys can be damaged through infection, or poor diet (especially high protein, which will result in more uric acid being produced), or by lack of water availability (which leads to dehydration). This can then lead to gout. Uric acid is not very soluble, even in the blood, and if the tortoise is dehydrated uric acid will form crystals (tophi) in organs (including the kidney, where it is in high concentrations) or joints. This condition is called gout.

Chronic kidney disease can be noticed when checking waste products passed from the bladder. For this reason, it is important to bathe tortoises regularly. When they are in their baths, they usually pass white urates. A change in colour or consistency of urine may be the first indication of kidney malfunction.

As a result of the removal of toxic products from the blood, the uric acid (urates) produced by the kidneys should be seen as soft and white within the urine. After hibernation/brumation it is normal for the urates to be very grey, or even brown in colour. Often described as milky, they should not be gritty or yellow in colour. Gritty hard urates may indicate dehydration, which contributes to the development of bladder stones.

Urinary or bladder stones (uroliths) are formed from uric acid in the bladder, sometimes during hibernation, when the tortoise is dehydrated, or on a too-high-protein diet. Sometimes the stones can be felt in the tail, as they move down into the cloaca. If too large they can become stuck in the cloaca. Passing these stones can be very painful for the tortoise. Any indication of a blockage should be treated as a veterinary emergency. Figure 7.22 shows a very large stone being surgically removed from the bladder itself.

A yellow colour, or sometimes even green colour, in the urates indicates significant problems with uric acid production, or liver disease (due to excessive biliverdin, which causes the green colour). This requires veterinary attention as a matter of urgency.

Tortoises do sometimes eat stones, which may also be passed out of the cloaca with faeces. This is

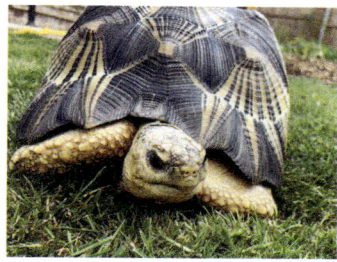
Fig. 7.20. Brian, a Radiated tortoise.

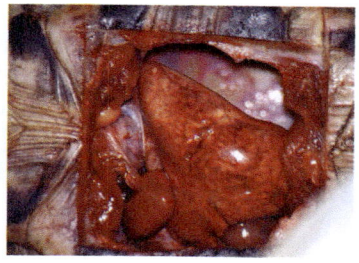
Fig. 7.21. Fatty liver seen during spay surgery of female tortoise (William Lewis).

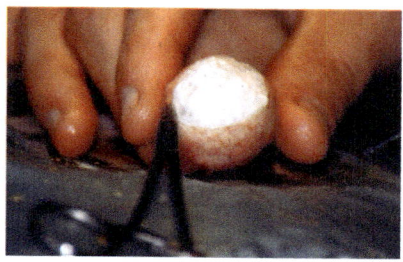
Fig. 7.22. Very large bladder stone being surgically removed (William Lewis).

normal behaviour for some species and as long as an obstruction is not caused, these stones may remain in the gut for long periods without creating any problems.

Lack of kidney function may lead to water retention and oedema, seen as general swelling of the limbs, particularly the hind limbs. Any signs of swelling of the limbs should be investigated, as this can be a general symptom of a number of underlying conditions.

7. Diseases due to hibernation duration

Traditionally hibernation/brumation has been too long in countries where the climate is cooler than the home range.

As stated in other chapters, identification of the species of your tortoise is essential before any attempt is made to hibernate/brumate. There are many species of tropical tortoise which do not hibernate naturally and hibernation would be fatal for these species. Examples include Leopard, Sulcata and Red-footed tortoises (see Chapter 12 on hibernation).

However, note that Horsfield's tortoises do naturally hibernate for longer periods of time than other species. Their home range is much colder than other species can tolerate. They are thought to hibernate for several months in the winter and may hibernate more than once in an annual cycle.

Hibernation for most temperate species, such as the Mediterranean tortoises, should be a maximum of 8 weeks (McArthur, 2003). Where hibernation is repeatedly longer than 12 weeks, over many years, the tortoise may find it increasingly difficult to recover. This is particularly true as they age, or where they are not supported with additional heat and light immediately post-hibernation. The consequences of this are that the tortoise becomes less active and feeds less well. The tortoise is physiologically compensating for less-than-optimal conditions for the rest of the year. There is a shortened feeding season and periods of very low temperatures to contend with.

Long hibernation/brumation periods may result in:

- Low blood glucose levels
- High blood urea and plasma proteins due to the build-up of toxins over too long a period of time
- Dehydration.

Post-hibernational anorexia

Overlong hibernations/brumations may lead to the development of post-hibernational anorexia (PHA). This syndrome of anorexia is the result of excessively long hibernation made worse by poor environmental provision and husbandry. Poor body condition, or being underweight before hibernation, can also contribute to this syndrome.

The diet may have been poor over a number of years. The tortoise may have been maintained at temperatures that are too low for much of the time. It may also be suffering from other underlying health issues, such as stomatitis, or other infections such as those of the upper respiratory tract.

If a tortoise is suffering from post-hibernation (brumation) anorexia it may need to be hand-fed in order to stimulate feeding, once any underlying causes have been treated. Sometimes chopping up food or liquidizing it so that the food is very soft and quite easy to swallow can be helpful. Use of commercial pellets that have been soaked in water may be enticing for some tortoises (although these are not advised as a suitable long-term diet for most species of herbivorous tortoises).

Cucumber can be appealing as a food for tortoises with little appetite. Putting the food into a corner of

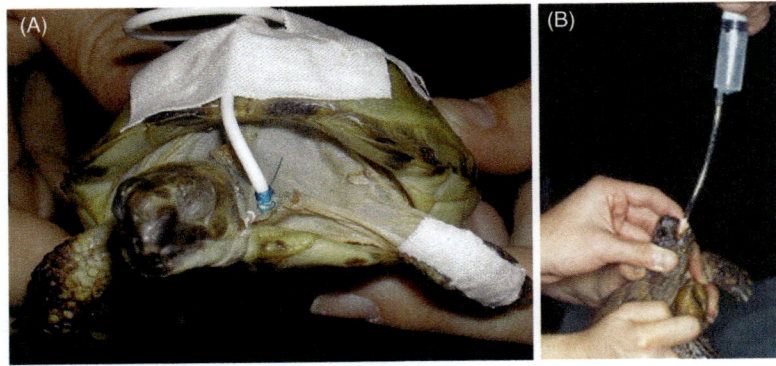

Fig. 7.23. (A) Pharyngeal tubes inserted to allow feeding and treatment with reduced stress for the tortoise (William Lewis). (B) A daily feeding tube is more stressful, as the tortoise's head has to be held out and the tube inserted (Eleanor Lien-Hua Tirtasana Chubb).

the enclosure so that the tortoise can easily take a bite or mouthful with very little effort or movement can be helpful. Putting the tortoise repeatedly near the food and using food with an odour (such as cucumber or sedum) is especially helpful for those with eye damage or blindness. Hand-feeding may also be required initially. For tortoises, smell is generally more important than vision.

It can take many months, or even years, to encourage an anorexic tortoise to feed completely independently again, and to take the full range of foods offered. Depending upon how ill they were when treatment started, how long they had been ill prior to this, and the severity of any other underlying conditions, a great deal of patience is needed to encourage them to take food again.

Treatment for anorexia may involve positioning of a pharyngeal feeding tube by a veterinary practitioner as shown in Fig. 7.23. This allows tube-feeding of liquid food, probiotics, supportive supplements such as Critical Care, Reptoboost (Vetark®) or antibiotics to be given without the repeated stress of inserting an oral feeding tube daily.

8. Injury and damage by predators, other tortoises and the environment

Damage by predators

Tortoises can be damaged by predators such as foxes, coyotes, racoons, rats or even large birds such as raptors and corvids (Fig. 7.24). They might encounter these predators when living in outdoor enclosures. For this reason, many keepers put their tortoises indoors at night.

I have seen many cases of injuries caused by domestic dogs, very occasionally an injury from a domestic cat and a case of injury from a pet parrot (Fig. 7.25). Dogs will gnaw on the shell as if eating a bone. If the dog has powerful jaws and teeth the damage can be extensive (Fig. 7.24). Similarly damage by rodents during hibernation may go undetected if the tortoise is not checked regularly, ideally every day. If the rodents cause damage over an extended period, without treatment, the effects may be severe. The resultant tissue loss and infection prove fatal.

Generally, predator injury involves damage to the shell and to the extremities of the limbs exposed at the edges of the shell. The wounds can be substantial and of course the flesh may be consumed by the predator rather than just resulting in tears or rips. There may be significant bleeding and exposure of internal organs (Fig. 7.26). The loss of tissue plus resulting blood loss can be fatal. The risk of infection is very high. Tortoises injured by predators should be seen by a veterinarian as a matter of urgency.

Damage by other tortoises

Damage by other tortoises can be due to repeated shell butting or hind-limb biting. This is usually done by males during mating (see Chapter 11 on breeding). The repeated trauma of the shell being bashed continuously in the same place can cause the shields, or scutes, to be damaged, weakened or loosened. Similarly repeated biting can bruise the skin and tissues, cause tears of the skin and damage the underlying tissues. This is common, resulting in injuries to the hind limbs and the tail area.

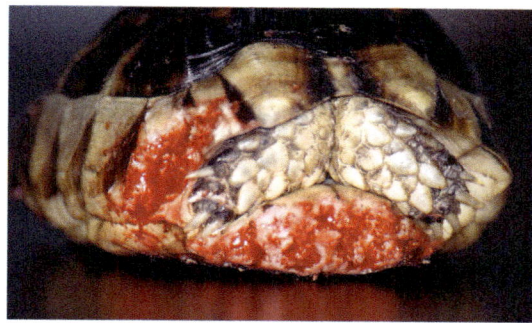

Fig. 7.24. Trauma and injury caused by fox or dog attacks (William Lewis).

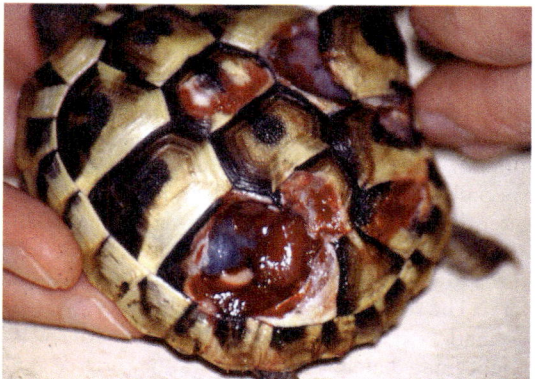

Fig. 7.25. Trauma from macaw bites (William Lewis).

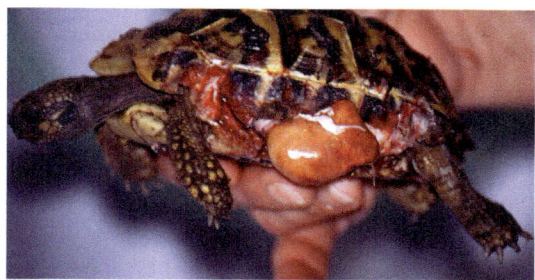

Fig. 7.26 Trauma can be very severe, exposing the internal organs and causing life-threatening injuries (William Lewis).

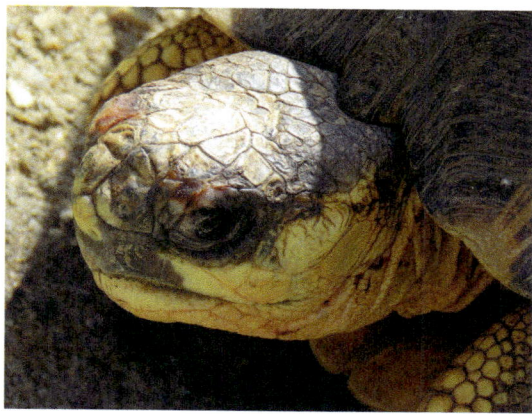

Fig. 7.27. Injury to the top of the eyes due to biting by other tortoises.

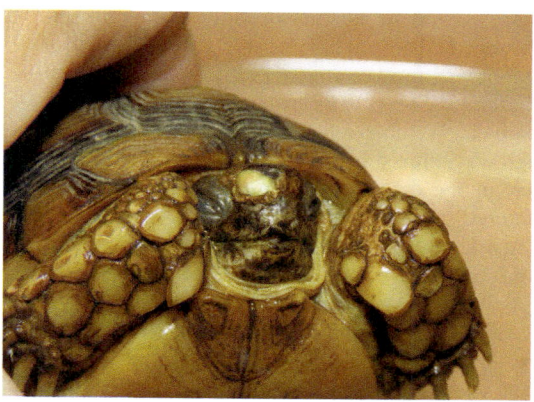

Fig. 7.28. Damage to the front of the face from an object in the enclosure.

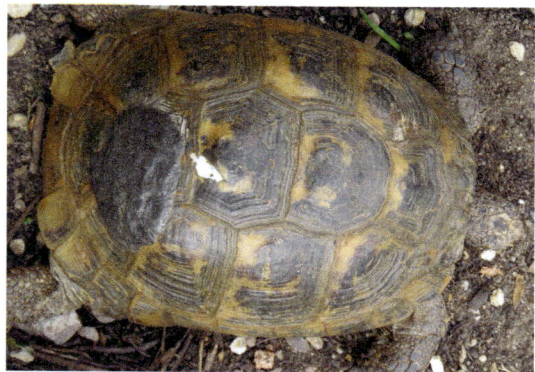

Fig. 7.29. Shell repair following injury from the point of a garden fork into the shell of Tarquin, repaired several years ago.

Some species, such as male Sulcatas, are territorial and show aggression towards each other when kept in groups (see Chapter 8 on behaviour and Chapter 10 on social interactions). Attempts may be made by one male to turn another onto its back, where it might overheat in the sun or be further injured.

Common Illnesses and Diseases

Damage by biting, clawing and climbing over other tortoises can cause skin damage. Delicate structures such as the eyes are especially vulnerable, as shown in Fig. 7.27 (see also eye diseases, below).

Environmental damage

(See also Chapter 19 on health and safety.)

Tortoises can be injured by barrier fencing. Wire should be avoided, as tortoises can easily rip scales from the skin of the head and front legs when attempting to get through a wire fence. Any sharp edges to fencing can also be a source of injury to the head, limbs or tail (Fig. 7.28).

Tortoises will walk through the glass side of greenhouses. Broken glass can cut and severely injure tortoises.

Tortoises can be injured by garden equipment. Care should be taken to ensure that a tortoise is removed from areas where spades, pitchforks, strimmers and lawnmowers are in use. All of these mechanical tools can cause severe shell and internal damage. We have a tortoise here which many years ago was injured by a garden fork, with a large hole left in the carapace where one prong of the fork entered right into the body cavity. The lesion caused was debrided and treated with antibiotics, and once infection was prevented the shell was repaired with epoxy resin (Fig. 7.29).

Extensive repairs of the shell that can be carried out by veterinarians might involve fixing metal ties and plates to stabilize the damage. Sterilized fibreglass or acrylic products (for repairing cars) can be used to cover the wound while the shell re-grows. Technovit® is a cattle and horse hoof-repair substance that is ideal and not permanent for the treatment of such injuries. Recently Kooliner® (a temporary lining for dentures) has been used to repair shell damage. It is now known that keeping the wound airtight is important to ensure that the tortoise can continue to breathe properly and to reduce any reinfection (Marschang and Chitty, 2019).

Burns from indoor heating sources are all too common where the set-up allows the tortoise to get too close to the heat source. These are seen as dark patches on the skin, or red, bleeding areas, possibly with blisters. Burns may also appear as whitened areas on the shell, which could take a number of years before the dead area of shell starts to slough off and new shell is seen.

Where unsuitable sources of UVB light are provided, UVB damage to skin and eyes is possible. This is a symptom of acute over-exposure to high UVB (photokeratitis). The cornea of the eye is usually affected first. Clouding (opacity) or damage on one or both corneas may cause intense pain. Affected animals will become immobile and depressed. The eyes will be permanently closed to reduce the pain. The eyelids often become swollen, and the skin of the limbs and head may appear burned. In young animals, especially, death may result from shock and dehydration following the debilitating blindness.

9. Drowning

Being submerged in water does not generally lead to death.

It is not unknown for tortoises to fall into garden ponds, particularly if the pond has vertical rather than sloping sides. The majority of species cannot swim and simply fall to the bottom of the pond. Even if they remain unnoticed in the water for 8 hours or more, tortoises can often survive. This is especially so if the water is cold, and the deeper the water the colder it is likely to be. This is due to ability of tortoises to lower their metabolic rate together with a low demand for oxygen, particularly in cold water. The tortoise may appear lifeless after such a traumatic experience, but if veterinary advice is sought immediately, in many cases the tortoise can be revived.

The tortoise may need help to breathe. The water must be drained from the lungs. Oxygen must then be provided using, for example, an oxygen tent. The tortoise may also need antibiotic treatment to prevent the development of pneumonia or other respiratory infections. Eye infections may also develop, which require treatment to avoid permanent eye damage. Other treatments to regain fluid balance may also be necessary. This is in addition to providing suitable warm temperatures and light indoors while a recovery is made.

I once helped a friend who had lost her tortoise in her garden. Tommy had not been seen all day. Having searched everywhere it was concluded that the only place that the tortoise could possibly be, was the koi pond, home to over 20 very large koi. The pond was enormous, and deep, which increased the chances of survival as it was more likely to be very cold at the bottom. Upon investigation, there did seem to be a large solid object at the bottom of the pond that could be moved with a broom handle. Its shape could not be made out as the bottom of the pond was so dark. In desperation the owner almost emptied the pond, using the very efficient filtration pumps. Her garden was entirely flooded with about 15 cm of lying water, while the koi flapped about in the bottom of what was left of the pond.

The object at the bottom of the pond, once assumed to be Tommy, was in fact a large rock that had fallen from the nearby rockery. Tommy had pushed out the rock whilst digging himself a very secure hiding place. Here he rested, blissfully unaware of the commotion and consternation he had caused. The pond was rapidly refilled to allow the koi relief. A repeat of this performance was avoided by the positioning of much more secure barriers around the pond.

10. Tumours

Tortoises do sometimes develop cancerous conditions. Large masses can form, sometimes undetected, for a number of months or years. Masses might not always be a cancerous tumour, however. A mass could be due to fluid build-up, or an infection causing an abscess, or might simply be a foreign body. Cancerous tumours are reported relatively rarely. While cancer can develop in a range of body tissues, life may be prolonged if surgical removal is possible (Fig. 7.30). If a cancer has had the opportunity to spread into a number of tissues and organs, sadly euthanasia may be the only option to prevent suffering.

11. Eye diseases

As discussed in the dietary section of this chapter, swollen eyelids or permanently closed eyes can be indicative of underlying disease not directly caused by a problem with the eyes themselves.

Problems with eyes can include swelling due to eye infections caused by viruses or bacteria. Hypovitaminosis A as a cause of eye disease is discussed in the diet section and UVB light photokeratitis is discussed in the section on environmental damage.

Eye abscesses are also seen, and ulcers and/or infection of the cornea can occur. Clouding over of the eye leading to blindness is not uncommon, especially in older individuals. One cause of this is freezing during hibernation/brumation. If the temperature of the location used for hibernation is not adequately monitored, and temperatures fall below 2°C for any period of time, the water in the eyes may start to freeze. This may lead to loss of vision as the cornea and lens become cloudy or opaque. Cholesterol and lipid (fat) deposits may also build up around the edges of the cornea as part of the ageing process. Similarly, cataracts can form in the lenses of older tortoises.

12. Reproductive diseases

(See also Chapter 11 on breeding.)

Female tortoises

Egg-retention (dystocia) or egg-binding – the inability to pass fully formed eggs

Female tortoises can have significant difficulty producing normal eggs in captivity.

If eggs are to be laid, first a suitable site to build a nest must be found (see Chapter 11 on breeding). If this is not provided the eggs may be retained for excessive periods. The tortoise may become egg-bound and then unable to pass the eggs without help.

Environmental conditions, including temperature, humidity and depth of substrate, also need to be suitable to stimulate egg-laying. These conditions can be challenging to provide outdoors in northern climates.

Females also need male tortoises around for short periods in order to be stimulated to produce eggs. It is thought that male pheromones play a part in normal egg production. In addition, the courtship and mating behaviours may play a part in stimulating ovulation, and therefore the production of fully formed eggs. A female, like hens, can produce eggs even if she has not been in contact with a male.

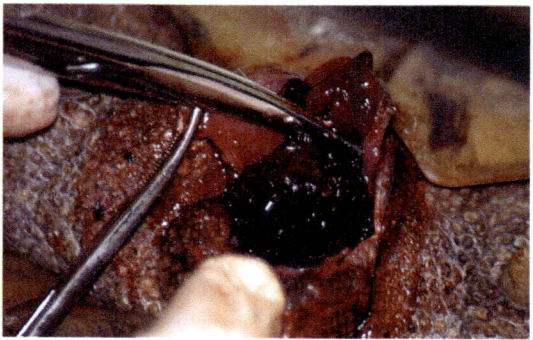

Fig. 7.30. Cloacal tumour being surgically removed (William Lewis).

Common Illnesses and Diseases

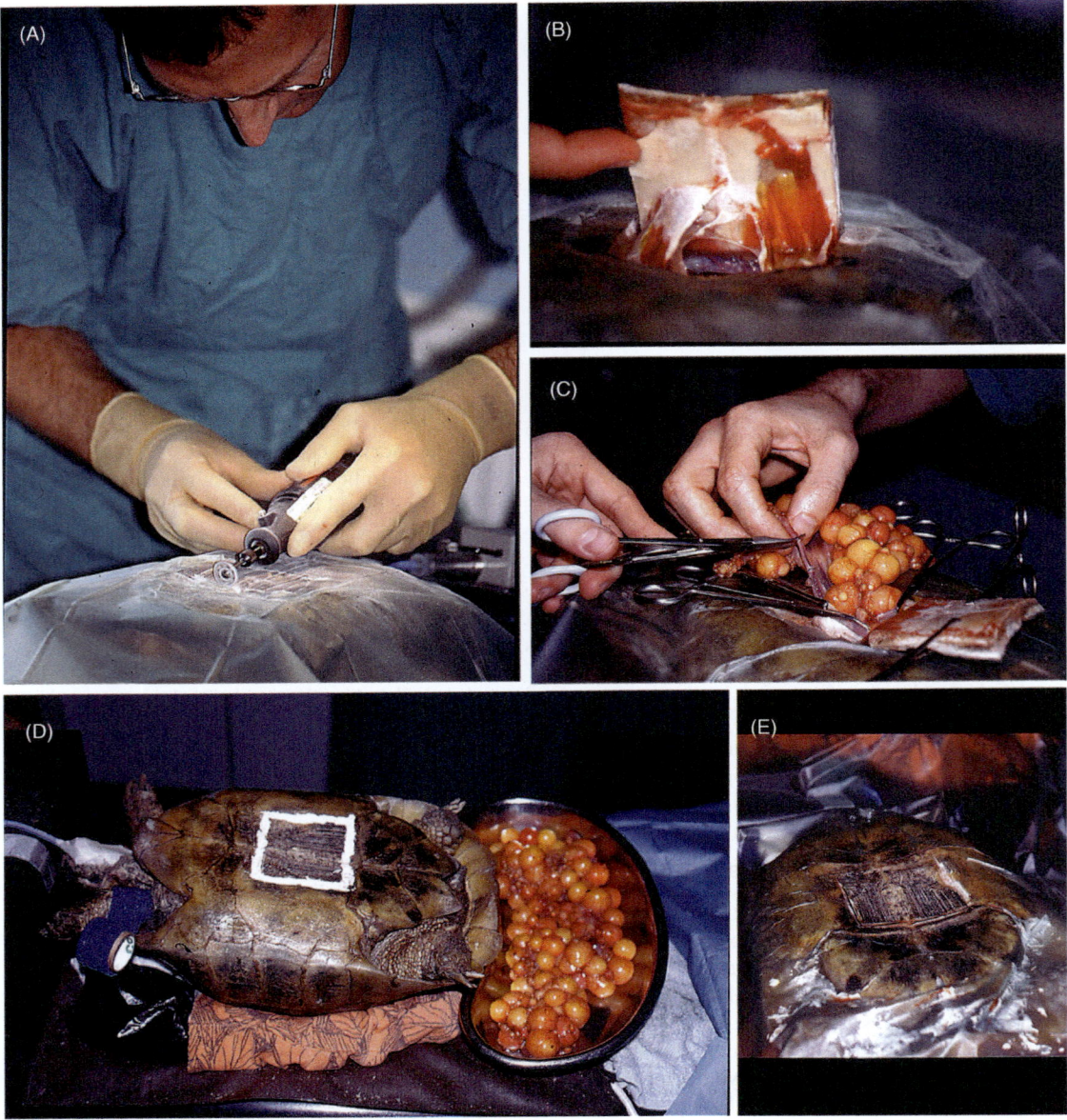

Fig. 7.31 A–E. Tortoise with follicular stasis being spayed (William Lewis) showing cutting a section plastron, opening the plastron, lifting the shell flap, removing the follicles, and replacing the flap.

Any lack of calcium in the diet may interfere with normal egg production, particularly the process of laying down the hard calcium carbonate shell. This is also needed for the uterus and cloaca to be able to expel the eggs. A clutch might contain 12 or more eggs, so a great deal of calcium will be required.

If the female is egg-bound treatment could include calcium supplementation followed by oxytocin to stimulate laying. If the tortoise is still unable to pass the eggs, they may need to be surgically removed along with the ovaries and fallopian tubes. This is called a spay (similar to the surgery carried out in cats and dogs) (Fig. 7.31).

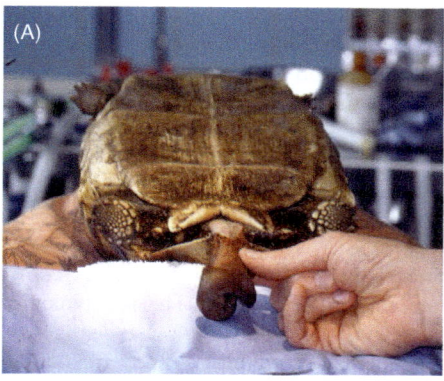
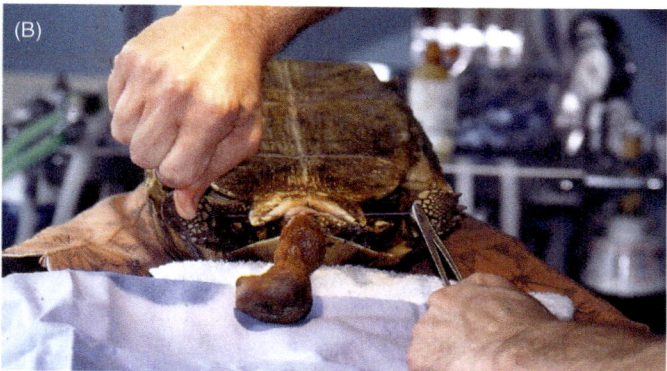

Fig. 7.32. Male penis amputation (William Lewis).

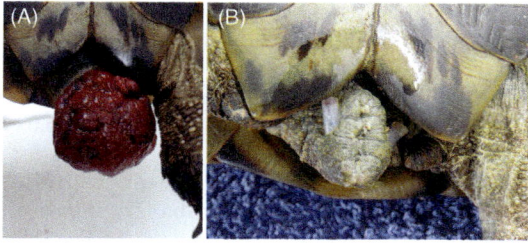

Fig. 7.33. (A) Female cloacal prolapse. (B) Treatment to try to hold the organ in place.

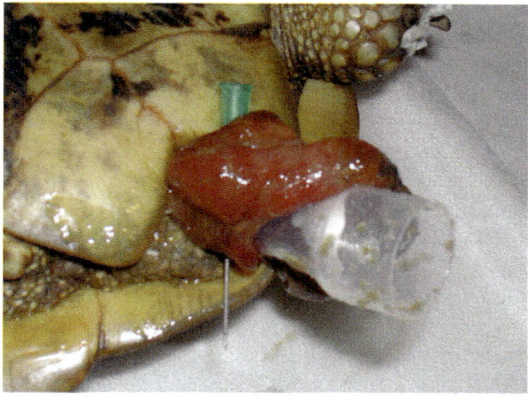

Fig. 7.34. Rectal prolapse and treatment to try to hold the organ in place (William Lewis).

Follicular stasis – pre-ovulatory ova stasis when follicles remain in the ovaries only partially developed

If the female is producing follicles in the ovaries, but they do not ovulate or go on to develop into fully formed eggs, the partially formed eggs will still be soft, as the hard shell has not yet been laid down on the surface. The term follicles describes eggs after they have been through the egg gland. If these follicles remain in the ovaries for a prolonged period, this is called stasis. Additional follicles may be added until the body cavity is full of follicles. The follicles may become infected and die. The then-necrotic tissue can cause serious infection or toxicity within the body cavity.

The cause of follicular stasis is largely due to poor husbandry. A rich diet may produce a fatty liver, which can also contribute to follicular stasis. Lack of a male to stimulate ovulation, along with low temperatures rather than a seasonal cycle, which includes a hot summer, may all contribute to this interruption to normal egg production.

Follicular stasis is a common cause of anorexia in elderly female tortoises living alone.

Treatment involves surgical removal of the ovaries and the follicles, and in some cases the uterus as well, as shown in Fig. 7.31. This is a permanent preventive treatment, as follicles cannot be formed again in the future. Alternatively, deslorelin may be given as an implant such as Suprelorin®F (Virbac) as an effective but much less traumatic treatment.

Stress-related disease in females

Females may become stressed by the presence of male tortoises, particularly if there are more males than females kept together, or if the males are particularly amorous or if the enclosure is too small for the females to get away. Repeated shell-butting or leg-biting can cause physical injury, and being subject to this behaviour repeatedly can cause enormous stress, especially if the female is trapped in the corner of an enclosure and cannot move.

Common Illnesses and Diseases

Male tortoises

During mating the tortoise will use the penis for copulation. There is the possibility of damage to the organ during that process.

13. Prolapses

Male tortoises may prolapse the penis, so that they are unable to withdraw the organ back into the cloaca. If this happens, damage may be caused to the organ as it is dragged along the ground. This may require amputation, as shown in Fig. 7.32, as the male can remove wastes and function without it.

Female tortoises may prolapse the oviduct, cloaca or clitoris (Fig. 7.33).

Tortoises may also prolapse their colon or part of the intestine such as the rectum, as shown in Fig. 7.34, for example through an intussusception.

In all cases, prolapse is a very serious veterinary emergency and help should be sought urgently.

First Aid

In many cases supporting the tortoise through illness involves improved husbandry. It is important to provide as near-optimal conditions as possible. As discussed in Chapter 3 on captive environment, suitable temperatures, lighting, substrate and humidity levels alongside a healthy diet can help a tortoise to cope with disease while recuperating.

One supportive measure we can offer is to ensure regular daily access to warm water in the form of a bath deep enough for the plastron to be covered. Allowing the tortoise to fully hydrate is very beneficial to disease management and treatment.

First aid for trauma leading to injury will involve applying pressure to stop bleeding, as for any other animal. Using sterile gauze and padding to apply pressure, held in place with vet wrap, would be a sensible practical step while seeking veterinary advice.

Prolapse from the cloaca of the penis in males or the oviduct in females can be contained and covered with clingfilm to try to reduce damage and water loss while getting the tortoise to a veterinarian.

Removal of foreign bodies in the eye can be achieved with a soft tissue or cotton bud but any damage should be followed up with veterinary treatment.

Cleaning of minor wounds can be achieved using products to remove bacteria and other pathogens such as Hibiscrub® and iodine-based products such as Tamodine (Vetark®). Cleaning the shell using a soft brush can be beneficial in removing dirt.

Conclusion

This chapter looks at diseases and illnesses commonly seen in tortoises in captivity. This is a dynamic state of affairs, as the types of disease change as conditions change. For example, there are newly identified infectious diseases being seen in species of tortoise that are being captive-bred in large numbers. This is an area where keepers need to be alert to potential new pathogens and to developments in prevention of disease. Available tests for disease are increasing all the time.

Overall, as we have a better understanding of our tortoises' needs and improvements in veterinary treatments continue to be made, the outcomes for our tortoises (should they become ill) will also improve. As some aspects of husbandry improve, illnesses caused by poor diet or lack of suitable lighting may decline.

Prevention is always better than cure. The information in this chapter focuses on the importance of our role as caregivers, in keeping our tortoises healthy through good husbandry and hygiene. Being aware of changes and acting quickly to support and treat a tortoise, before disease becomes established, is vital in maintaining our tortoises through a long life.

This chapter is no substitute for veterinary treatment, and you should seek advice from a qualified professional at the earliest opportunity if you are concerned that your tortoise is unwell. Making contact with a local veterinarian, and being prepared should anything go wrong, is good practice for tortoise keepers.

Acknowledgments

I am very grateful to the UK veterinary surgeon, Martin Lawton, for reviewing this chapter. (Dr M.P.C. Lawton BVetMed; CertVOphthal; CertLAS; CBiol; MRSB; DZooMed; FRCVS; RCVS Recognized Specialist; RCVS Advanced Practitioner in Veterinary Ophthalmology). I am also grateful to the UK veterinary surgeon, William Lewis BVSc, CertZooMed, MRCVS for allowing the use of his photographs.

References and Further Reading

Bardi, E., Manfredi, M., Capitelli, M., Lubian, E., Vetere, A., Montani, A., Bertoni, T., Talon, E., Ratti, G. and Romussi, S. (2021) Determination of efficacy of single and double 4.7mg Deslorelin acetate implant on the reproductive activity of female pond sliders (*Trachemys scripta*). *Animals* 11(3), 660.

Brown, S.J.L., Naylor, A., Machin, R. and Pellett, S. (2019) Ch 17 Gastrointestinal disease. In: Girling, S.J. and Raiti, P. (eds) *BSAVA Manual of Reptiles*, 3rd edn. BSAVA, Quedgeley, UK, pp. 284–308.

Capitan, S. (2022) The use of invertebrates as alternatives to vertebrates in food production: opportunities and challenges. Introductory Research Essay, Swedish University of Agricultural Sciences. Available at https://pub.epsilon.slu.se/29226/1/capitan-s-20221013.pdf

Chitty, J. and Raftery, A. (2013) *Essentials of Tortoise Medicine and Surgery*. Wiley Blackwell, Chichester, UK

Deane, K. and Valentine, A. (2022) Ch 2 Assessment and recording methods tool kit. In: Rendle, M. and Hinde-Megarity, J. (eds) *BSAVA Manual of Practical Veterinary Welfare*. BSAVA, Quedgeley, UK, pp. 18–70.

Eatwell, K. and Hedley, J. (2019) Ch 24 Parasitology. In: Girling, S.J. and Raiti, P. (eds) *BSAVA Manual of Reptiles*, 3rd edn. BSAVA, Quedgeley, UK, pp. 411–422.

Ebenhack, A. (2012) *Health Care and Rehabilitation of Turtles and Tortoises*. Turtle and Tortoise Preservation group. Living Art Publishing.

Ellerd, R., Saleh, M.N., Luksovsky, J.L. and Verocai, G.G. (2022) Endoparasites of pet reptiles and amphibians from exotic pet shows in Texas, United States. *Veterinary Parasitology: Regional Studies and Reports* 27, 100671.

Highfield, A. (1996) *Practical Encyclopaedia of Keeping and Breeding Tortoises and Freshwater Turtles*. Carapace Press, London.

Hofmannova, L., Kvicerovo, J., Bizkova, K. and Modry, D. (2019) Intranuclear coccidiosis in tortoises – discovery of its causative agent and transmission. *European Journal of Protistology* 67, 71–76.

Jacobson, E.R., Brown, M.B., Wendland, L.D., Brown, D.R., Klein, P.A., Christopher, M.M. and Berry, K.H. (2014) Mycoplasmosis and upper respiratory tract disease of tortoises: a review and update. *The Veterinary Journal* 201(3), 257–264.

Johnson, J.G. (2013) Therapeutic Review: Deslorelin Acetate Subcutaneous Implant. *Journal of Exotic Pet Medicine* 22, 82–84.

Johnson, J.D. (2019) Ch 20 Urogenital system. In: Girling, S.J. and Raiti, P. (eds) *BSAVA Manual of Reptiles*, 3rd edn. BSAVA, Quedgeley, UK, pp. 342–352.

Kolesnik, K., Obiegala, A. and Marschang, R.E. (2017) Detection of *Mycoplasma* spp., herpesviruses, topiviruses, and ferlaviruses in samples from chelonians in Europe. *Journal of Veterinary Diagnostic Investigation* 29(6), 820–832.

Marschang, R.E. (2011) Viruses affecting reptiles. *PubMed* 3(11), 2087–2126.

Marschang, R. and Chitty, J. (2019) Ch 25 Infectious diseases. In: Girling, S.J. and Raiti, P. (eds) *BSAVA Manual of Reptiles*, 3rd edn. BSAVA, Quedgeley, UK, pp. 423–442.

Marschang, R.E. and Hyndman, T. (2023) Ch. 65 Emerging Infectious Diseases of Reptiles. In: Miller, R.E., Lamberski, E. and Calle, P.P. (eds) *Fowler's Zoo and Wild Animal Medicine Current Therapy, Volume 10*. Elsevier.

McArthur, S. (2003) Post hibernation anorexia (PHA) Testudo species. In: *BCG Symposium*, 29 March 2003

McArthur, S., Wilkinson, R. and Hernandez-Divers, S. (2004) *Medicine and Surgery of Tortoises and Turtles*. Blackwell, Oxford, UK.

Rendle, M. and Calvert, I. (2019) Ch 22 Nutritional problems. In: Girling, S.J. and Raiti, P. (eds) *BSAVA Manual of Reptiles*, 3rd edn. BSAVA, Quedgeley, UK, pp. 365–396.

8 Tortoise Behaviour and Learning

Abstract
Tortoises are vertebrates with a central nervous system (CNS) and a peripheral nervous system (PNS), which connects the CNS to the other parts of the body. The nervous system is the control centre for behaviour and learning. Behaviours are either innate (inborn) or learned.

The types of reflex, or innate, behaviour we see in tortoises are considered, together with those behaviours that can be learned. Learned behaviour is based on experience throughout the stages of life. Examples of training within the captive setting are examined. The purposes of training for welfare purposes are also considered.

The types of daily behaviours we see in tortoises are described, along with seasonal behaviours related to reproduction and levels of activity.

Tortoises are capable of learning through classical and operant conditioning. This chapter looks at the basic principles of learning in tortoises and includes the types of environmental stimuli that are relevant to them. The aspects of their environment that tortoises need to remember are considered. The types of activities and behaviours that they can learn are considered, along with the factors influencing their ability to learn.

What do we mean by behaviour?

Behaviour is an action carried out by an animal in response to a change in the environment. The environment can be external – is it too cold to be wearing shorts, for example? Alternatively, there could be an internal change. If you have just eaten a heavy meal, an increased amount of blood is sent to the intestines to aid digestion. This leaves less blood for the rest of your body. The behavioural response to this is to rest while the meal is broken down. Sometimes the response may be to take no action. If a young bird recognizes the shadow of a predatory raptor overhead, the best behavioural response might be to freeze as a way of hiding. The raptor cannot then detect any movement.

Changes in the environment are called **stimuli** and can include anything that an animal can perceive. Sounds, smells, sights, tastes, sensations of touch, pain, heat or cold are all stimuli. In order to respond, we need sense organs to detect changes – eyes to see, ears to hear, a nose to smell, a tongue to taste and skin to detect touch, pressure and temperature. Animals can also respond to internal changes by showing certain behaviours. For example, changes in the levels of reproductive hormones drive the desire to mate and produce offspring.

Information gained has to be fed into the central system, which then processes the information. Like all other vertebrates, tortoises have a central nervous system (CNS) consisting of brain and spinal cord to process information. As a result of processing, the CNS sends information back to the parts of the body (such as muscles and glands), which can bring about changes, or carry out actions, that we call behaviours (McBride and Hinde-Megarity, 2022).

Some behaviours are automatically controlled, such as heart and breathing rate fluctuations, or the release of hormones and neurotransmitters. Such behaviours are called **reflex** or **innate** behaviours. We do not have to think about them; they happen automatically.

Other behaviours involve choice, allowing an animal to make decisions on the best course of action. These are **learned** behaviours and are based on an animal's experience of similar situations that have happened in the past. The animal must have the ability to learn from these previous experiences and to remember them. Behaviours can be a blend of instinct and learned responses. For example, tortoises are pre-programmed to feed, but will learn how to feed more effectively with experience,

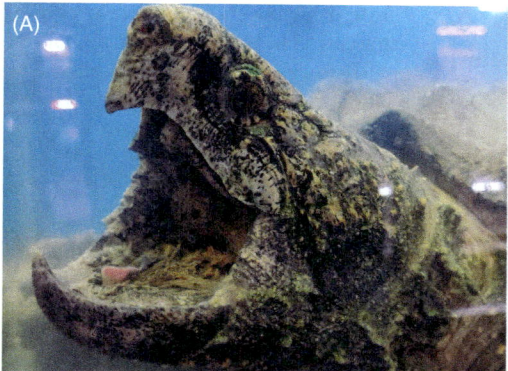
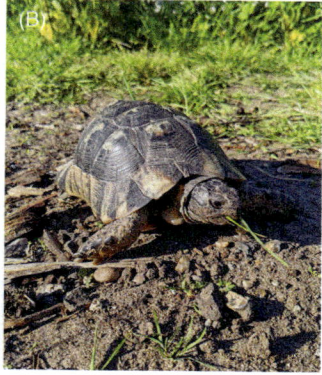

Fig. 8.1. (A) Snapping turtle and (B) terrestrial tortoise to show the very different beaks linked to feeding behaviours (Dillon Prest).

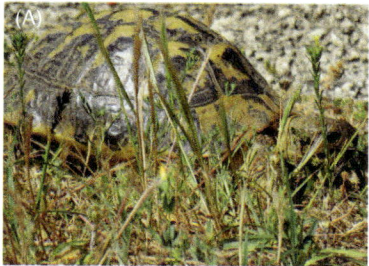
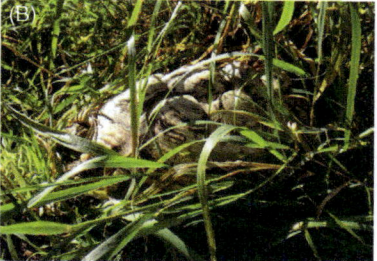
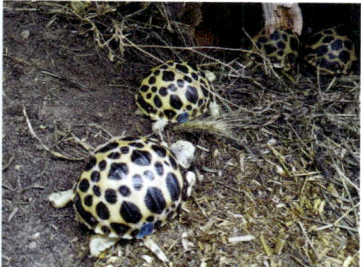

Fig. 8.2. (A) Hermann's tortoise camouflaged in natural habitat in Majorca. (B) Leopard tortoise camouflaged in grass.

Fig. 8.3. *Geochelone platynota* hatchlings seeking shelter (Andy Lewis).

and may develop favourite foods, which they select over other foods.

In all cases, normal behaviours are carried out in order to improve the chances of survival. Abnormal behaviours may be described as pathological (often driven by disease, they are not rational) as they do not promote survival. Survival is best achieved by eating, and avoiding being eaten. The other main behavioural driver is to reproduce, in order to further the continuation of the species (see Chapter 11 on breeding).

These survival adaptations are influenced by whether an animal is a predator or a prey species (McBride and Hinde-Megarity, 2022). While there are some predatory aquatic turtles (such as the carnivorous snapping turtles *Chelydra serpentina* (Fig. 8.1A) and soft-shelled turtles that form the Trionychidae), the terrestrial tortoises (Fig. 8.1B) are herbivorous or omnivorous and are therefore potential prey animals.

Prey animals need strategies and adaptations to avoid being eaten. In the case of tortoises, their shell patterns provide camouflage, making them very difficult to see in their natural habitat (Fig. 8.2).

The shell itself is a superb adaptation for survival. It has been effective in the continual existence of tortoises since their evolution around 200 million years ago. The shell is hard and strong and so it is the best possible defence against being eaten (McArthur *et al.*, 2004). The shell of some species is very thick in order to provide a defence against large naturally occurring predators. Leopard and Sulcata tortoises, for example, have much thicker shells (even taking account of size differences) than their counterparts in North Africa. This is because they live in sub-Saharan Africa where there are leopards and lions that could eat them.

Tortoises, especially when hatchlings and juveniles, will always seek out shelter (Fig. 8.3). They are rarely seen out in the open, as they can be relatively easily predated when young (see Chapter 19 on health and safety).

How is behaviour controlled?

The behaviour seen in an animal in any given situation will be a result of three factors:

1. Genetic make-up (described as the genotype).
2. The environment acting on the animal at any given time.
3. The combined effects of (1) and (2) based on past experience and learning.

In tortoises, the genetic make-up will include all the essential information any given species requires to survive in its natural environment. All baby tortoises are born with the knowledge of how to feed, what to eat, which are the most favourable environmental conditions and how to seek out shelter and refuge. The knowledge needed for courtship, mating and reproduction will also be present but used only after sexual maturity is complete, when the juvenile matures and becomes an adult.

The environment to which each tortoise is adapted is very specific in terms of temperature, light intensity, humidity, vegetation and availability of food plants and water. In captivity (as described in Chapter 3 on the captive environment) we take responsibility for trying to recreate the natural environment. It is impossible for us to achieve this completely. This immediately creates a mismatch between the tortoise's natural pre-programmed behaviours and its artificially created environment.

The tortoise will always be trying to achieve the most favourable conditions (as determined by its genetic make-up) for feeding and breeding. These may not be available. The tortoise can learn to respond to the captive environment, however. It is very common for tortoises kept in gardens to quickly learn where their shelter or house is to be found, for example: Timmy has put himself to bed in his outdoor shelter every evening for the past 33 years.

Thus, there are three parts to the nervous system that control behaviour:

1. The sense organs and internal monitors to perceive change.
2. The CNS to coordinate responses and make decisions where needed.
3. The motor systems or muscles and glands to allow the animal to respond and show behaviours.

The sense organs collect environmental information (along with internal monitoring systems) and pass it into the CNS, which consists of the brain and spinal cord. The information is processed; decisions are made from available choices where needed. As a result, the muscles, glands and other tissues take action.

Tortoises are thought to have a well-developed sense of smell, with sniffing of food items, the ground and other tortoises a commonly seen behaviour (Fig. 8.4).

Tortoises can see well (Fig. 8.8), and colour discrimination is possible from the presence of more cones than rods in the retina. Colour preference is observable in many species, with red, yellow and orange food items such as flowers often selected (Fig. 8.5) (McArthur et al., 2004).

I heard a story many years ago from a vet who had taken in a Red-footed tortoise overnight as an urgent rehoming case, and ended up with the tortoise in her kitchen prior to finding suitable accommodation the next day. The tortoise had been housed in a large box temporarily, but during the night she had broken out of that and had spent part of the night eating the large red flowers off the wallpaper which covered the kitchen walls. As a result, there were bare patches in the wallpaper where the tortoise had stripped pieces of red away, as a potential source of food!

Taste buds on the tongue provide a sense of taste. From observing food item selection, it seems likely that taste and smell are important triggers in stimulating appetite and feeding (Fig. 8.7) (McArthur et al., 2004).

Hearing is thought to be limited in terrestrial species, but much more effective in aquatic turtles as sound transmits more efficiently in water. The eardrum is seen as an external membrane on the side of the head, with no external ear present. Tortoises can only detect low tones. This is linked to their ability to detect vibrations on the ground (McArthur et al., 2004). This alerts them to approaching threats. Tortoises can also detect touch and temperature using sensors in their skin and shell, to enable them to move away from damaging stimuli such as excess heat.

Naturally occurring tortoise behaviours

If a tortoise is in good health, you should expect to see the following daily behaviours:

- Walking
- Feeding
- Basking
- Drinking
- Sheltering
- Urinating
- Defecating

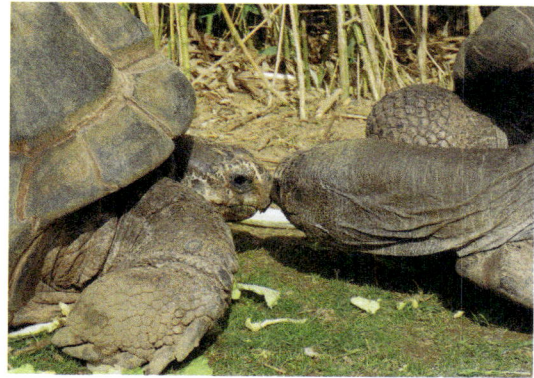

Fig. 8.4. Aldabran tortoise (*Aldabrachelys gigantea*) sniffing another Aldabran tortoise.

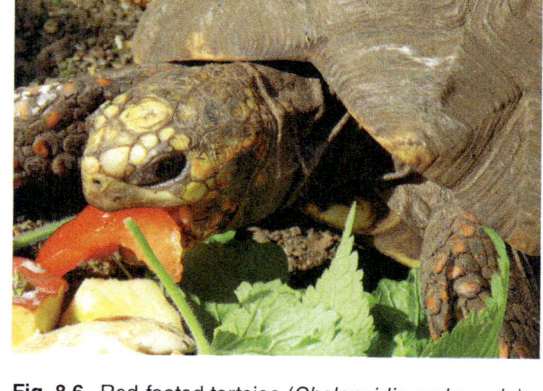

Fig. 8.6. Red-footed tortoise (*Chelonoidis carbonaria*) choosing a red food item.

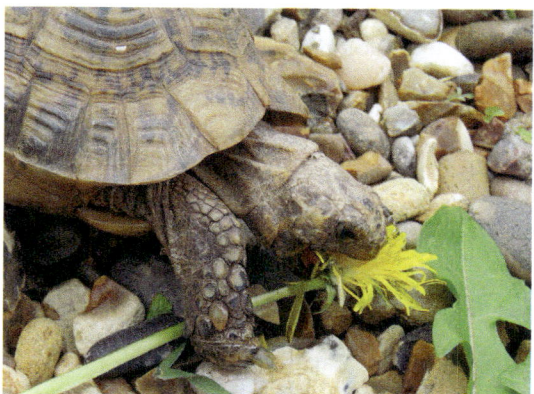

Fig. 8.5. Spur-thighed tortoise (*Testudo graeca* spp.) choosing a yellow dandelion flower over the green leaves available.

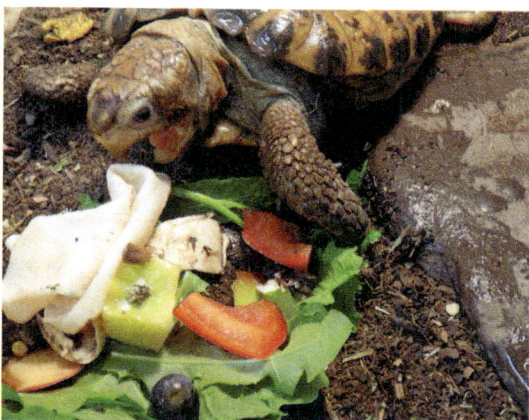

Fig. 8.7. Sulawesi tortoise (*Indotestudo forstenii*) selecting particular food items from a mixture, in this case a small amount of meat provided in mixed leaves and fruits.

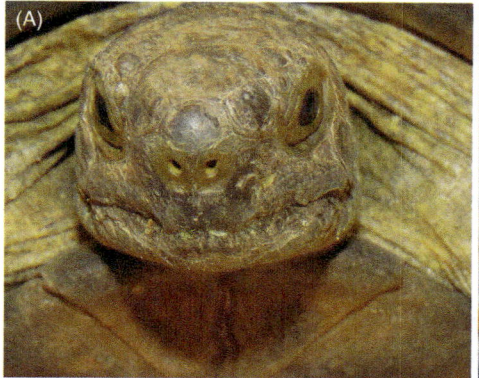
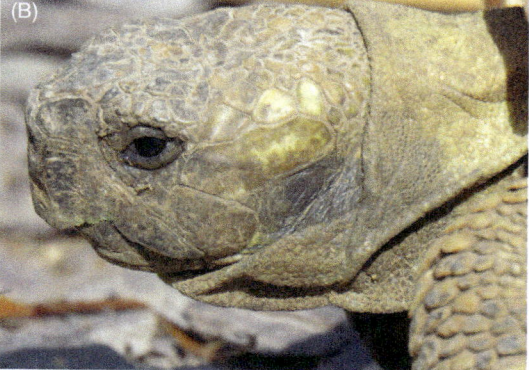

Fig. 8.8. (A) Spur-thighed tortoise's eyes are on the sides of the head, as in many prey species. (B) Hermann's tortoise's ears are a flat scale on the side of the head.

Tortoise Behaviour and Learning

Additional seasonal behaviours include:

- Courtship
- Mating
- Nest building/egg-laying in females

Body temperature is regulated behaviourally by:

- Basking in the sun to gain as much heat as possible. Limb extension or lying at the best angle to gain most sunshine can amplify this.
- Seeking shade from plants or other objects in an enclosure (Fig. 8.9).
- Burrowing into the substrate. The soil is used to reduce temperature and to increase humidity. Digging burrows and tunnels is an essential survival behaviour in very hot climates where the tortoises aestivate during the summer (Fig. 8.10).
- Sitting in puddles or trays (Fig. 8.11).
- Nocturnal or diurnal activity to avoid extremes of heat or cold, in tropical or environments with very variable temperatures.
- Mouth gaping and gular fluttering (flapping the skin of the neck, below the chin) for cooling purposes. Seen by giant tortoises in very hot climates.
- Assuming positions whereby the body is extended, giving more surface area for the sun to warm, or lifting the body away from a surface that is too hot.

Normal behaviours indicating good health and mental well-being

The range of normal behaviours shown on a daily basis by tortoises is indicated below (Chitty and Raftery, 2013; Williams, 2017). The main cycle is:

BASK → FEED → BASK → SHELTER → FEED → BURROW

This cycle is a repeating pattern and is largely related to temperature regulation and the need for food. The cycle may occur many times in a single day with walking, climbing and digging behaviours seen as the tortoise continuously seeks physiological homeostasis, when the body conditions are optimal.

Basking/sheltering

Basking and sheltering are seen throughout the day to maintain the preferred body temperature (PBT) within the preferred optimum temperature zone (POTZ) (McArthur *et al.*, 2004).

Walking

Land tortoises spend a great deal of time in the wild walking to find food, which is not always abundant or accessible. Mediterranean tortoises (Wegehaupt, 2009b), Egyptian tortoises (*Testudo kleinmanni*), Leopard (*Centrochelys pardalis*) and African Spurred tortoises (*Centrochelys sulcata*) are all known to walk several kilometres daily, having territories of very large sizes. Biedenweg and Schramm (2019) recorded territories for *T. kleinmanni* of up to 16 ha for males and 7 ha for females. Cleary this is a huge area for a very small species, and an indicator that we can never provide too much space for any species in captivity (Fig. 8.12).

Provision of appropriately sized enclosures, as large as we can make them, is therefore essential (Divers, 1996; Varga, 2019) and can be challenging in captivity, especially for larger species such as Leopard and Sulcata tortoises (Fig. 8.13).

Exploratory behaviour

When in a suitable-sized enclosure (Varga, 2019), tortoises will walk around, climb over obstacles, and check out the boundaries and other features such as a water bath, plants, shelters, slopes and different substrates (Fig. 8.14). They will sniff the ground and any objects such as plant pots. Failure to show this type of behaviour may be indicative of poor health.

Feeding

Land tortoises that are herbivorous will spend much of the day grazing and browsing on edible plants. Omnivores will seek out small animal food items, such as snails, which move slowly enough to be eaten.

Drinking/bathing/defecating

Tortoises drink by sitting in water and pumping water into the throat. They must be partially submerged in order to do this. Opportunities for drinking are limited in the wild and are taken up whenever available. Waste urates and faeces are often produced while the tortoise is bathing. This gives keepers an opportunity to check the physical appearance and consistency of both. The state of the urates and faeces produced will give a good indication of the tortoise's overall health (see Chapter 6 on health checks).

Mating/breeding

Mating behaviour takes place throughout the year in tropical species. In Mediterranean tortoises, and other more temperate species, courtship and mating are seasonal (see Chapter 11 on breeding).

Vocalizations

Vocalizations are rare in chelonians. One exception is the 'brrrr-brrrr-brrrr' of male *Testudo kleinmanni* during mating (see Chapter 11 on breeding). Other species do vocalize during breeding with chirruping, grunting or squeaking noises. Vocalizations have been observed when chelonians are in extreme pain (Chitty and Raftery, 2013) (see Chapter 9 on emotional states).

Territorial behaviour

Some species show territorial behaviours. These include Galapagos tortoises, Leopard tortoises and Sulcata tortoises. The males want to keep the best areas for finding females so that they have the best opportunities to breed (see Chapter 11 on breeding). They will show aggression towards other males in an attempt to prevent them accessing females (Fig. 8.15). Females will try to keep other females away from the best nesting sites by physically pushing them away or trying to turn the other female away. Social hierarchy exists in some species of tortoise (see Chapter 10 on social interactions). The presence or absence (depending on the species) of other tortoises is an essential aspect of maintaining well-being, avoiding excessive stress (see Chapter 7 on common illnesses and diseases).

Social behaviour

Chapter 10 on social interactions looks at this aspect of tortoise behaviour. Interactions between animals and with human caregivers and keepers is discussed. There is evidence that tortoises are aware of individual familiar humans and that this affects their behaviour (Ward and Melfi, 2015).

Innate or instinctive behaviours in tortoises

Reflex or unconditioned behaviours do not need any learning. They happen in response to a stimulus without any control by the tortoise. For example, if you poke your finger towards a tortoise's face, the tortoise will instinctively withdraw its head. This rapid survival response is designed to prevent the head being grabbed or damaged.

These behaviours tend to be simple and quick to perform, as they are imperative for survival. The tortoise might not survive if thought and decision making were required, as these actions significantly slow response time.

The types of reflex behaviours seen in tortoises include:

- Withdrawal into the shell of head and limbs.
- Frantic head and limb flicking if they are turned over onto their backs.
- Movement away from toxic substances.
- Courtship and mating behaviours have elements of reflex behaviours.

Learning can take place linked to instinctive behaviours, so that tortoises can learn to feed more efficiently, for example through selection of the most nutritious plant material, which is found in young leaves. Tortoises can learn to be more effective when eating animal material such as invertebrates. In these examples, instinctive behaviours are developed through learning.

What kind of behaviours can be learned by tortoises?

Tortoises learn the topography or layout of their environment and are thought to have long-term memory of this aspect of their territory. Tortoises will repeatedly use the same paths and walkways through their habitat (Wegehaupt, 2009a). They can learn where different food plants and water can be found in different seasons of the year.

In captivity they can be taught stationing and targeting, as described in the examples below. Some of this training has shown how important the familiarity of the surroundings is when learning is taking place.

Positive reinforcement training (PRT) involves operant conditioning in which an animal is rewarded for responding in a particular way to a stimulus. This encourages the animal to show the same response if presented again with the same stimulus. Something the tortoise finds rewarding, such as a favoured foodstuff, acts as a reinforcer of the behaviour (Gutnik *et al.*, 2020). Tortoise memory is therefore essential for this learning to take place.

There are examples of long-term memory being shown in tortoises. Gutnik *et al.* (2020) found that Galapagos and Aldabran tortoises in Vienna and Zurich zoos (10 animals), when given the tasks of biting a target and then going to another target, could remember these tasks after 3 months. A task requiring

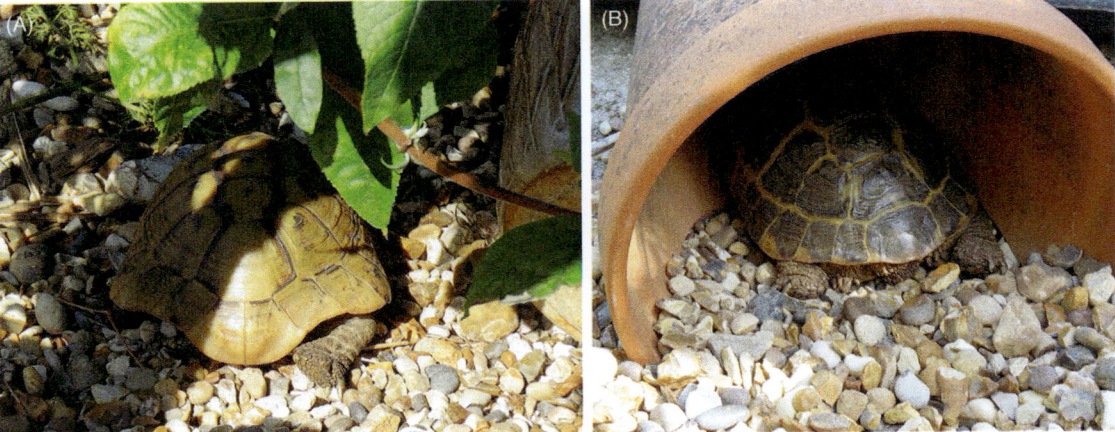

Fig. 8.9. Seeking shade from shrubs and bushes, shelters and hides. From partial shade to full shade using a variety of environmental opportunities and depending upon thermoregulatory needs in that situation.

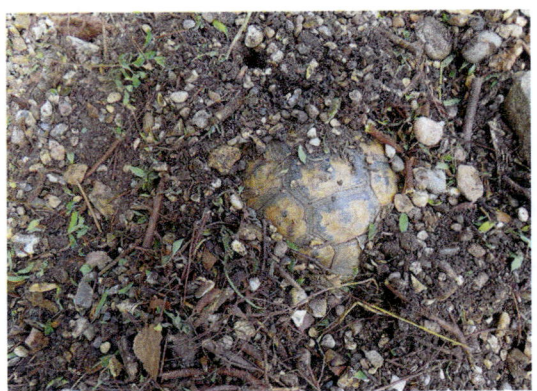

Fig. 8.10. Burrowing into the substrate to thermoregulate and to access higher humidity in the microclimate. This picture shows how difficult it may be to see a tortoise that digs in for hibernation (see Chapter 12 on hibernation) in an unsuitable location in the garden where the weather may be too cold and wet for safe hibernation.

the memory of a coloured target was then trained. The tortoises were asked to discriminate between two colours. The tortoises who had been previously target trained learned to discriminate between the two coloured targets up to three times faster than animals not previously target trained. Some animals that were tested 9 years after the initial training retained the operant conditioning to a target. This is clearly an indication of very long-term memory. Their memory of the discrimination task was not initially retained but they could relearn the task more rapidly than tortoises that had never been trained at all. Gutnik *et al.* (2020) suggest that the go-to target task is related to implicit memory, and that more specific recall of the coloured target is indicative of explicit memory. Table 8.1 explains the difference between these two types of memory and why implicit memory may allow recall more easily in the long-term (Table 8.1).

How do tortoises learn?

In order to learn, tortoises need to be able to do two things:

1. Link or associate two events.
This is the basis of **classical conditioning**, where one event predicts another, and **operant conditioning**, where a trained cue or signal stimulates a behaviour which can either be reinforced with something positive (making it more likely to occur again) or punished (making it less likely to occur again).

2. Remember previous events and associations.
Remembering what the consequences of an event were the last time and remembering whether they were pleasant or unpleasant.

Tortoises are capable of learning through both classical and operant conditioning. This means that they can be taught to link two events through classical conditioning. For example, the presence of a target stick with a large round red paddle predicts a favourite food being given (classical conditioning). Once this relationship is established, the target can be used to cue, or stimulate a desired behaviour (operant conditioning) (Mackie and Patel, 2022).

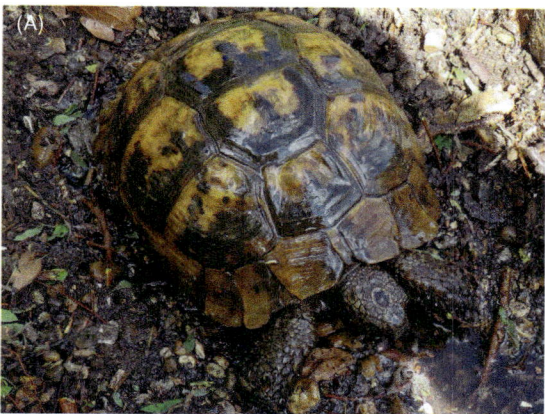 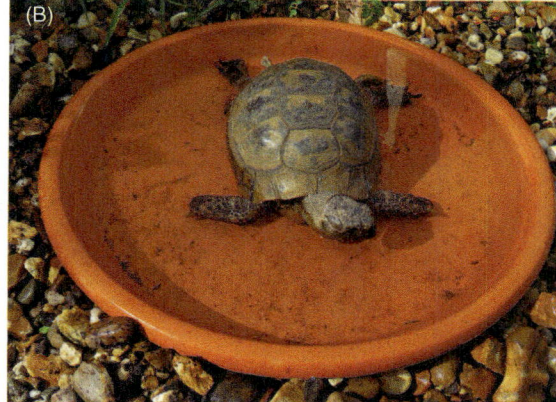

Fig. 8.11. (A) Sitting in water such as puddles. (B) Accessing other reservoirs of water to drink, excrete waste products and to thermoregulate.

Table 8.1. Long-term implicit and explicit memory (Gutnik *et al.*, 2020).

Implicit memory	Explicit memory
An example of an implicit memory could be our learning to ride a bike. Even if we do not ride the bike again for years, we would still find it easier (if we later took it up again) than someone who had never previously learnt.	Explicit memory requires us to make a conscious effort to recall facts or information. It is not always easy to recall what we learnt in school history lessons (historical dates and events, for example). We have to try to remember that information when recalling that period of our lives.

Teaching learned responses to tortoises in captivity can have a number of benefits. These include training tortoises to position themselves for preventive health checks and care, such as vaccinations, blood tests, or trimming of nails and beaks. In addition, preparation for handling and transportation is of benefit in zoo animals where there is a need to move animals from one collection to another for breeding and conservation purposes.

General principles when training

These principles apply to all reptiles.

- The animal should be maintained at a suitable temperature.
- Body position should be as natural as possible.
- Minimal handling and inversion of the body – keeping at least two limbs on a surface.
- Training through positive reinforcement (PRT) is essential – reward-based training.
- The most positive, least intrusive methods should be used – previously least invasive, minimally aversive (LIMA) or more recently the LIFE model - least inhibitive, functionally effective (Fernandez, 2023).

- Voluntary participation by the animal improves welfare and avoids force.
- Positive reinforcement improves human–animal interactions (HAI).
- Training encourages the development of coping skills for being in captivity.
- Training encourages the development of coping skills when being in the presence of humans.
- Training should take place in a familiar environment, with familiar humans (caregivers).

What are the general techniques used in training tortoises?

Desensitization, or classical conditioning, involves learning that two events are always linked. This means that the first event always predicts the second. So, if you are using a clicker, the click predicts food; ringing a bell predicts food; a bright red circle on a target stick predicts food, etc. This helps the tortoise to cope with potentially intrusive experiences because they predict something pleasant such as food. Holding a foot for examination or taking a blood draw for testing could be associated with being given a tasty treat, for example.

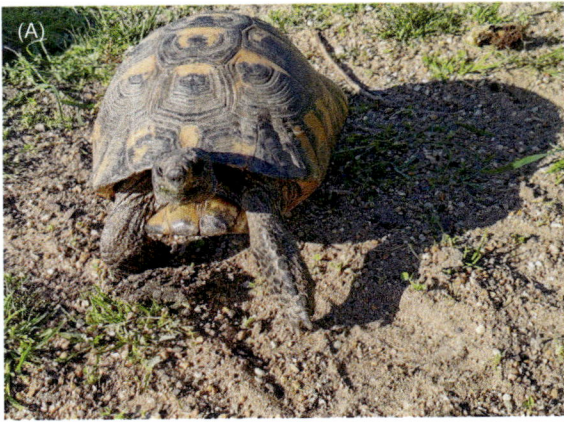
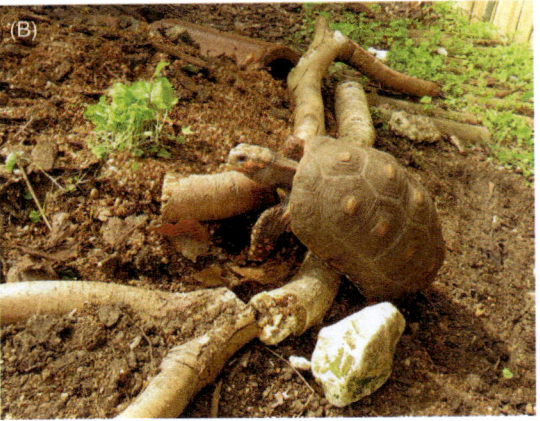

Fig. 8.12. (A) Walking and (B) climbing over obstacles is an essential behaviour taking up much the tortoise's daily activity, moving locations to find food or a mate or to thermoregulate.

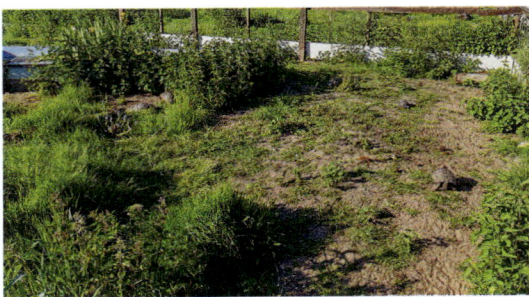

Fig. 8.13. Large enclosures provide the most suitable accommodation, given that in the wild the tortoises roam over very large areas in their daily lives.

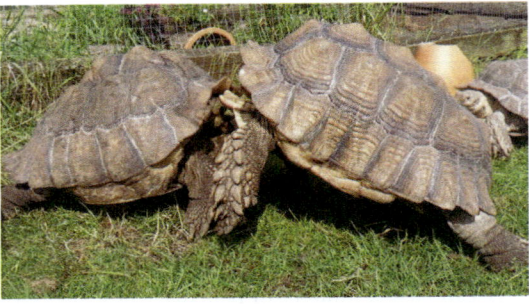

Fig. 8.15. Two Sulcata tortoises engaged in physical pushing, which may escalate into trying to turn each other over in defence of space or during competition for a female (Eleanor Lien-Hua Tirtasana Chubb).

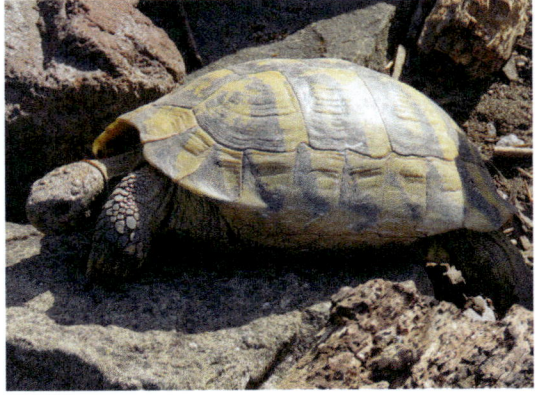

Fig. 8.14. Hermann's tortoise moving around in enclosures engaging with the environment.

It is important that the behaviour being stimulated is not a reflex response over which the tortoise has no control (see Galapagos tortoises example below).

Operant conditioning or training using three-stage model

The three stages are (A) Antecedent; (B) Behaviour; and (C) Consequence (Mackie, 2021; Varga, 2019).

- **A = Antecedent**

This is usually called the cue. It may be a visual cue such as a target stick, or the sound of a bell. It has been discovered that the environment and preparation for training are crucial when setting the animal up for success and to give the greatest opportunity for learning.

- B = Behaviour

This is the desired response, or action. It is reinforced by rewarding the behaviour with something the animal likes and wants, e.g. food.

Choice should be given between A and B so that the animal chooses to show the behaviour rather than being coerced, or forced, in any way.

- C = Consequence

This is the reinforcer (e.g. food) that rewards the desired behaviour and therefore increases the frequency with which the behaviour is shown.

When planning training for success, the following should be undertaken (Mackie, 2021):

- Set the scene in a familiar environment.
- Create calm conditions that meet environmental needs.
- Familiar caregivers should be the only people present if possible. This ensures that the people have a good knowledge and understanding of the species and of the individuals being trained.
- The goals for the training should be clearly set out in a plan.
- Offer something that the animal wants and is motivated to try to obtain (e.g. a favourite food).

What behaviours can be trained in tortoises?

Some basic behaviours can be taught.

1. Targeting – showing the tortoise a visual signal or cue, such as a target stick, which the animal is encouraged to touch. The target can also be moved to teach movement from one place to another without handling (Fig. 8.16).

2. Recall – to a visual signal or a sound (less useful in terrestrial tortoises) or vibration on the floor. This encourages the animal to come to the visual or auditory signal.

3. Stationing – using a visual signal, such as a coloured cone. The tortoise can be trained to take up a position near the signal and to stay there. This position could be on a weighing-scales, for example (Fig. 8.17).

4. Transportation – teaching familiarity with a crate or box for transportation over distances (Fig. 8.18). This encourages the tortoise to enter the small space willingly without anxiety or stress.

Examples of tortoise cognition and learning

There is evidence that newly hatched tortoises (and reptiles generally), or neonates, who are exposed to large, complex environments as soon as they are born, are more likely to develop the survival behaviours that they need for life in the wild. This includes locating routes through the environment, food and water sources and places to seek shelter in retreats (Wright and Raiti, 2019).

In the zoo setting, to minimize use of anaesthesia or restraint, stationing and target training can be used to teach large tortoises to place themselves onto weighing scales, or to follow a target stick out of their enclosure or into a travel container. Fieschi-Meric *et al.* (2022) gave the example of moving Galapagos tortoises from one enclosure to a new location at the zoo, using target training. The animals walked to the new enclosure following an operantly conditioned target, rather than manual restraint having to be used.

The desensitization to processes involving veterinary and husbandry interventions, which can be created by repeated reward-based training sessions, allows a positive association to be built up with types of handling (Freeland *et al.*, 2020). Activities needed for health checks, preventive and veterinary care, such as vaccinations, imaging and scanning, examination, sampling blood, or giving medication, can all be mitigated by training.

By training the tortoises to follow cues, handling and restraint can be kept to a minimum to reduce stress (Weiss and Wilson, 2003; Williams and Beck, 2021). The Galapagos tortoises example below from Zoological Society of London (ZSL) London Zoo shows how increasing agency for the animals, thus giving them choices about participation in procedures, improves learning. This can also improve welfare (Kish, 2018; McBride and Hinde-Megarity, 2019; Mackie and Patel, 2019).

The use of feeding stations within the enclosures to build a 'target area' can also be used to improve staff safety with some species (Mackie, 2021).

Research with giant tortoises – Aldabran tortoises (Learmonth *et al.*, 2021) and at ZSL London Zoo with Galapagos tortoises – has shown the impact of social interactions with humans (see Chapter 10 on social interactions) in the zoo setting (Fieschi-Meric *et al.*, 2022).

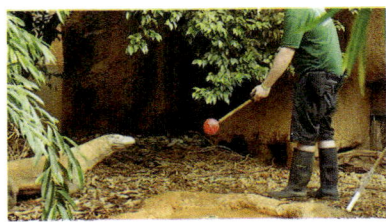

Fig. 8.16. Target training with a Komodo Dragon at ZSL London Zoo (Jim Mackie, ZSL).

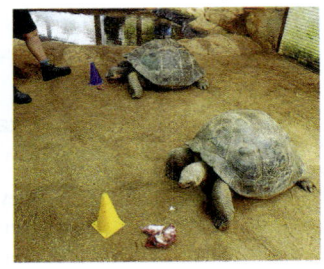

Fig. 8.17. Station training with Galapagos tortoises at ZSL London Zoo (Jim Mackie, ZSL).

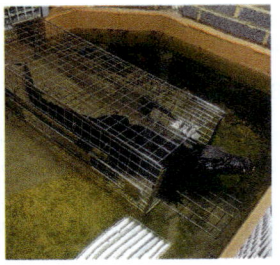

Fig. 8.18. Training to go into a crate for transportation with a crocodile at ZSL London Zoo (Jim Mackie, ZSL).

Red-footed tortoises

Tortoises have been shown to be able to learn the route through a simple Y-shaped maze. One recent study by Bridgeman and Tattersall (2019) tested Red-footed tortoises on their ability to learn to recognize and approach visual cues within a Y-maze.

The tortoises learned the visual discrimination between the two sides of the maze. They were then able to successfully learn four reversals, when the visual cue was moved from one side of the maze to the other. The previously rewarded cue was reversed, and the reward placed in the other side of the maze. Performance improved as the cues were reversed. This provided insights into the visual proficiency and behavioural flexibility of the tortoises and revealed previously unrecognized cognitive abilities (Bridgeman and Tattersall, 2019).

Mueller-Paul *et al.* (2014) demonstrated the ability of Red-footed tortoises to learn to target a touchscreen. Two of the tortoises also learned to use the touchscreen to solve a spatial two-choice task and were able to transfer their knowledge from the touchscreen to a physical arena. The researchers chose Red-footed tortoises as a highly visual species, with good colour vision and who would use vision to solve a task.

Galapagos tortoises

Many thanks are due to Jim Mackie, Laura Freeman, Charli Ellis and Chris Michaels and ZSL London Zoo, for allowing this inclusion to the chapter (full acknowledgements are at the end of the chapter). The training examples below demonstrate very effectively a degree of cognition in Galapagos tortoises, hitherto completely unknown. (There are further examples of ZSL London Zoo work in Chapter 10 on social interactions in tortoises.)

Galapagos tortoises have a mutualistic relationship with Darwin's finch. In this mutualistic relationship there is benefit for both tortoises and finches. When a finch stands near a leg of a tortoise the 'finch response' is stimulated. This response involves the tortoise stretching out its limbs and extending its neck. This allows the finch to go under the tortoise's carapace, to feed on skin parasites without being crushed by the tortoise.

This reflex response had been used in ZSL London Zoo for some time to draw blood from the necks of their Galapagos tortoises (Bryant *et al.*, 2016). The advantage is that manual restraint of these large animals is no longer necessary. The keeper stimulates the reflex by touching the tortoise's legs. This mimics finch behaviour. The behaviour being stimulated is a reflex response, however, so the tortoise initially responds automatically. Once stimulated, the tortoise extends the neck and limbs, allowing the blood-draw procedure to take place. Food was used as a reinforcer, and food was used to move the tortoise into position for the blood-draw (lure and reward training). This is considered to be a modal action pattern (MAP), which, although in-built (innate), is shaped by experience. 'Over time the tortoise would actually drop the carapace to the floor if the conditions were not right, which would prevent the action of the tactile stimulation happening at all' (Mackie, personal communication).

The training for the procedure was carried out in a temperature-controlled, familiar environment, with the familiar keeper and one member of the veterinary team, in as calm a situation as possible.

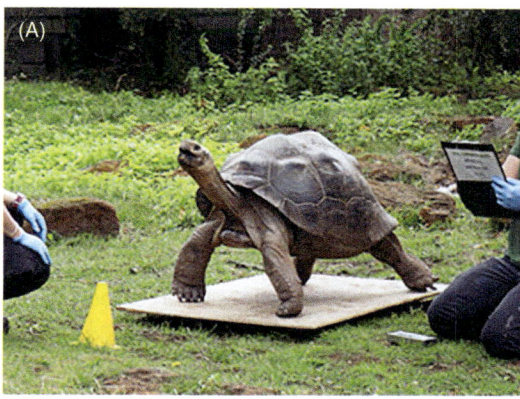 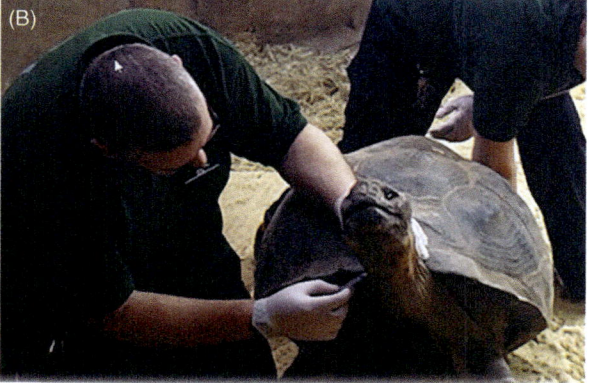

Fig. 8.19. ZSL training set-up (A) for weighing and health checks, and (B) for a blood draw (Jim Mackie).

The staff wanted to give the tortoises the choice to participate, or not, and therefore to be able to choose whether the blood was to be taken, or not. Choice was given to participate before the stimulation of that largely reflex behaviour.

The tortoises were given the opportunity to take up a position – stationing – at either a yellow or a purple cone, thus giving them choice. The cone was the cue used to station individuals, which acted like a 'start button'. 'If they approached the cone, that was taken as an indicator that the tortoise wanted to participate to gain valued food reinforcers. The keeper would be standing up during the stationing and once the tortoise was in the correct position, the action of the keeper crouching beside the tortoise was the cue for the tortoise to extend the neck (like the finch that lands next to the tortoise in the wild).' Only if the neck began to be extended would the keeper begin the tactile work on the base of the neck or the rear under the carapace, in the hope that this was the moment greater agency was being offered to the animal. The keepers' conclusion from this work is that, as well as being a reflexive response, there is a reinforcing value to the tactile stimulus (Mackie, personal communication).

'In addition to these processes, more time was spent gradually exposing (through desensitization) the tortoise to the various equipment needed for blood draws, radiograph, nasal and eye swabs as well as the extra veterinary personal. If at any time, the neck retracted, the trainer took this as a signal that the tortoise was not comfortable and removed the stimulus. Over time, the trainer became more aware of the precursors to the withdrawal and was able to remove the stimulus before retraction. This constitutes a form of non-coercive negative reinforcement (increasing neck extension behaviour by removing stimulus).' (Mackie, personal communication). The complexity of training demonstrated through positive and negative reinforcement, graduated exposure therapy, classical conditioning and modal action patterns, illustrates just how complex the learning processes are in these tortoises.

The behaviour being recreated is therefore much more like the natural situation. In the Galapagos, the finch stands beside the tortoise to stimulate the response and then waits until the tortoise starts to stretch before going under the carapace. Trained behaviours can therefore be used to give animals choice or agency. As a result of giving choice, welfare is improved (Fig. 8.19).

Conclusion

In domestic settings we rarely consider the sorts of training activities described here with our tortoises. We are all aware, however, of the need to provide enrichment and choice within the environment (see Chapter 3 on the captive environment). The results of these training activities in zoos demonstrate a higher level of cognitive function and sentience than was previously realized. The ability to learn complex tasks has been clearly established in tortoises. There is much more work to do in researching other aspects of tortoise behaviour in relation to memory (long- and short-term), together with the impact on learning of environment and the impact of the presence of other tortoises and humans on learned behaviour.

A useful summary of considerations for provision made for our captive tortoises (and reptiles as a whole group) comes from Wilkinson and Burman (2022), who suggested the following.

1. A cognitively enriched environment should be a default for all reptile species.
2. Reptiles can, and do, learn to navigate around space to meet their needs and remember salient experiences – often for long periods of time. The design of their enclosures and husbandry regimes should therefore reflect this.
3. Personality/temperament differences between individuals of the same species may necessitate the 'tailoring' of housing and husbandry to match individual needs.
4. Observing both generic and species-specific behaviour can tell us about reptile welfare.
5. Reptiles should have sufficient space to perform their natural behaviours.
6. Reptiles can experience both moods and emotions; they are therefore capable of suffering but also experiencing positive mood states. This should be taken into account in all aspects of their housing and husbandry.

These considerations are important when making decisions for our tortoises regarding environmental provision, living alone or in groups, and opportunities for learning as part of enrichment.

In the future, as we understand more about learning in tortoises, training may become a much more common activity carried out with captive tortoises, potentially leading to greater enrichment and mental stimulation in the lives of captive tortoises in all settings.

Acknowledgements

Sincere thanks to Jim Mackie for making me aware of this work in a number of presentations and personal communications, and to his colleagues at the Zoological Society of London (ZSL) and London Zoo. The staff involved in this pioneering work to be thanked, along with ZSL London Zoo, are: Luke Harding (Blue Iguana Conservation); Grant Kother (Animal Behaviour Consultant); Charli Ellis (ZSL); Joe Capon (ZSL); Jim Mackie (ZSL); Thomas Maunders (ZSL); Iri Gill (Chester Zoo); Laura Freeland; Chris Michaels; and Matthew Rendle (RVN).

References and Further Reading

Biedenweg, F. and Schramm, R. (2019) *The Egyptian Tortoise* Testudo kleinmanni *Lortet 1883: A Fascinating Little Beauty*. Tartaruga-Verlag, Germany.

Bridgeman J.M. and Tattersall G.J. (2019) Tortoises develop and overcome position biases in a reversal learning task. *Animal Cognition* 22(2), 265–275.

Bryant, Z., Harding, L., Grant, S. and Rendle, M. (2016) A method for blood sampling the Galápagos tortoise, *Chelonoidis nigra* using operant conditioning for voluntary blood draws. Zoological Society of London, London Zoo, UK. *The Herpetological Bulletin* 135, 7–10.

Chitty, J. and Raftery, A. (2013) *Essentials of Tortoise Medicine and Surgery*. Wiley Blackwell, Chichester, UK.

Divers, S. (1996) Basic reptile husbandry, history taking and clinical examination. *Veterinary Record In Practice* 18(51), 51–65.

Fernandez, E.J. (2023) The least inhibitive, functionally effective (LIFE) model: A new framework for ethical animal training practices. *Journal of Veterinary Behavior* 71, 63–68.

Fieschi-Meric, L., Ellis, C., Servini, F., Tapley, B. and Michaels, C.J. (2022) An improvement in enclosure design can positively impact welfare, reduce aggressiveness and stabilise hierarchy in captive Galapagos giant tortoises. *Journal of Zoological and Botanical Gardens* 3, 499–512.

Freeland, L., Ellis, C. and Michaels C.J. (2020) Documenting aggression, dominance and the impacts of visitor interaction on Galápagos tortoises (*Chelonoidis nigra*) in a zoo setting. *Animals* (Basel) 10(4), 699. DOI: 10.3390/ani10040699.

Gutnick, T., Weissenbacher, A. and Kuba, M.J. (2020) The Underestimated Giants: Operant conditioning, visual discrimination and long-term memory in giant tortoises. *Animal Cognition* 23, 159–167.

Kish, C. (2018) Choice control and training for ectotherms. *IAABC Foundation Journal*, Issue 8.

Learmonth, M.J., Sherwen, S. and Hemsworth, P.H. (2021) Assessing preferences of two zoo-housed Aldabran giant tortoises (*Aldabrachelys gigantea*) for three stimuli using a novel preference test. *ZooBiol* 40(2), 98–106.

Mackie, J. (2021) Animal Behaviour Management Officer at Zoological Society of London (ZSL) London Zoo, as part of the work of BIAZA (British and Irish Zoos and Aquariums Association) Animal Behaviour and Training Working Group, Reptile Training in Zoos RAWG presentation and personal communications.

Mackie, J. and Patel, C. (2022) Ch 6 Welfare-focused animal training. In: Rendle, M. and Hinde-Megarity, J. (eds) *BSAVA Manual of Practical Veterinary Welfare*. BSAVA, Quedgeley, UK, pp. 146–165.

McArthur, S., Wilkinson, R. and Hernandez-Divers, S. (2004) *Medicine and Surgery of Tortoises and Turtles*. Blackwell, Oxford, UK.

McBride, A. and Hinde-Megarity, J. (2022) Ch 3 Animal behaviour. In: Rendle, M. and Hinde-Megarity, J. (eds) *BSAVA Manual of Practical Veterinary Welfare*. BSAVA, Quedgeley, UK, pp. 71–103.

Mueller-Paul, J., Wilkinson, A., Steurer, M., Hall, G. and Huber, L. (2014) Touchscreen performance and knowledge transfer in the red-footed tortoise (*Chelonoidis carbonaria*). *Behavioural Processes* 106, 187–192.

Varga, M. (2019) Ch 3 Captive maintenance. In: Girling, S.J. and Raiti, P. (eds) *BSAVA Manual of Reptiles*. BSAVA, Quedgeley, UK, pp. 36–68.

Ward, S.J. and Melfi, V. (2015) Keeper–animal linteractions: differences between the behaviour of zoo animals affect stockmanship. *PLoS ONE* 10, e0140237

Wegehaupt, W. (2009a) *Mediterranean Tortoises, Where and how they live in the wild*. Kressbronn, Germany

Wegehaupt, W. (2009b) *Naturalistic Keeping and Breeding of Hermann's Tortoises*. Kressbronn, Germany

Weiss, E. and Wilson, S.J. (2003) The use of classical and operant conditioning in training Aldabra tortoises (*Geochelone gigantea*), for venipuncture and other husbandry issues. *Applied Animal Welfare Science* 6(1), 33–38.

Wilkinson, A. and Burman, O. (2022) *Cold-blooded care: How reptile behaviour and cognition research can inform our understanding of reptile welfare*. Prof. Anna Wilkinson and Prof. Oliver Burman (University of Lincoln). Contact: awilkinson@lincoln.ac.uk; oburman@lincoln.ac.uk

Williams, J. (2017) Stress in Chelonia (tortoises, terrapins and turtles). *The Veterinary Nurse* 8(5)

Williams, J. and Beck, D. (2021) Stress, anxiety, fear and frustration in different reptile species: How to reduce these negative emotional states during veterinary procedures. *Veterinary Nursing Journal* 36.

Wright, K. and Raiti, P. (2019) Ch 5 Breeding and neonatal care. In: Girling, S.J. and Raiti, P. (eds) *BSAVA Manual of Reptiles*. BSAVA, Quedgeley, UK, pp. 70–88.

9 Emotional States in Tortoises

Abstract
This chapter is a discussion of the potential emotional states of tortoises, and includes ways of identifying those emotional states. The impact of mental well-being, and emotional well-being, is as important as physical health when considering welfare. The physical features of tortoises that make the identification of emotional states challenging are described. Identifying a happy, stressed or anxious tortoise is very difficult. These emotional states are as yet undefined in terms of appearance or behaviour in most reptiles.

Stress, distress and anxiety are extremely difficult to identify in tortoises. In order to avoid stress, good environmental conditions, husbandry and health are essential. Maintaining tortoises in captivity with their welfare and well-being as the priority is key to reducing poor mental health. Acute stress may be seen as a result of handling, veterinary treatment and transportation, especially if done badly. Stress is, however, more likely to be chronic, due to long-term poor environmental conditions or bad practice in husbandry.

Maintaining tortoises in a good emotional state is vital to maintain overall well-being and welfare.

What are the main indicators of emotional state?

There are two main indicators:

- Physical health – without disease or illness and with normal body form, shape and structure (no deformities due to abnormal growth and development).
- Showing normal behaviours – as seen in ectotherms, including thermoregulatory behaviours, basking, burrowing, seeking shade, walking, climbing, digging, hiding.

Additional indicators:

- Feeding with good appetite
- Reproductive behaviours

Behavioural changes in tortoises are the first signs of stress, distress, injury or disease. Similarly physical signs and symptoms may indicate a behavioural problem (Warwick *et al.*, 2013). This article notes that using behavioural indicators of well-being and welfare is important but should always be contextualized. For example, in captivity is the enclosure space so small and the environmental provision so lacking in enrichment and opportunity that normal behaviour for a wild tortoise, such as walking many kilometres in a day, is seen as a repetitive, pacing behaviour, indicative of stress and frustration?

What is a 'happy' tortoise?

Identifying the emotional state of a tortoise at any given time is challenging for a number of reasons. The physical features of a tortoise tend to limit signalling opportunities (Williams and Beck, 2021). They also limit the opportunities for clear behavioural signals.

Lambert *et al.* (2019) looked into sentience, which is the ability to have feelings, to perceive fear or joy, in reptiles. His study found 'at least eight different aspects of sentience in the scientific literature. These are anxiety, distress, excitement, fear, frustration, pain, stress, and suffering.' None of these refer to happiness or contentment. There are only a small number of studies identified by Lambert *et al.* (2019) that have explored, and found evidence of, emotions and a state of pleasure in reptiles. Recently, however, more studies examining emotional states appear to be taking place in zoo collections and in field research (Doody *et al.*, 2021).

Identifying a 'happy' tortoise is very difficult and is as yet undefined in terms of appearance or behaviour. Often in this field, it is negative emotions that can be more clearly identified. Identification of anxiety and fear is often more clearly defined than the absence of these emotions. When considering a contented tortoise, it would be logical to think that one that has its physical needs met is more likely to be in a positive emotional state than one that is lacking in some basic need. Figure 9.1 shows examples of tortoises in different emotional states.

A tortoise that has choices in its environmental provision, which allow the animal to achieve physiological homeostasis, is one that is more likely to be calm, relaxed and content (to use these human descriptors of emotional states). Feeling happy as a tortoise is something we can largely only imagine, but if we apply human criteria and consider when we feel happy this is most likely to be when we are well fed, comfortable, relaxed and not in danger; perhaps with other humans whose company we enjoy. This aspect of human health has been very well examined with the work of Maslow (1943) identifying the levels of human need. This work has been developed to examine needs from a non-human perspective (McBride and Hinde-Megarity, 2022). The revised pyramid refers to being in physiological homeostasis as the starting point for well-being and includes, at higher levels, references to the Five Freedoms (now Five Domains) (Deane and Valentine, 2022).

Identifying happy, or at least comfortable, relaxed tortoises has not been researched to any extent. The criteria for the assessment of these emotional states have yet to be defined in these animals. If we can define fear and frustration, we also need to try to define the opposite emotional states. We should also remember that lack of ability to demonstrate emotional state does not mean that those states do not exist. Kabelik's work (2021) in lizards demonstrated similar brain physiology to that of mammals, with regard to release of hormones linked to stress responses (e.g. corticotropin-releasing factor, or CRF). The lizards may not have been able to demonstrate stress in a way that humans can perceive, but the physiological and emotional responses were present.

How do tortoises express their feelings?

The types of behaviour, facial expression and body language that could be used to express emotional states could include the following (McBride and Hinde-Megarity, 2022).

- Vocalizations – some tortoises vocalize during mating (e.g. 'brrrr' in *T. kleinmanni*) but a tortoise's physical structure limits the opportunity for sound creation as well as volume.
- Mouth open or closed – gaping is associated with temperature regulation and may be an indicator of thermal stress due to overheating.
- Change in body position or posture – holding the body clear of the ground or flattening to the ground.
- Degree of relaxation – difficult to define but could relate to willingness to extend head and limbs and whether limbs are extending out or resting on the ground.
- Walking away – from perceived threat or aversive stimulus.
- Pushing/nudging objects – perceived as threats.
- Sniffing – of the ground, food, objects or other tortoises as a sign of exploratory behaviour.
- Staring – eyes focused and in fixed position orienting towards the ground, food, objects or other tortoises.
- Chasing, circling, biting, head-butting – sexually driven courtship and mating behaviours in different species, indicative of sexual arousal and excitement.
- Biting, charging, butting, flipping – directed at other tortoises in competition for a mate, nesting site or for territory in agonistic (aggressive) species.
- Scrabbling of limbs – to try to gain purchase on a solid surface when some or all limbs are raised off the ground.
- Repetitive head and limb flicking – in response to being upside down (a very stressful position for any tortoise, potentially life-threatening).
- Defensive reaction to handling or a strongly aversive stimulus – generally seen as withdrawal into the shell with a reluctance/refusal to come out again.

As Figs 9.2 and 9.3 indicate, changes in emotional state are not easily communicated by tortoises, due to their fixed faces.

Wilkinson and Burman (2022) suggested that as reptiles can experience both moods and emotions, they experience positive mood states, as well as negative emotions. They reported that tortoises are faster to move and extend their necks further when they are more relaxed. These behavioural indications of emotional state are relatively easy for us to identify as keepers.

I own a male Spur-thighed tortoise called Tommy, who many years ago developed URTD or runny nose syndrome. He was taken to a vet for treatment, and it was decided that, as the infection had persisted for some time and the nasal discharge was changing from a clear free-flowing liquid into cloudy more viscous mucus, he needed antibiotics.

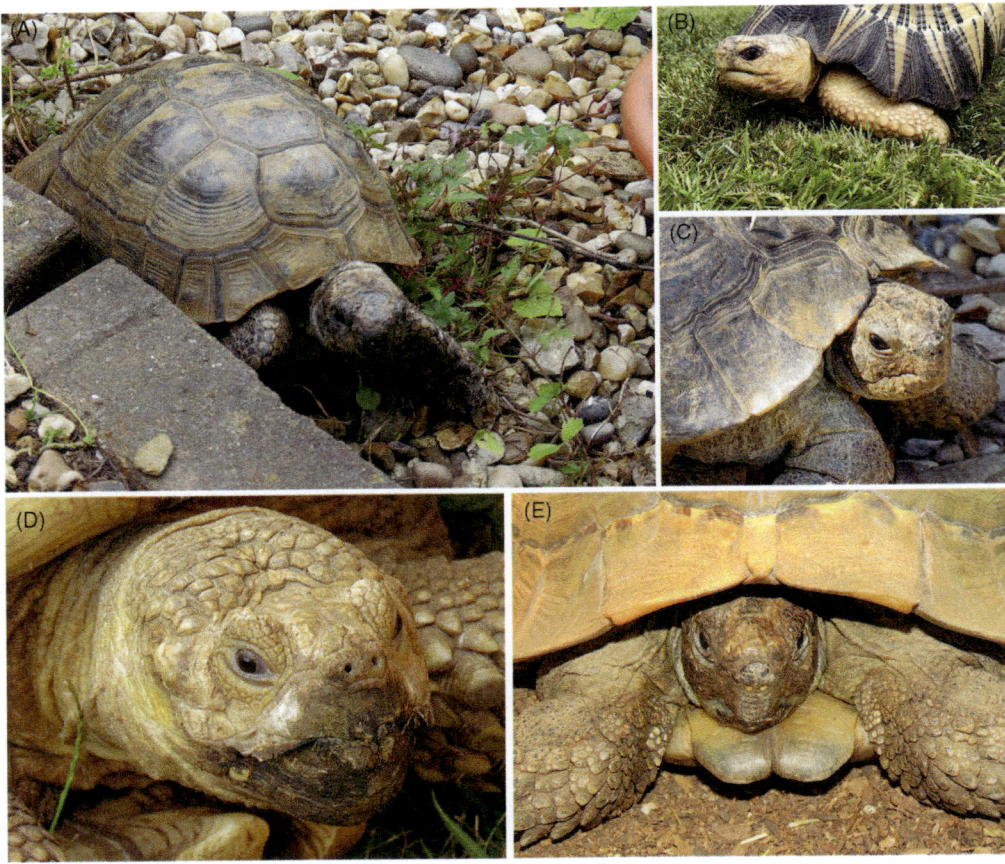

Fig. 9.1. Are these happy, contented tortoises? This is very difficult to determine; the context and circumstances are essential in order to determine likely emotional state. (A) Spur-thighed male resting in enclosure. (B) Radiated tortoise resting on lawn. (C) Spur-thighed female who has been digging and eating. (D) Male Sulcata very interested in what is happening around him in an unfamiliar environment. (E) Very unwell female Spur-thighed tortoise with a painful condition called gout.

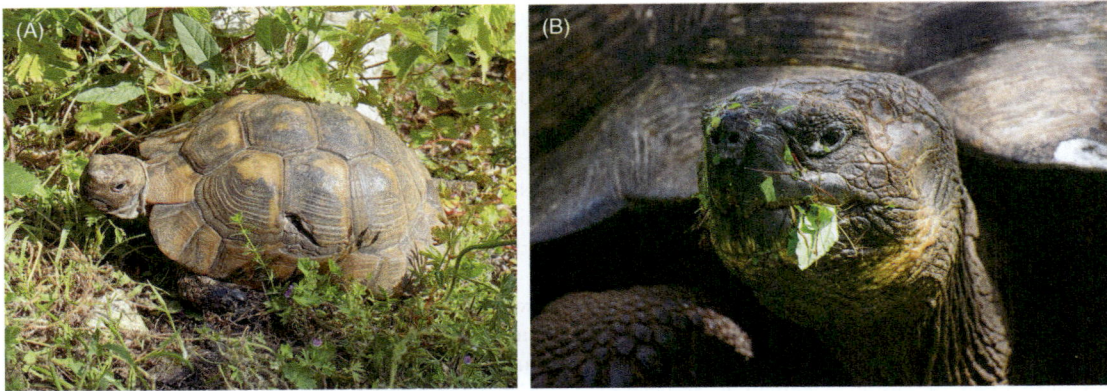

Fig. 9.2. (A) Relaxed-looking female Spur-thighed tortoise resting in a sea of edible plants. (B) Alert Galapagos tortoise (Gary Franklin).

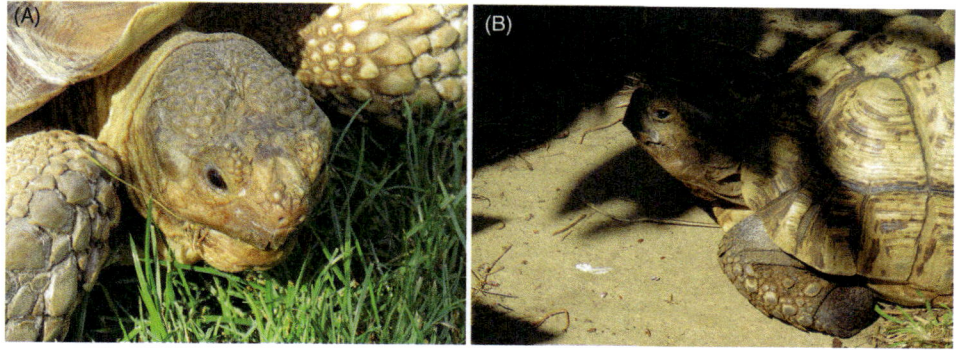

Fig. 9.3. Tortoises feeding and moving showing more signs of alertness and interest. (A) Male Sulcata eating on a newly available piece of grass. (B) Male Leopard tortoise alert to novel movement (me) in the enclosure.

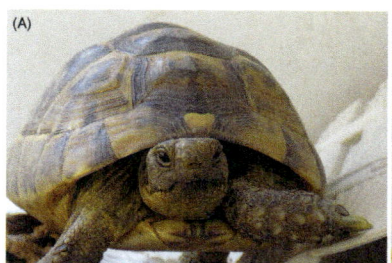
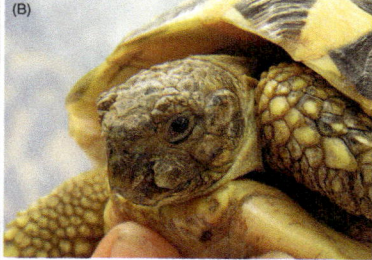
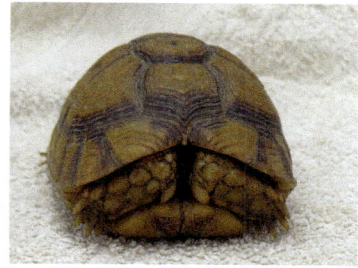

Fig. 9.4. (A) Happy tortoise in indoor enclosure. (B) Unhappy tortoise being held for a health check.

Fig. 9.5. Tortoise completely withdrawn into shell with head and all four limbs protected.

These were to be given by injection in the limbs every other day, alternating between all four limbs. The vet gave the first injection into the right front leg. Tommy had been quite prepared to walk on the examination table prior to the vet holding onto his leg and restraining it to insert the needle. Following the injection, he refused to put that leg out on the table and, although he continued to move about, showed clear signs of distress and discomfort in that leg. He refused to put the leg outside of the shell for some hours, preferring to walk with three legs rather than expose it. The same behaviour was shown when the injections were repeated at home as directed by the vet, with his refusal to extend the limb that had received the injection for several hours after treatment.

Veterinary examinations, health checks and clinical treatments are all experiences that are likely to be very stressful for tortoises. The transportation, handling and exposure to unfamiliar people are all stressors, over and above any examination or treatment required (Divers, 1996; McArthur *et al.*, 2004; Chitty and Raftery, 2013; Fazio *et al.*, 2014; Ward and Melfi, 2015; Rayment-Dyble, 2019, p. 34; Williams and Beck, 2021).

Definitions

Without good health and welfare, a tortoise will not be able to avoid stress and distress. Stress is a term widely used as a negative emotional state – we all sometimes feel stressed, as we would describe it, and we often link it to anxiety. In fact, stress is an essential part of life for all species, created by the environment as a result of change (Gray, 1987). This is something that all living organisms have to be able to respond to if they are to survive. Problems occur when those stress levels rise, and remain elevated, for extended periods. Then stress becomes distress.

In the same way, we use anxiety and fear interchangeably but as terms they do have different meanings as is indicated in Table 9.1.

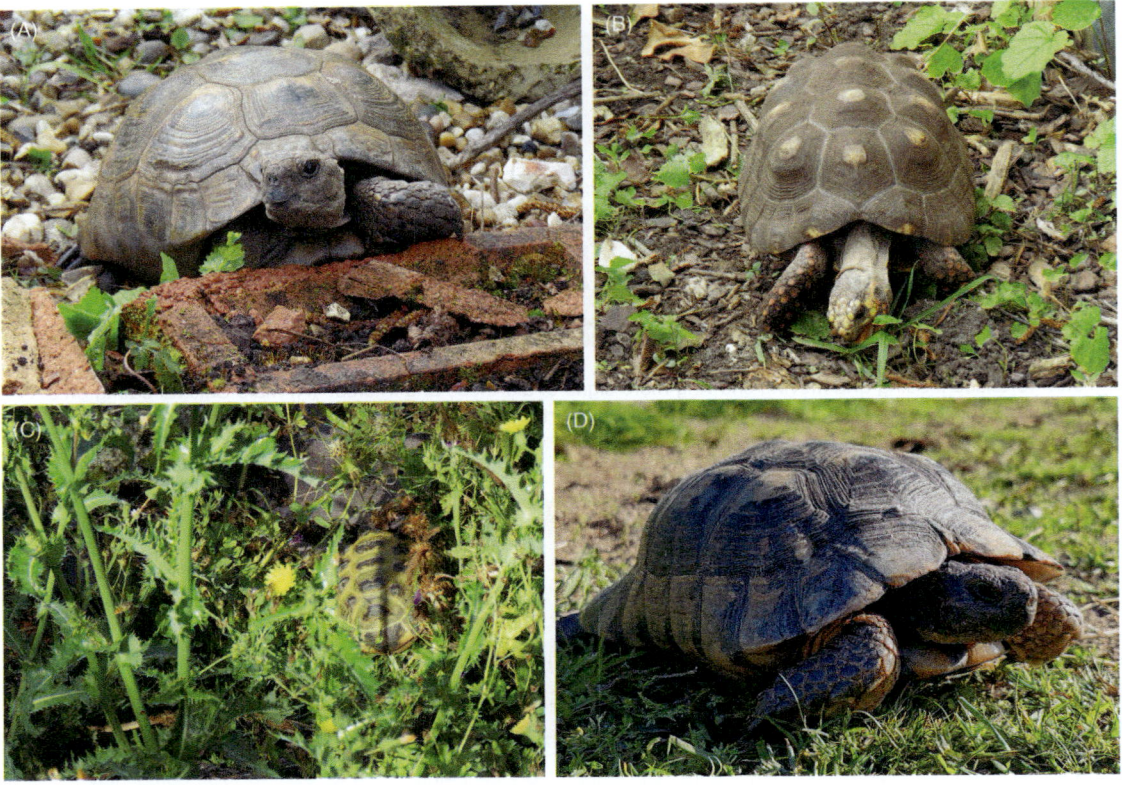

Fig. 9.6. Tortoises behaving normally in their enclosures. (A) Spur-thighed female. (B) Red-footed female. (C) Horsfield's in enclosure. (D) Marginated tortoise (Dillon Prest).

What are the signs of stress, distress, anxiety and fear in tortoises?

Tortoises have hard scaly skin, covered in shields or scutes. A large part of their body is encased in a hard immobile shell. Tortoises cannot show facial expressions, due to the fixed scales of the head – they cannot smile, grimace or frown. They cannot therefore show these clear indicators of emotional state (Fig. 9.4) (Williams and Beck, 2021).

Tortoises also have limited limb movements because of the fixed nature of the shell, which largely encloses their body. The articulation between head and limbs and the shell is limited and restricts movement, thus reducing the opportunity to demonstrate body language or posturing. Tortoises do not vocalize to any significant extent. Emotional expressions of relaxation or pleasure, distress, fear, frustration or pain are therefore difficult to identify. This does not mean that they are not feeling these emotions, but communicating and signalling of them to others is not easy (Deane and Valentine, 2022; McBride and Hinde-Megarity, 2022).

Identifying fearful behaviours is not easy in tortoises, although there are some clear indicators in extreme situations. For example, when tortoises withdraw into their shell and will not protrude their head or legs, it is a sign that their environment has become so alarming that they feel obliged to withdraw completely from it and the potential threat (Fig. 9.5) (McArthur et al., 2004).

Warwick et al. (2013) identified a number of behavioural signs of stress in captivity, including the summary in Table 9.2, which identifies signs and causes particularly relevant to tortoises.

Sudden forced ejection of large volumes of urine is commonly seen on handling or veterinary treatment or during transportation. This is an indication of high levels of stress and fear in tortoises. Defecation is not uncommon in these situations, for similar reasons (Williams and Beck, 2021). The proximity of unfamiliar humans, restraining the tortoise's body, or

Table 9.1. Definitions of emotional states (Gray, 1987; Panksepp, 1998).

Term	Definition
Sentience	Ability to experience feelings and sensations.
Emotional states	Mental states associated with feelings, thoughts, concepts, moods brought about by neurophysiological change.
Stress	Mental and emotional state created by adversity or challenging situations, leading to anxiety and a heightened state.
Distress	Extreme feelings of anxiety, worry, grief, pain may lead to distress
Anxiety	Mental and physical state of negative expectations leading to a heightened state of readiness, increased arousal and anticipation. An anticipation of something unpleasant or frightening happening based on past experience.
Fear	The presence of a frightening stimulus – object, person, or situation, leads to physiological changes, such as increased adrenaline levels. This causes increased heart and breathing rate, which readies the animal to take action in order to survive the perceived threat. Fear is an essential survival mechanism, allowing organisms to react to potentially life-threatening situations. The response is referred to as the FLIGHT, FIDDLE ABOUT, FREEZE, FIGHT mechanism.
Excitement	An emotional state characterized by arousal, heightened anticipation, enthusiasm and desire. This can be perceived in a pleasurable way or in a predatory or sexual way.
Frustration	Arises from an inability to achieve desired goals or aims, because these have been thwarted and prevented from being fulfilled. For example, being able to see a delicious food but not being able to reach it. These feelings are closely linked to anger and disappointment.
Pain and suffering	Pain is a physical sensation due to neurological changes caused by information sent to the brain. It is generated as a result of any part of the body experiencing tissue damage, disease or infection. Pain is therefore linked to physical and mental discomfort and distress. Suffering is the emotional expression of this pain and distress.

Table 9.2. Signs of stress in captive tortoises.

Behaviour signs	Potential causes
Repeated attempts to get out through transparent barriers, including glass and wire	Failure to recognize abstract invisible barriers. Attempts to escape enclosures that are too small. Attempts to find a mate for breeding.
Hyper- or hypo-activity	Very active/inactive due to over-crowding or too small an enclosure. Disease or illness may lead to reduced activity. Low temperature may lead to inactivity. May be found hiding in colder locations within the enclosure for extended periods due to disease, injury or pain.
Hesitancy of movement, jerky limb movements	Fear, pain, too small an enclosure, which is restrictive of movements.
Failure to respond to novel stimuli or food	Fear, pain, disease, stress.
Prolonged withdrawal of head, tail and limbs	Fear, pain, disease, stress.
Aggression towards other tortoises	May be defensive or aggressive if related to competition for territories, resources or mates. Courtship may involve biting, chasing, shell ramming as normal parts of the mating ritual.

moving its head or limbs into unnatural positions may all contribute to fear-based responses.

Training the tortoise to cope with this can be done as part of carrying out regular health checks. Such training may help reduce the negative effects felt by the tortoise (see Chapter 8 on behaviour and learning).

In severe circumstances, stress may lead to distress as a result of pain. Chitty and Raftery (2013) identified pain indicators developed from observations, as shown in Table 9.3 (Chitty and Raftery, 2013; Williams, 2017).

Fazio et al. (2014) found that in a study of 23 healthy juveniles (*Testudo hermanni*) cortisol levels were greatly increased for more than 4 weeks after handling and a short transportation experience. Cortisol is often referred to as the stress hormone, as it helps an animal to cope with stress. Here the cortisol levels may have been increased to allow the animals to return to physiological homeostasis following stressful experiences.

Table 9.3. Pain indicators in Chelonia.

Indicator	Comments
Anorexia	Failure to feed is always an indicator of poor health or stress. This frequently occurs post-hibernation or during normal hot summer months.
Resentment of palpation	Reluctance to have limbs held or manipulated may indicate pain due to medical condition, e.g. gout, swelling or injury.
Dragging limbs or body	Indicates loss of muscle strength or nerve function to control and move limbs and/or body. Often seen as a result of metabolic bone disease.
Failure to raise body from surface	Tortoise lacks muscle strength or nerve function and/or feels too unwell to raise itself.
Raising body abnormally	Tortoise is raising its body away from a surface that may be too hot; or may be feeling pain or distress in lower abdomen, limbs or due to reproductive problems.
Urination	Loss of urine in hibernation indicates a stress event (tortoise must be woken up immediately) or sudden forced ejection of large volume may indicate stress/distress/pain.
Ataxia	Inability to move at all, suggests very significant health issue or very high distress or pain levels.
Biting/rubbing lesion	Pain or discomfort within limbs or shell due to damage.
Withdrawal of head or limb(s)	A clear indicator of a sense of threat from the environment – a reflex defensive survival mechanism.
Rapid rocking of front limbs (due to respiratory distress)	Rapid rocking of front limbs (due to respiratory distress) Indicative of serious health issue caused by respiratory distress, but may be indicative of wider health issues.
Head and front leg flicking – repeatedly side to side	Occurs when tortoise is held vertically off a surface and wants to be set down onto a flat surface, or is held upside down on its back.
Lameness	Damage to limbs, disease in limbs, lack of strength in limbs, due to vitamin or mineral deficiency.
Defecation	A reflexive response in many animals associated with extreme fear levels
Closed eyes	Often indicative of general poor health due to vitamin or mineral deficiency or some generalized condition.
Reduced/no activity	As a tortoise becomes increasingly unwell, often due to poor environmental conditions or husbandry, activity is reduced. May be seen over many years, for example due to excessively long hibernation periods.
Neck stretching	Pushing the head out and extending the neck to its fullest length can indicate pain and distress in other areas of the body.
Vocalizations – screaming in extreme pain	Very few species vocalize – some males during mating e.g. 'brrrr-brrrr-brrrr' of male *T. kleinmanni*. Observed only rarely in animals in extreme pain.
Gaping	Used to temperature-regulate, but may sometimes indicate respiratory or other distress as the tortoise struggles to increase oxygen intake.

What are the signs of calmness and comfort?

Identification of signs of quiescence and comfort are more difficult to determine, as discussed above. Warwick *et al.* (2013) suggested that the following behaviours, which are possible in tortoises, may indicate these relaxed states:

- Relaxed breathing, feeding, drinking.
- Unhurried body movements and walking.
- Body posture and orientation indicate calmness and relaxed pose within the environment.
- Relaxed interest in nearby or novel objects.
- Calm sniffing and smelling of nearby objects, other tortoises.

What are the welfare implications of stress, distress, anxiety and fear in tortoises?

Long-term or chronic distress and fear are detrimental to the health of any animal. In captive tortoises, we have a responsibility to ensure that the way in which we keep them minimizes these negative emotional states. Anything that can be done to reduce distress will be helpful. This will largely be achieved through adequate environmental provision, good husbandry and appropriate social grouping for species that live in groups in the wild.

Long-term distress and anxiety will contribute to poor health and well-being and may result in physical illness. There is also a negative impact on the ability to learn if welfare considerations are poorly maintained (see Chapter 8 on behaviour and learning).

Reduction of negative emotions such as fear and frustration can be achieved through environmental enrichment and by offering choice and control in the tortoise's enclosure. Adequate space for movement, and to access thermal gradients for thermoregulation, will enable tortoises to maintain their preferred body temperature and so improve welfare. This can be aided by the provision of microclimates created to provide opportunities to hide and bask in warm and cold areas.

How can the effects of handling and treatment be reduced?

Teaching tortoises to target objects and to stand at a station can help to reduce the negative effects of regular health checks and treatments such as vaccinations, or beak, feet and nail trims. The training process prepares the tortoise to cope with the handling and sensations associated with these procedures. Illustrations of this type of training are shown in Chapter 8 on behaviour and learning.

Diagnosis and treatment may well require invasive techniques. Blood analysis, endoscopy and biopsy are all commonly used techniques. Ultrasound and radiography have the advantage of not being invasive and are often possible without sedation.

Sometimes a procedure such as inserting an oesophagostomy feeding tube, instead of repeated handling and manipulation of the head and limbs for gavage tubing of a sick tortoise, may be much less stressful to the tortoise. This is always going to be an ethical dilemma and ultimately a decision to be taken with your veterinarian.

More recently, techniques have been developed for the sampling of cortisol levels from faecal samples. This totally removes the stressful handling required for blood sampling (Carbajal *et al.*, 2019). Developments such as these will continue to improve welfare by making sampling much more straightforward and less invasive.

If tortoises are to be transported (to the vet, for example), heat pads or hot-water bottles should be used to maintain the preferred body temperature. This will reduce thermal stress (McArthur *et al.*, 2004; Chitty and Raftery, 2013, 2014; Williams and Beck, 2021).

Conclusion

There is a great deal of further research and investigation needed if we are to improve our understanding of tortoise learning, behaviour and emotional states. Research in this field remains in the very early stages.

Until recently the mental and emotional states of tortoises was not even considered in most situations. Physical health has always been the focus. Moving forward, there is greater emphasis on the holistic perspective of health and well-being, and a greater understanding of the need to consider environmental enrichment and stimulation. There is also work going on in the field of learning and training (see Chapter 8 on behaviour and learning). Social interaction between tortoises as a source of either stress or fulfilment, depending upon the species, is now also being considered (see Chapter 10 on social interactions).

Keeping tortoises well includes them having a positive mental state and being emotionally calm and in a state of comfort. Careful daily observations of behaviour and habits are essential in achieving this. Keeping tortoises well in captivity is much more demanding than most people realize. These tortoises appear to be 'happy' and emotionally well; objectively defining and measuring such mental states is a more challenging proposition altogether (Fig. 9.6).

As ever, the limitations of this work relate to the ability of humans to perceive communications of other species and to understand their meaning. We find this even more difficult when considering animals so very different from ourselves. We inevitably anthropomorphize when trying to understand other species. There is a very big divide in trying to make sense of why tortoises behave in the way that they do, and the extent to which they have feelings and emotions.

References and Further Reading

Carbajal, A.L., Casas-Díaz, E.L., Rodríguez, S.L., González-Fernández, M., Palencia, G., Monreal-Pawlowsky, T. and Lopez-Bejar, M.L. (2019) Two novel matrices for non-invasive monitoring of glucocorticoids in loggerhead sea turtles (*Caretta caretta*). In: Benhaiem, S., Berger, A., Honer, O., Landgraf, C. and Radchuk, V. (eds) *Conference proceedings wildlife research and conservation*. Leibniz Institute for Zoo and Wildlife Research, p.150.

Chitty, J. and Raftery, A. (2013) *Essentials of Tortoise Medicine and Surgery*. Wiley Blackwell, Chichester, UK.

Deane, K. and Valentine, A. (2022) Ch 2 Assessment and recording methods tool kit. In: Rendle, M. and Hinde-Megarity, J. (eds) *BSAVA Manual of Practical Veterinary Welfare*. BSAVA, Quedgeley, UK, pp. 18–70.

Divers, S. (1996) Basic reptile husbandry, history taking and clinical examination. *Veterinary Record In Practice* 18(51), 51–65.

Doody, J.S., Dinets, V. and Burghardt, G.M. (2021) *The Secret Social Life of Reptiles*. John Hopkins University Press, Baltimore, Maryland.

Fazio, E., Medica, P., Bruschetta, G. and Ferlazzo, A. (2014) Do handling and transport stress influence adrenocortical response in the tortoises (*Testudo hermanni*)? International Scholarly Research Notices. *ISRN Veterinary Science* 2014, Article ID 798273.

Gray, J.A. (1987) *The Psychology of Fear and Stress*. Cambridge University, Cambridge, UK.

Kabelik, D. (2021) Corticotropin-releasing factor distribution in the brain of the brown anole lizard. *bioRxiv*. Doi: 10.1101/2021.02.16.431399

Lambert, H., Carder, G. and D'Cruze, N. (2019) Given the cold shoulder: a review of the scientific literature for evidence of reptile sentience. *Animals* 9(10), 821.

Surgery of Tortoises and Turtles. Blackwell, Oxford, UK.

Maslow, A.H. (1943) A theory of human motivation. *Psychological Review* 50(4), 370–396.

McArthur, S., Wilkinson, R. and Meyer, J. (2004) *Medicine and Surgery of Tortoises and Turtles*. Blackwell, Oxford, UK.

McBride, A. and Hinde-Megarity, J. (2022) Ch 3 Animal behaviour. In: Rendle, M. and Hinde-Megarity, J. (eds) *BSAVA Manual of Practical Veterinary Welfare*. BSAVA, Quedgeley, UK, pp. 71–103.

Panksepp, J. (1998) *Affective Neuroscience: The Foundations of Human and Animal Emotions*. Oxford University Press, Oxford, UK.

Rayment-Dyble, L. (2019) Ch 2 Reptile pet trade and welfare. In: Girling, S.J. and Raiti, P. (eds) *BSAVA Manual of Reptiles*, 3rd edn. BSAVA, Quedgeley, UK, pp. 26–35.

Ward, S.J. and Melfi, V. (2015) Keeper–animal interactions: differences between the behaviour of zoo animals affect stockmanship. *PLoS ONE* 10, 20140237.

Warwick, C., Arena, P., Lindley, S., Jessop, M. and Steedman, C. (2013) Assessing reptile welfare using behavioural criteria. *In Practice* 35, 123–131.

Wilkinson, A. and Burman, O. (2022) *Cold-blooded care: How reptile behaviour and cognition research can inform our understanding of reptile welfare*. Prof. Anna Wilkinson & Prof. Oliver Burman (University of Lincoln). Contact: awilkinson@lincoln.ac.uk; oburman@lincoln.ac.uk

Williams, J. (2017) Stress in Chelonia (tortoises, terrapins and turtles). *The Veterinary Nurse* 8(5).

Williams, J. and Beck, D. (2021) Stress, anxiety, fear and frustration in different reptile species: How to reduce these negative emotional states during veterinary procedures. *Veterinary Nursing Journal* 36.

10 Social Interactions in Tortoises

Abstract

Tortoises can be solitary animals with little interaction with others of their species, or they can be more gregarious, gathering together at water sources, for example, and interacting on a more regular basis. This chapter considers interactions related to hierarchies in groups of tortoises, agonistic (aggressive) behaviour towards conspecifics (animals of the same species) and the impact of environment on interactive behaviours. The chapter also discusses examples of environmental impact on levels of aggressive behaviour in zoo animals.

The ways in which tortoises communicate with each other as part of social interaction is also described. Field studies of tortoise and turtle behaviour are discussed in relation to social interactions. Interactions linked to courtship and mating are discussed. This is linked to Chapter 11 on breeding.

The impact of human interactions is also discussed from studies at Zoological Society of London (ZSL) London Zoo, together with the impact of humans on learning ability. This is linked to Chapter 8 on behaviour and learning and to Chapter 9 on emotional states in tortoises, and how they may be defined.

The research in this area is limited but the studies that have been made suggest that social interactions are much more common in many species of tortoise (and chelonians generally) than previously thought. It is also clear that the interactions are very species-specific, linked to lifestyle and biological adaptations. This has implications for the ways in which we house them in captivity, not just in terms of breeding, but also in welfare terms.

How do tortoises communicate with each other?

Communication in tortoises can be visual, acoustic, chemical or tactile. There are few studies into the impact of different types of stimuli on tortoise behaviour and interactions. This is a recent field of study, with research into noise volume and its effects on behaviour being a very new area (Freeland et al., 2020).

Tortoises have good colour vision and use sight to move around, feed, drink and interact with other tortoises. It is not surprising, therefore, that signals concerned with visual communication have been identified as important when establishing relationships such as hierarchies (Freeland et al., 2020). These visual signals include raising the head, moving it and air-biting. Many tortoises and turtles have distinct and very attractive shell and skin patterns. While some patterning is for the purposes of camouflage, some tortoises have patterns that are important in courtship and mating (Fig. 10.1) (see Chapter 11 on breeding).

Body posture may also be used to signal intentions. The height of the body raised from the ground can be significant. So too can the position of the head at its maximum height. Attempts to physically displace other tortoises are seen in species such as Sulcatas. A Sulcata tortoise may move towards another one, giving threat signals and then ultimately barge it out of the way, or try to turn the other animal over onto its back.

Height is one of the factors identified by Fieschi-Meric et al. (2022) and Freeland et al. (2020) in determining position in the dominance hierarchies of Galapagos tortoises. Physical size is also important, with bigger animals being more dominant and therefore able to access more resources. Levels of aggression also play a large part in establishing and maintaining hierarchical position. Aldabran tortoises will also show competition for resources (Fig. 10.2).

Pheromones are used for communication in reptiles. Gopher tortoises, for example, have huge glands in the throat that enlarge during the breeding season. These are thought to produce secretions as chemical signals (Doody et al., 2021). The tortoises rub their throat glands with the front legs and then wave their forearms as part of sexual signalling.

Tactile interactions can also be identified. This does not just concern courtship or mating behaviour,

---

© CAB International 2025. *Tortoise Husbandry and Welfare.* (J. Williams)
DOI: 10.1079/9781800623736.0010

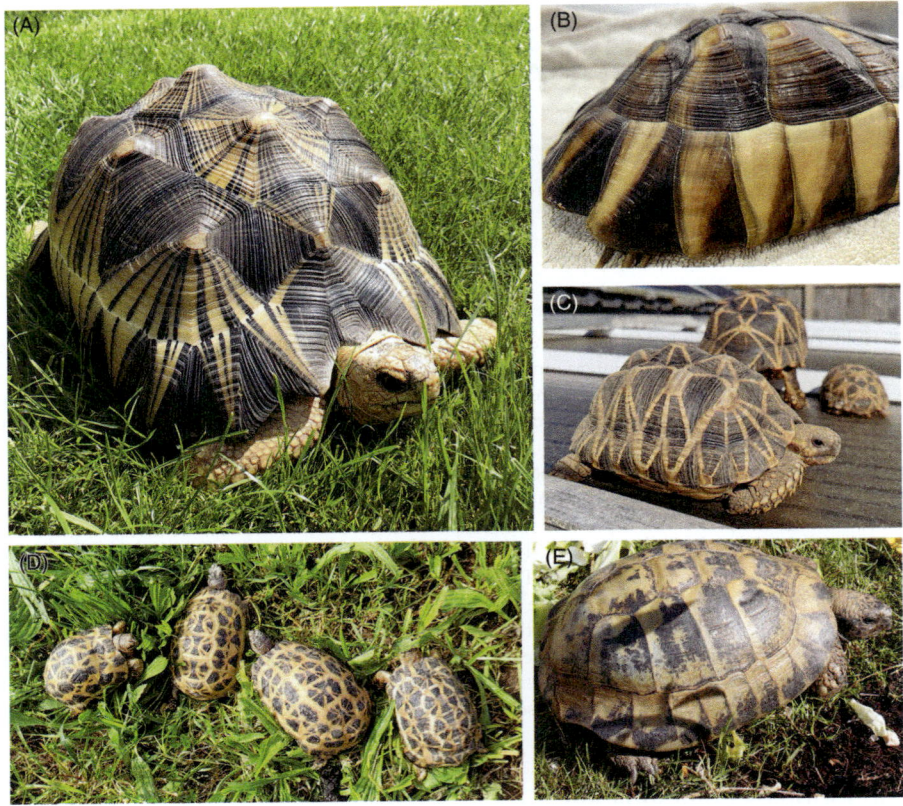

Fig. 10.1. Tortoise shell patterns vary significantly with species. Some species have more uniform colorations, whereas other species are beautifully patterned. The patterns are often much more distinct and brighter in young animals. (A) Radiated tortoise (*Astrochelys radiata*) with highly patterned shell. (B) Some Marginated tortoises (*Testudo marginata*) have very distinct dark and light areas on their scutes. (C) The very beautiful and rare Burmese Star tortoise (*Geochelone platynota*) (Dillon Prest). (D) Variations in shell patterns of *Pixys arachnoides* (Andy Lewis). (E) The less distinctive markings of a Hermann's tortoise (*Testudo hermanni*).

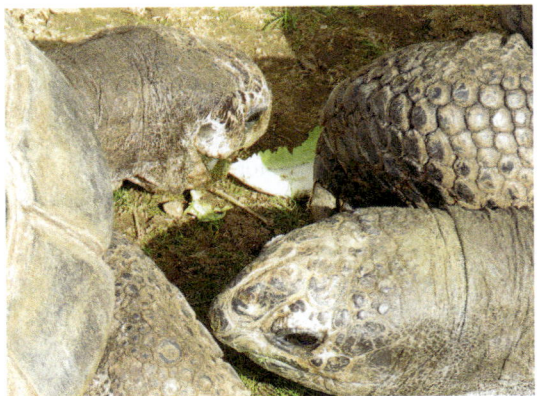

Fig. 10.2. Aldabran tortoises interacting to access food in their enclosure.

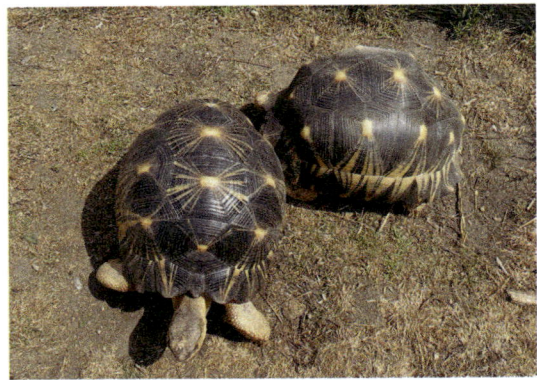

Fig. 10.3. Radiated tortoises touching and sniffing each other.

although they are important in some species in this reproductive context. I have observed nose-to-nose sniffing and touching in newly introduced animals (Fig. 10.3).

What types of interactions do tortoises have with each other?

Many tortoises are solitary species – they live alone, coming across another tortoise occasionally as they walk and forage for food. These tortoises do not need the company of other tortoises, and in some cases the presence of others may cause them problems in captivity. However, the presence of tortoises of the same species may play an important part in the normal seasonal cycles, largely related to reproduction. However, there are instances when tortoises group together for survival, for example hatchlings emerging together. In Mediterranean tortoises, animals will behave in similar ways to the animals around them, such as emerging from hibernation in spring (Wegehaupt, 2009a), due to environmental stimuli and seeking water or food items as they become available through the seasons (Fig. 10.4).

When living together in groups, tortoises may compete for specific regions. For example, females may seek out and compete for the same nest-building site if there is only one suitable area. They can damage each other when trying to push each other out of the way. They will also continuously ram the shell of any tortoise who is in a location they want. This causes stress and potential shell damage.

Similarly, if there is only one basking area, tortoises may climb on top of each other to reach a suitable temperature. Figure 10.5 illustrates a group of female Horsfield's tortoises basking together in one location.

A thesis study (Rife, 2007), which investigated the social behaviour of juvenile Northern Diamondback terrapins (*Malaclemys terrapin terrapin*) while they were basking, found that familiar kin (related animals) were found to bask in larger groups and were more willing to share the limited basking site. This was in comparison with unfamiliar kin, and familiar non-kin. These results suggested that this species of terrapin forms social groups based on both familiarity and relatedness (Rife, 2007).

Gutnik *et al.* (2020) reported that there is flexibility in learning in tortoises and a growing body of evidence of 'the significance of social interaction and social learning in reptiles'. Their trials were impacted by the presence of other tortoises within the enclosure in the two zoo studies. They reported that some tortoises were unable to perform in trials due to the presence of other more dominant individuals who were allowed to remain in their enclosure during training and testing.

Tortoises have a more complex social environment than has been previously realized. Some species show agonistic behaviours, including the Sulcata tortoises as previously mentioned. When juvenile Hermann's or Spur-thighed tortoises are kept together in pairs, in my experience, one will grow more quickly. I have observed the larger individual driving the smaller tortoise away from food in what appears to be competition for available food.

As previously described, female Spur-thighed tortoises will ram each other when trying to gain access to nesting sites if kept in small enclosures. All these examples suggest that more interaction and competition for resources is taking place than we have previously understood. This emphasizes the importance of adequate resource provision and large enclosures in captivity, especially where groups of animals are housed together (Freeland *et al.*, 2020; Fieschi-Meric *et al.*, 2022 as illustrated by the ZSL London Zoo studies) (see Chapter 8 on behaviour and learning).

Non-social Red-footed tortoises (*Chelonoidis carbonaria*) were reported by Wilkinson *et al.* (2010) as being able to learn from the actions of a conspecific in a detour task. The results indicated that the animals who were not able to watch and learn failed in the task. This evidence suggests that social or visual cues observed can be used in learning.

Aggregation is seen in some species for mating and during annual cycles. For example, in Red-eared terrapins (*Trachemys scripta elegans*) and other species of terrapin, such as the Northern Diamondback terrapin, female terrapins aggregate prior to mating and nest in clusters (Rife, 2007). They have also been seen to gather around ponds, and not just in the mating season (Doody *et al.*, 2021). Social bullying may be seen between males, most probably in competition for the best locations and feeding opportunities, suggesting a possible hierarchy within the males. Aggregations around ponds in the Galapagos are also seen, for bathing and drinking opportunities, as well as when finding a mate for breeding.

Reproductive behavioural interactions

Many interactions between tortoises do relate to courtship and mating rituals. Head bobbing is commonly seen in males, whose aim is to attract and stimulate females to mate. In aquatic species, vibrating the water near the female, using claws to attract her, has been observed in the Red-eared terrapin, *T. scripta elegans*. Use of chemical communication and vocalizations have also been identified as part of courtship (Doody *et al.*, 2021).

In terrestrial tortoises, head bobbing, nose touching and sniffing are common mating behaviours as shown in Fig. 10.6. Butting the rear of the female's shell or biting at her back legs is seen in Spur-thighed and Hermann's tortoises, respectively. Ritualized walking and circling are also common behavioural signals in courtship.

Male tortoises will pester females (or other males if there are no females) in search of a partner to mate with. If the enclosure does not allow the tortoises to get away from each other, the mating behaviour can cause injury and shell damage to other tortoises due to repeated shell-bashing in some species, such as Spur-thighed tortoises. In other species, such as Hermann's tortoises, the male may bite the back legs of the female as he attempts to get her to stand still and allow mating to take place.

This can cause stress, and negatively impact welfare, where groups of tortoises are kept together. Having said that, small groups of female tortoises, and in some cases groups of males, who are not particularly driven to mate can live together in captivity as long as the enclosure is large enough. Some species are more social and can live in harmony in groups. These include Red-footed tortoises, which I have encountered living in groups in captivity on a number of occasions. Similarly, groups of Horsfield's can live together as shown in Fig. 10.5 above. I have kept groups of Spur-thighed females together and I have a group of three male Hermann's tortoises who live together in harmony, as shown in Fig. 10.7A. I have also previously kept a group of three Hermann's females together without problem behaviours developing, as shown in Fig. 10.7B.

These anecdotal examples, and those of other keepers, suggest that although there are species-specific behaviours to be considered, the nature of the individual tortoise will vary and influence their degree of willingness to share resources and cohabit amicably. The influence of enclosure size and availability of resources are also very relevant, as discussed here.

A recent study (Le Balle *et al.*, 2021) of two populations of the species of Red-footed and Yellow-footed Brazilian tortoises, *Chelonoidis carbonarius* and *C. denticulatis*, recorded behavioural responses to stress, novel environments, novel objects and social encounters. Their results indicated that *C. carbonarius* showed a higher frequency of risk-taking behaviours, which they related to the availability of resources and predator pressures in their two habitats.

If females are kept separately from males there may be negative impacts on health of the females over the long term (see Chapter 7 on common illnesses and diseases). This is because the presence of a male is needed to stimulate normal egg production (Fig. 10.8).

Mating sounds include grunts, brrrs, hisses, clicks and chirrups (Doody *et al.*, 2021). The sounds may be used for approach and attraction as well as during the mating process itself. The information conveyed by the sounds may include information about the male's size, body condition and previous reproductive success. Figure 10.9 shows some vocalization during copulation in this pair of Aldabran tortoises.

What types of interactions do tortoises have with humans?

As tortoise keepers and caregivers, we feel that we have established a relationship with our animals. As humans, we tend to anthropomorphize relationships with animals as an inevitable consequence of being human. We see the world and the other living creatures from a human perspective. However, it is only recently that evidence has been produced to show that tortoises can recognize individual humans (Ward and Melfi, 2015). The degree to which we interact with our tortoises on a daily basis, through handling and husbandry for example, will be impacting their welfare. To what extent and whether positively or negatively for individual tortoises in a given situation and setting is unclear.

In the past, when long-term tortoise owners have told me that their tortoise recognizes them when they go into the garden, I have been inclined to dismiss this notion as unfounded. However, more recent studies (Ward and Melfi, 2015) have shown that animal–keeper relationships, human–animal interactions (HAIs) or dyads, are formed. The most important factors in forming these relationships are the keeper's attitude towards the animals and the keeper's knowledge and experience of the animals in their care. The data from this study in zoos showed that these dyads influenced behaviour.

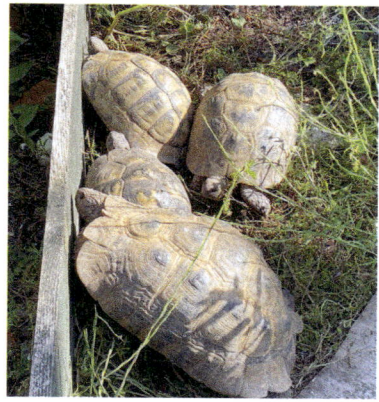

Fig. 10.4. Group of Spur-thighed tortoises basking together in large enclosure.

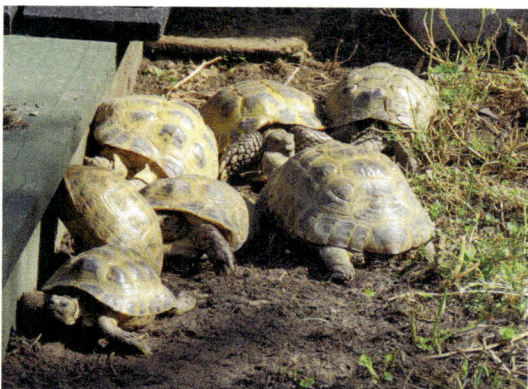

Fig. 10.5. Horsfield's tortoises crowding together for basking in a large outdoor enclosure. Note that there are other potential basking sites, but this group have chosen the same location.

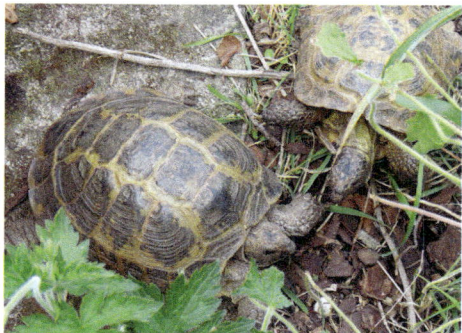

Fig. 10.6. Male Horsfield's sniffing and head bobbing in front of the female.

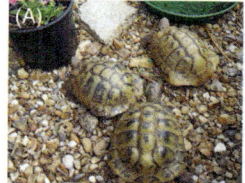 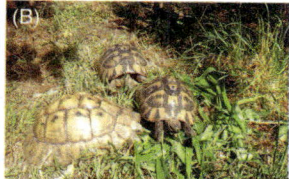

Fig 10.7. (A) Group of three male Hermann's tortoises living together. (B) Group of three female Hermann's tortoises living together.

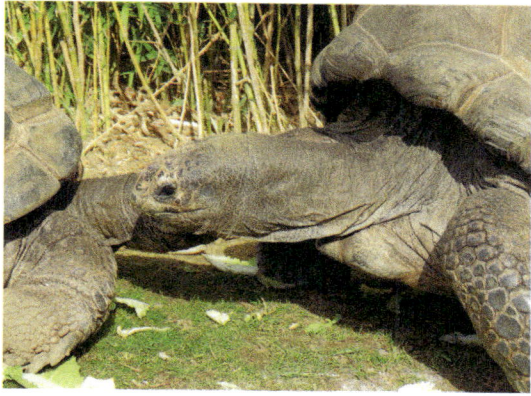

Fig. 10.8. When female and male tortoises are living in the same enclosure, reproductive behaviours are often inevitable, as in the case of these two Aldabran tortoises sniffing each other. In some species, seasonal changes are required – for example species that do not reproduce unless hibernation has taken place.

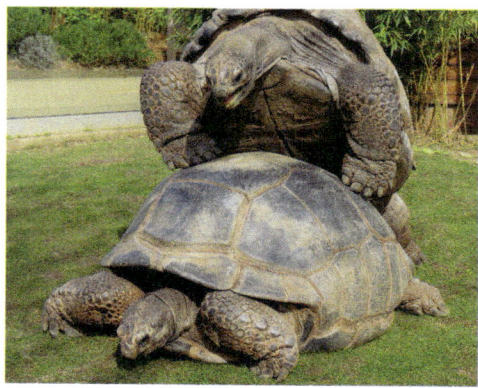

Fig. 10.9. Courtship rituals carried out by males are intended to gain the female's interest and then to get her to stand still and allow him to mount the back of the shell for copulation to take place, as shown by this mature pair of Aldabran tortoises.

Social Interactions in Tortoises

The presence of familiar keepers allowed the animals to respond more rapidly to cues in training. This improved their ability to learn. The original notion of 'stockmanship' with livestock animals shows that good management of animals, with a person who operates in a safe, effective and low-stress manner, increases productivity and welfare standards.

Where we keep one or a small number of tortoises at home, the opportunity to develop very strong bonds exists. This is something that we need to be aware of, as the relationship between us and our tortoises may well be impacting their welfare.

Learmonth *et al.* (2021) showed that for some giant tortoises, human interaction acts as a preferred reinforcer or reward. Some of the tortoises actively prefer this interaction with keepers to being given food or an enrichment toy. However, the importance of human interaction as a reward is influenced by many other factors. An individual's preference may change over time and as the context changes. This is an area requiring a good deal more research, in order to develop our understanding of the factors that may make interactions with humans reinforcing.

Research in zoos indicates that tortoises will seek out humans. It was believed that physical contact as a way of establishing a relationship may be beneficial. This is not always the case, however. It depends on who the humans are and their relationship with the tortoises. Research at ZSL London Zoo showed that the larger a visitor group, the greater was the increase in aggression in Galapagos tortoises following the visits. This has led to the zoo stopping 'Keeper for a Day' events with Galapagos tortoises. Nor are visitors allowed to have physical contact with the tortoises, as this was also identified as a factor leading to increased aggression (Freeland *et al.*, 2020).

How can the environment affect tortoise interactions?

Noise levels were identified as impacting upon aggression levels in the ZSL London Zoo Galapagos tortoises (Fieschi-Meric *et al.*, 2022). Their research indicated that increased noise levels made it more likely that interactions would escalate into a fight. The researchers also suggested that high noise levels may impair communication channels between individual tortoises, which would otherwise be used to mitigate aggressive interactions.

Given the impact that noise levels can have on us and other mammals, this is an important consideration in terms of enclosure location in captivity. We all know how annoying a loud repetitive noise such a siren can be. Might living near a busy road, for example, impact on our tortoises when they are outdoors? These aspects of tortoise sensory perception, sentience and cognition have not even begun to be considered for tortoises in captivity.

The more space and resources available, the less interaction the tortoises at ZSL London Zoo had with each other (Freeland *et al.*, 2020; Fieschi-Meric *et al.*, 2022). Aggression was frequently associated with the proximity of resources such as food, and competition for basking or bathing areas and mud wallows. Competition for resources, and the potential for resource guarding in tortoises, is therefore a potential influence on interactions and significantly affects the desire for social engagement.

This links again to the need for choice for tortoises in captivity. Given a suitable environment they can choose when to engage with each other, and when they do the interaction is more likely to be peaceable. Where they are too close together, in groups that are too large, or where resources are limited, they lose choice, and are forced into interactions with the consequent increase in aggression levels noted in the ZSL London Zoo studies.

What is the impact of social behaviour on well-being and welfare?

Although research into this area of behaviour is limited, it is likely that interactions can lead to positive behavioural outcomes, even though many interactions between giant tortoises in captivity were shown to be based on the desire to gain and hold onto valuable resources. It is probable that the suitability of the tortoise's environment is as important in terms of mental health, as measured by appropriate and desired social interactions, as it is to physical health.

Dominance-based hierarchies exist in groups of individual Galapagos tortoises (Freeland *et al.*, 2020; Fieschi-Meric *et al.*, 2022) and are established through displays of aggression and by controlling access to resources. The stability of any hierarchy will be influenced by environmental change and change in the individuals of the group. The greater the stability, the lower were the levels of aggression noted in the ZSL London Zoo studies. This is something to be considered not just in the zoo setting but for all of us who care for more than one tortoise. This should be considered when grouping animals together: the numbers and gender ratios, along with the amount of space available. The differences in personality and temperament seen in individuals of the same species may require adaptations to housing provision and husbandry to meet those needs (Wilkinson and Burman, 2022).

The importance of observing and recording interactions between our tortoises, when kept in groups, is emphasized through the zoo studies. We should take that on board as keepers with private collections, in rescue, and in all locations where tortoises are to be found in captivity. Are the tortoises getting on and what signs should we be looking for of contentment, or alternatively stress? Are the tortoises gaining benefits from being together, or are they losing out from this situation? These questions are new to us as tortoise keepers in different settings. We potentially have much to contribute to levels of understanding. The observations of many thousands of tortoise keepers could be gathered and put to good use in this very new field of research and study.

Conclusion

The reasons for tortoises gathering together are poorly understood. Apart from groupings related to reproduction, or because of limited nesting sites, other social interactions have not been well studied. The research examples here are mainly from small zoo populations of giant tortoises. Relatively little research has been carried out in the natural environment. Wegehaupt (2009a,b) provided an insight into the behaviour and interactions of Mediterranean tortoises but, because of the degree of interference and environmental disruption caused by humans in the habitats of such tortoises, it is becoming more difficult to be sure that observed behaviours are completely 'natural'. Combined with the increasing impact of climate change and global warming, for any analysis of time-budgets in the wild, which are created from studies of the proportion of time that naturally occurring behaviours contribute to daily routines, identification of 'normal' behaviour patterns is very difficult. The time spent basking or feeding, resting or hiding, for example, as normal behaviour patterns in the natural environment is becoming increasingly challenging to identify and record. We may lose this information before we have even established the baseline data.

It is becoming increasingly clear that tortoises do have social lives and that they have a complex repertoire of behaviours. We need to understand these much more. Lambert et al. (2019) found 37 studies reporting reptiles to be capable of emotional states of anxiety, stress, distress, excitement, fear, frustration, pain and suffering and 'four articles that explored and found evidence for the capacity of reptiles to feel pleasure, emotion, and anxiety'. Research covered the 20 years 1999–2018. This is a very small number of studies – on average two per year. The more we study this area, the more evidence we find of sentience and emotional capacity, including the significance of social interactions and social relationships in tortoises (and reptiles as a whole).

References and Further Reading

Doody, J.S., Dinets, V. and Burghardt, G.M. (2021) *The Secret Social Life of Reptiles*. John Hopkins University Press, Baltimore, Maryland.

Freeland, L., Ellis, C. and Michaels, C.J. (2020) Documenting aggression, dominance and the impacts of visitor interaction on Galápagos tortoises (*Chelonoidis nigra*) in a zoo setting. *Animals* 10, 699.

Fieschi-Meric, L., Ellis, C., Servini, F., Tapley, B. and Michaels, C.J. (2022) An improvement in enclosure design can positively impact welfare, reduce aggressiveness and stabilise hierarchy in captive Galapagos Giant tortoises. *Journal of Zoological and Botanical Gardens* 3, 499–512.

Gutnick, T., Weissenbacher, A. and Kuba, M.J. (2020) The Underestimated Giants: Operant conditioning, visual discrimination and long-term memory in giant tortoises. *Animal Cognition* 23, 159–167.

Lambert, H., Carder, G. and D'Cruze, N. (2019) Given the cold shoulder: a review of the scientific literature for evidence of reptile sentience. *Animals* 9(10), 821.

Le Balle, R., Cote, J., Antonio, F. and Fernandez, S. (2021) Evidence for animal personalities in two Brazilian tortoises (*Chelonoidis denticulatus* and *Chelonoidis carbonarius*) and insights for their conservation. *Applied Animal Behaviour Science* 241, 105400.

Learmonth, M.J., Sherwen, S. and Hemsworth, P.H. (2021) Assessing preferences of two zoo-housed Aldabran giant tortoises (*Aldabrachelys gigantea*) for three stimuli using a novel preference test. *ZooBiol* 40(2), 98–106.

Mackie, J. (2021) Animal Behaviour Management Officer at Zoological Society of London (ZSL) London Zoo, as part of the work of BIAZA (British and Irish Zoos and Aquariums Association) Animal Behaviour and Training Working Group, Reptile Training in Zoos RAWG presentation and personal communications.

McArthur, S., Wilkinson, R. and Hernandez-Divers, S. (2004) *Medicine and Surgery of Tortoises and Turtles*. Blackwell, Oxford, UK.

Rife, A. (2007) Social and basking behaviors in juvenile, captive-raised Northern Diamondback terrapins (*Malaclemys terrapin terrapin*). BS Thesis, Boston College.

Ward, S.J. and Melfi, V. (2015) Keeper–animal interactions: differences between the behaviour of zoo animals affect stockmanship. *PLoS ONE* 10, 20140237.

Wegehaupt, W. (2009a) *Mediterranean Tortoises, Where and how they live in the wild*. Kressbronn, Germany.

Wegehaupt, W. (2009b) *Naturalistic Keeping and Breeding of Hermann's Tortoises*. Kressbronn, Germany.

Wilkinson, A., Kuenstner, K., Mueller, J. and Huber, L. (2010) Social learning in a non-social reptile (*Geochelone carbonaria*). *Biological Letters* 6, 614–616.

Wilkinson, A. and Burman, O. (2022) *Cold-blooded care: How reptile behaviour and cognition research can inform our understanding of reptile welfare*. Prof. Anna Wilkinson and Prof. Oliver Burman (University of Lincoln). Contact: awilkinson@lincoln.ac.uk; oburman@lincoln.ac.uk

11 Breeding Tortoises

Abstract

This chapter looks at tortoise reproductive systems and the procedures involved in breeding tortoises. Male and female reproductive processes are outlined. Husbandry requirements for successful breeding are discussed, along with preparation for mating and egg production. The maintenance of sexually mature tortoises is discussed for a range of chelonian species. This includes consideration as to whether multi-sex groups should be kept together, or housed as individuals with groups only being allowed to come together for mating purposes.

The potential benefits and drawbacks of breeding are highlighted together with the likely consequences for adults in both the long and short term. Courtship and mating rituals are outlined along with egg production. Methods of incubation leading to successful neonate hatching are described. Care from the early stages of life is described in these precocial animals, which upon hatching immediately live independently as miniature adults. The ethics and purposes of breeding are discussed in terms of the welfare impact on both adults and hatchlings.

The ethics of breeding – what are the reasons for breeding tortoises?

Breeding tortoises in captivity can fulfil a number of purposes. Once adult and sexually mature, reproductive behaviour is part of normal behaviour. It could be argued that the opportunity to mate and propagate should always be provided if we are to fulfil the requirements set out in the Five Freedoms (Mellor, 2016; Yeates, 2022) and Five Domains, as they are now described. The 'freedom and opportunity to express normal behaviour' is the fourth Freedom listed.

There may be individual situations where other considerations are significant, however. An elderly female tortoise, for example, who has lived alone in captivity for 40 years, may be too old to safely mate and produce eggs. The potential risk of disease, resultant from being introduced to another tortoise (see Chapter 7 on common illnesses and diseases) may outweigh any potential benefits of breeding.

The opposite may be true for a fit and healthy adult female tortoise whose reproductive system is active, but which needs the presence of a male tortoise to be stimulated to function. Lack of a male may lead to health risks such as partial egg production (follicular stasis – see Chapter 7 on common illnesses and diseases) or egg retention. Egg retention may also result when husbandry provision does not offer suitable egg-laying sites, or when temperatures are too low for the female to lay. Reproductive processes continue even in isolated females. I have cared for female tortoises who continue to lay eggs, despite not having been in contact with a male for many years.

Males that live alone are often very frustrated due to the lack of opportunity for courtship and mating. Courtship and mating behaviours are normal and innate. All living organisms have a pre-programmed biological drive to reproduce and continue the species. Males are driven to find a female particularly in the springtime, post-hibernation/brumation. Lack of a female, when the drive to mate and breed is so strong, may lead to loss of appetite and depression. It is also common to see distressing repetitive behaviours linked to attempts to escape the enclosure to find a mate. For example, a male tortoise may repeatedly turn himself over onto his back as he tries to climb the sides of the enclosure. Inappropriate sexual behaviours may be directed at tortoise-like objects, such as shoes, boots, large rocks or garden ornaments (Fig. 11.1).

I was once contacted about a juvenile male Hermann's tortoise who was starting to show inappropriate sexually driven behaviours. He would chase after people moving around the garden, biting at their feet. This was particularly painful for anyone without shoes on. It was assumed that the tortoise was being aggressive and, knowing little

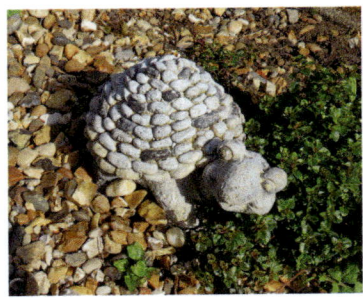
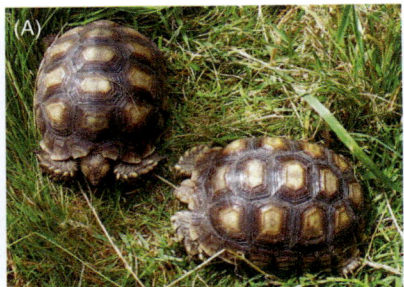
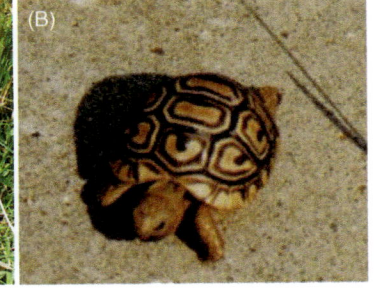

Fig. 11.1. Stone tortoise garden ornaments can often be the focus of attention for a male in the absence of any females.

Fig. 11.2. (A) Baby Sulcatas, which are very cute when small but increasingly difficult to accommodate when adult. (B) Hatchling Leopard tortoise, with such a beautiful shell pattern.

about tortoise behaviour, the owner sought advice from social media. One respondent advised 'alpha-rolling' the tortoise onto his back, then spraying his face with water to 'teach' him not to bite at feet.

Rarely have I heard such ridiculously ineffective advice. As it shows no comprehension of the reason for the tortoise's behaviour, it has no hope whatsoever of changing the unwanted behaviours. For male Hermann's tortoises, biting the legs of females is part of the courtship ritual. The aim is to slow the female down until she eventually stands, allowing mating to proceed. In this instance, because a female was not present, the male tortoise had transferred this behaviour onto people's feet, a substitute that, like a female, also moved away when the tortoise bit at them.

As courtship and mating behaviours are innate, it is not possible to train an alternative behaviour – even if rolling the tortoise onto his back and spraying water into his face could be described as a form of training (which it is not). Actions such as this are simply an attempt to punish, causing distress and fear, without any possibility of bringing about a cessation of this normal, although misdirected, reproductive behaviour.

After thinking about individual tortoise health and welfare concerns, the other main consideration that must be borne in mind is how the breeding of captive animals can be of potential benefit to the species as a whole. The ethics of this are examined in Chapter 20, but it is certainly the case that many species of tortoise are now threatened with extinction in the wild, as listed by the International Union for Conservation of Nature (IUCN) and by the Convention on International Trade in Endangered Species (CITES).

Captive breeding to provide animals for the pet trade and other uses is preferable to taking wild-caught animals, which would further diminish already threatened populations. Commercial-scale breeding takes place across Europe, North America and in parts of Asia for the pet trade and in some countries for food. These animals are farmed purely for financial gain, but not always in sustainable ways (see Chapter 20 on tortoise keeping in the past, present and future). Some species are so endangered in the wild that there are coordinated programmes to breed them in captivity (see Chapter 17 on Egyptian tortoises). Examples include the European Studbook Foundation (ESF) and the European Endangered Species Programme (EEP).

Conversely, in Europe and the UK there are many unwanted tortoises looking for homes, their owners being no longer able to care for them for a number of reasons. The breeding of excessive numbers of tortoises, which the market cannot sustain, or breeding species that are unsuitable as domestic pets, such as the giant tortoises (e.g. Sulcatas), is causing many welfare problems (Fig. 11.2). Large tortoises are often rehomed as they grow and reach unmanageable sizes, as they need enclosure sizes measured in acres or hectares rather than feet or metres. This is a huge dilemma in welfare terms and raises the question of the sustainability and suitability of some species to be pets (see Chapter 20 on tortoise keeping in the past, present and future).

Each of us must make decisions on breeding, therefore, based on the individual animals we care for and the particular circumstances in which we find ourselves. Being responsible when breeding; considering the suitability of any given species as pets; finding suitable homes for hatchlings; providing prospective owners with accurate information on care and husbandry – all are essential considerations in any ethical breeding enterprise. As mentioned previously, the sale and purchase of tortoises is restricted in many countries. Legal requirements should be researched and the current position understood before the sale of any hatchlings takes place.

It is of course possible to allow the breeding processes to take place and for eggs to be laid but not incubated, thus preventing the growth of embryos and subsequent birth of hatchlings. This allows the adults the potential beneficial opportunities provided by reproductive behaviours and normal reproductive cycles without the ethical concerns of what the future holds for any offspring produced.

Having said all that, for those of us who love tortoises there are fewer things on the planet cuter than a hatchling baby tortoise. They are so small and yet so perfectly formed, independent from the moment they escape the egg, as to leave one in no doubt as to the incredible feat of nature that has led to this lovely creature (Fig. 11.2B).

How do I distinguish between males and females?

Generally speaking, the colours and patterns on the shells of male and female tortoises of the same species are very similar. There is no distinction between facial or body features either. Males are not more brightly coloured or marked, as is common in birds, for example.

For all except the giant Galapagos and Aldabran species, the females are significantly larger than the males. They may be up to one-third bigger. This is to allow the body to accommodate the bulk of the eggs when formed. In the giant species this is not necessary as the body size is already so large – males and females are similar sizes (Fig. 11.9).

As can be seen in Figs 11.3, 11.4, 11.5, 11.6, 11.7 and 11.8, in most species female tortoises are significantly larger than males. For example, an adult Spur-thighed female (*T. graeca graeca/whitei*) could weigh 3500 g and have a straight carapace length (SCL) of 300 mm. The male of the same species may be only 1200 g and 200 mm SCL. In *T. kleinmanni*, the adult male could weigh 150 g and be 90 mm SCL, while the largest females are 130 mm SCL and weigh 480 g.

A more reliable indicator of gender is often the length of the tail. In the males of many species the tail is much longer than that of the female, and is often wrapped around the hind leg to hold it close to the body. This is particularly obvious in species such as Hermann's, Horsfield's and Leopard tortoises. The position of the opening, or cloaca, in the tail is usually closer to the body in females.

In many species the differences in tail length, position of the vent, or cloaca, and the way the tail is held are the most obvious ways to identify males and females, as shown in Figs 11.3, 11.4, 11.5, 11.7 and 11.8 for different species. In Spur-thighed tortoises the difference in tail length is much less significant so in this species gender identification can be more difficult, especially in younger animals that are not yet fully grown. Figure 11.10 shows the differences diagramatically.

In some species the plastron of the male has a much more pronounced upward dome shape, so that underneath it is concave. This is so that the carapace of the female can be accommodated when the male mounts her during mating. This is the case in Red-footed tortoises, for example (Fig. 11.11).

In other species both males and females have a concave plastron, while in the Leopard tortoise the plastron is flat in both males and females (see Fig. 11.7).

In some species the female's body is wider and rounder, or oval in shape. Males may have a more elongated body, or be more triangular in shape with the body widening at the hips/pelvis. This is very obvious in Hermann's tortoises.

In young tortoises, identification of sex can be difficult. McArthur *et al.* (2004) suggested that sexual differences are not very apparent in many species before the age of 5 years. In some species, such as Spur-thighed tortoises, it may take 10 years for clear male or female characteristics to be seen.

Reproduction in tortoises

Tortoises reproduce sexually using internal fertilization. Sperm from the male must be placed into the female reproductive tract during the mating process. Figure 11.12 shows the reproductive tracts of females and males. The sperm will swim to fertilize the eggs. Once the fertilized eggs have developed and embryos formed, the female will deposit the eggs into a 'nest' and leave the young to incubate and then hatch unattended. Tortoises show no parental care. Once hatched, the baby tortoises are ready to live independently and unsupported, as miniature adults.

The female reproductive system – how does this work?

The female reproductive tract consists of a pair of ovaries attached to paired oviducts, as shown in

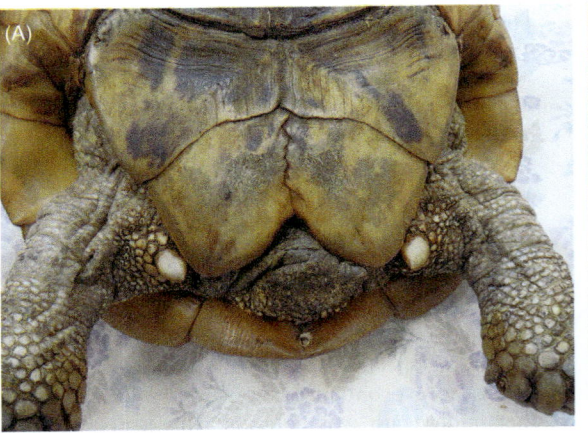
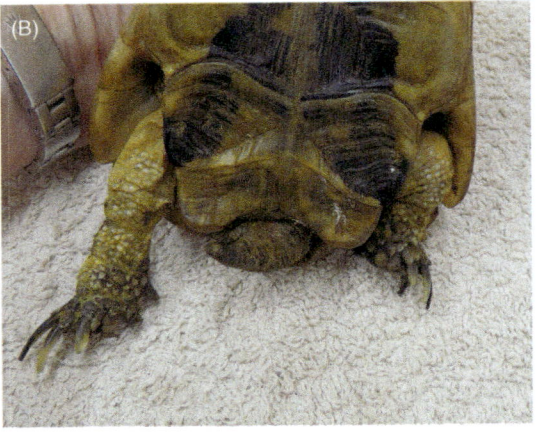

Fig. 11.3. (A) Female and (B) male Spur-thighed tortoises.

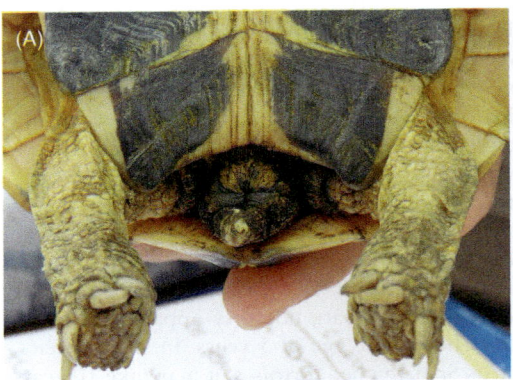
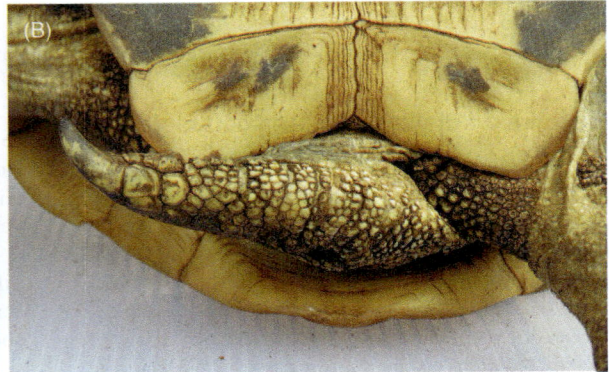

Fig. 11.4. (A) Female and (B) male Hermann's tortoises.

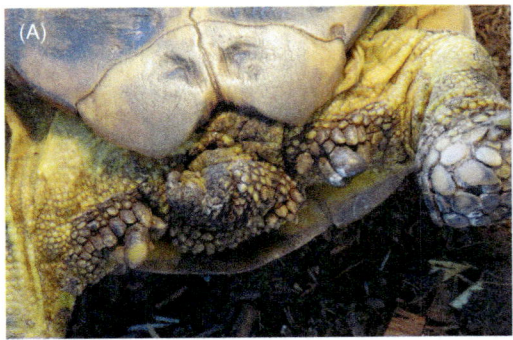
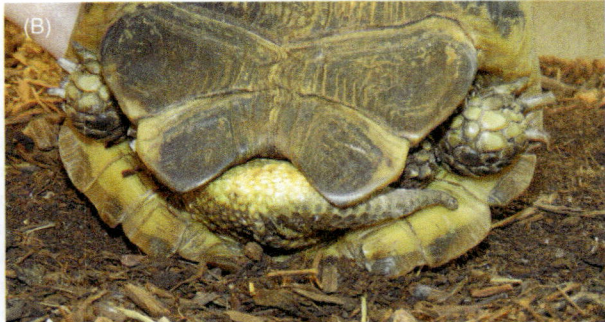

Fig. 11.5. (A) Female and (B) male Horsfield's tortoises.

Fig. 11.12. Raised oestrogen levels stimulate the release of ova, or eggs, from the ovaries. These travel down the oviducts as follicles. Here they begin the process of maturing. If sperm is present the egg will be fertilized. Once the egg is fertilized, yolk and a hard calcium-based shell is added. The shell provides waterproof protection against dehydration together with protection against physical

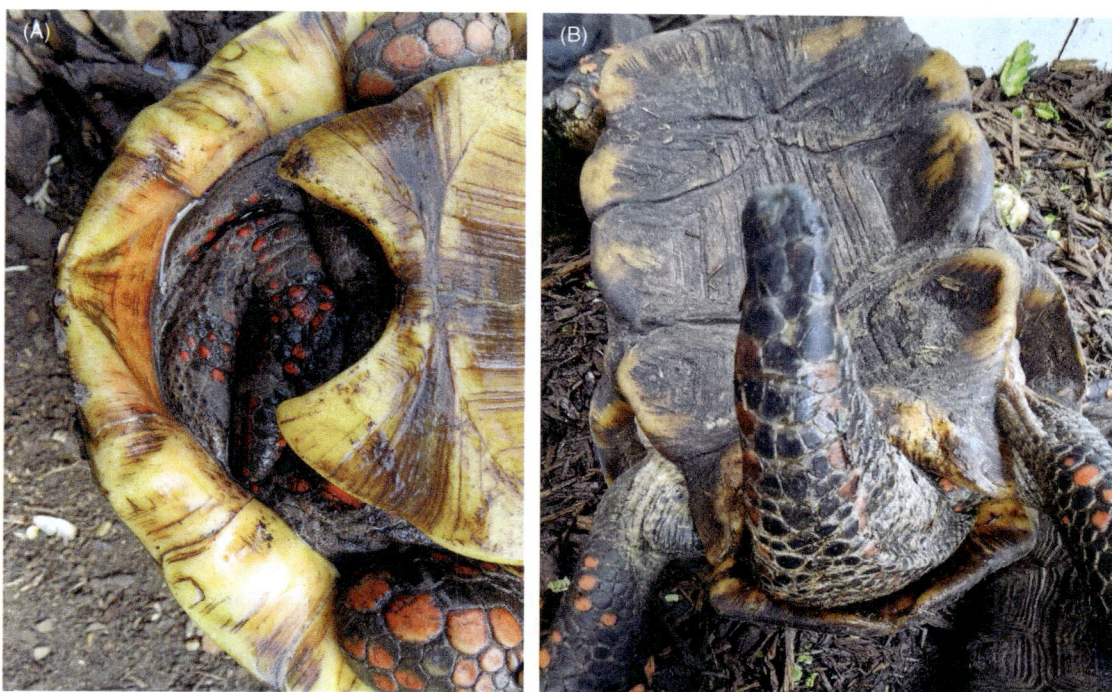

Fig. 11.6. (A) Female and (B) male Red-footed tortoises (James Sullivan).

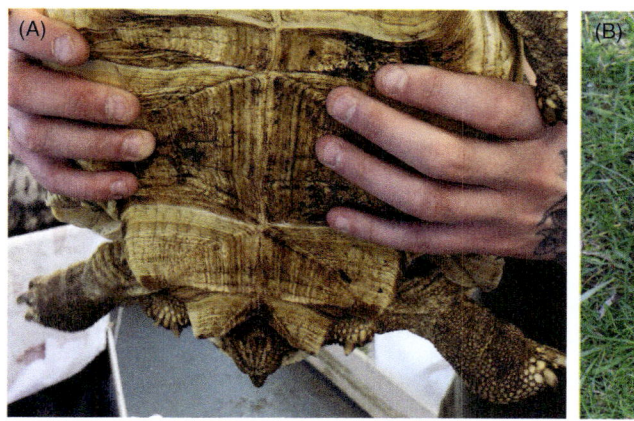 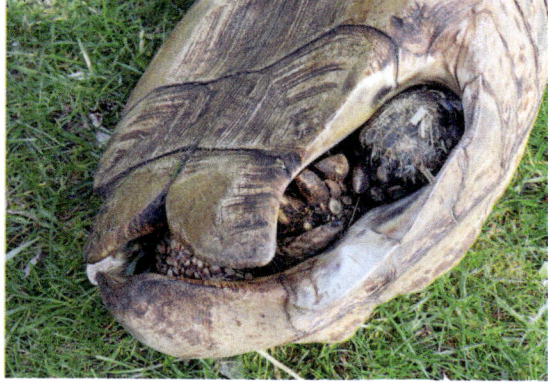

Fig. 11.7. (A) Female and (B) male Leopard tortoises.

damage (McArthur *et al.*, 2004; Jepson, 2006), which may result when the eggs are being laid.

The number of eggs and therefore follicles produced will depend upon the species of tortoise. This can range from one in the smaller species such as Gopher tortoises, to over 30 in larger Sulcatas. Giant species can lay 20–25 eggs, and the large marine turtles can produce over 100 eggs in one clutch.

Female tortoises start to produce eggs once mature and this can take 20 or more years in the wild. In captivity tortoises often grow much more quickly and reach maturity within 8 years. Size and weight will determine when the female is ready to reproduce.

Egg production and development are stimulated by a number of environmental factors, such as temperature and daylength, but also the presence of

Breeding Tortoises

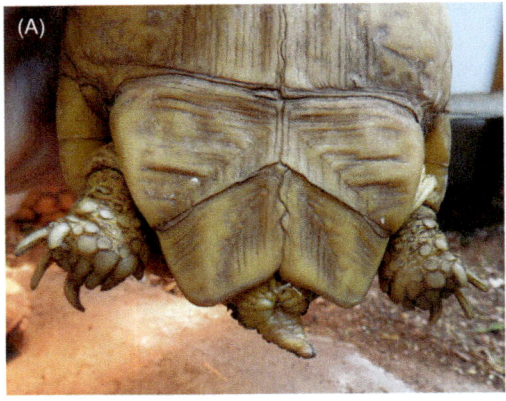 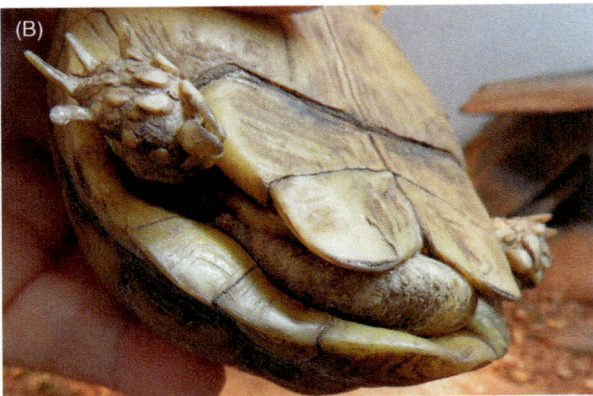

Fig. 11.8. (A) Female and (B) male Kleinmann's tortoises.

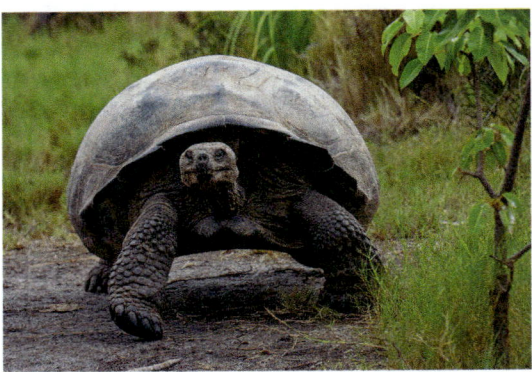

Fig. 11.9. Galapagos tortoises of both sexes are the same size (Gary Franklin).

male tortoises. In more temperate species, for example, seasonal spring changes bring about increased temperatures, longer daylength and increased food availability – some of the factors leading to stimulation of the reproductive tract. It is thought that male presence and pheromones, together with mating behaviours, may also be needed to stimulate the follicles to deposit the hard calcium-based shell required for complete egg formation (Fig. 11.14) (McArthur et al., 2004; Johnson, 2019).

The eggs are laid in clutches into a 'nest' dug by the female (Fig. 11.15). Once they are laid the female will cover the eggs with soil so that the location of the nest site becomes virtually impossible to identify. In captivity, in most cases, the eggs will need to be removed from the nest and incubated at suitable temperatures if the eggs are to have any chance of hatching (Highfield, 1996). If the captive tortoise is being kept in its native country (as a pet) or somewhere warm like the natural habitat, it may be possible for the eggs to hatch in the nest.

Eventually female tortoises stop producing eggs. The ageing process means that their organs become less able to function effectively (McArthur et al., 2004). This is likely to happen over the age of 80 years but will vary with individuals. Females will pass infertile eggs if there are no males present as long as the other environmental conditions are suitable to stimulate the process.

It is thought that females can retain viable sperm for 2 or more years in situations where there are adverse environmental conditions, or no males present. This means that females can lay fertilized eggs for years after their last mating (Highfield, 1996; Biedenweg and Schramm, 2019). Female tortoises will also lay unfertilized eggs in the absence of a male, as egg production is a normal part of the annual cycle.

The male reproductive system – how does this work?

The male reproductive system is simpler. Sperm production takes place in the testes. Sperm then travel down a tube called the vas deferens into the cloaca.

After courtship, the male mates by climbing onto the back of the female. Spurs, which are present on the hind legs or tail of some species, are used to hold onto the female for the few minutes this mating takes. The male uses his penis to introduce the sperm into the female during mating. The structure of the penis is often described a heart-shaped and is purple in colour. I have received calls from many owners over the years worried that their tortoise has passed

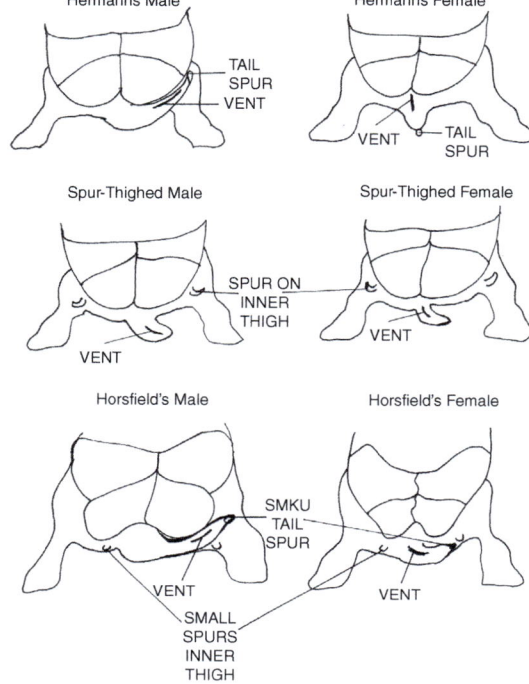

Fig. 11.10. Diagram of tails of males and females for comparison of length and position of vent.

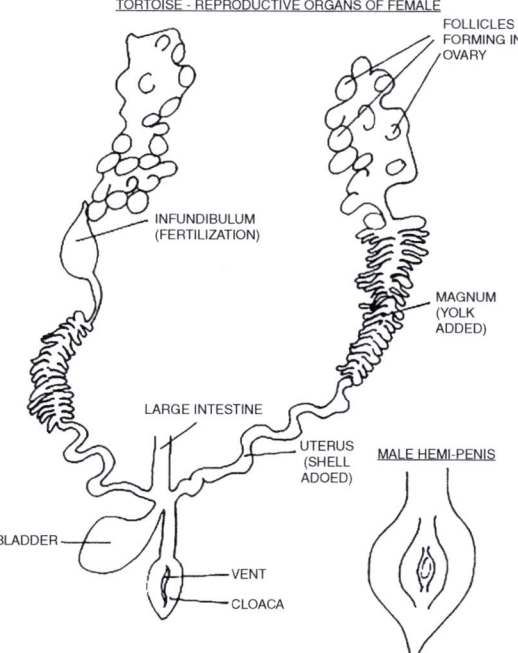

Fig. 11.12. Diagram of female reproductive system and the male penis.

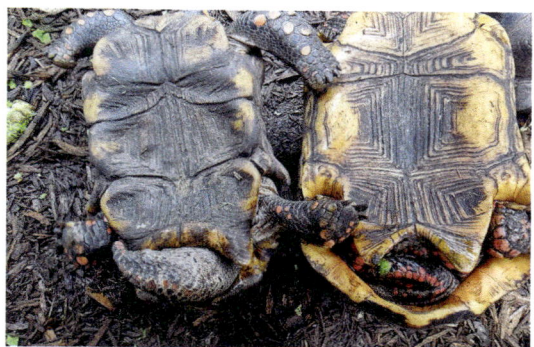

Fig. 11.11. Underside of male and female Red-footed tortoises (James Sullivan).

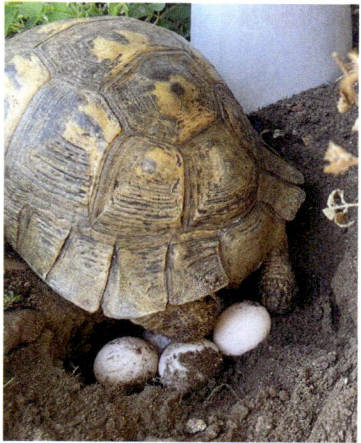

Fig. 11.13. Female building a nest and laying a clutch (Caroline Sumeray).

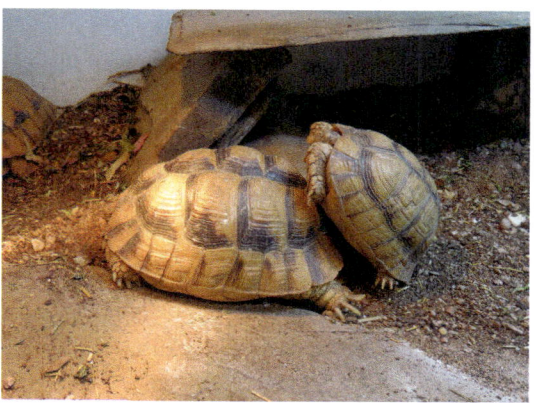

Fig. 11.14. Male and female Kleinmann's tortoises mating.

Breeding Tortoises

some horrid purple object like liver. In male tortoises, this is the penis being extruded.

The sperm pass out of the male's cloaca and into the female's cloaca. From there the sperm swim up into the oviducts in order to fertilize any ova (eggs) present.

The production of sperm continues throughout the male's adult life. Testosterone levels have been shown to rise prior to mating in some species (McArthur et al., 2004). There is little data concerning this for the range of tortoise species mentioned in this book.

Males produce sperm throughout their adult lives. The penis, which is also used for the passage of urine out of the urinary tract (Chitty and Raftery, 2013), is used to introduce the sperm into the female tract.

Note that in both male and female tortoises the urinary, reproductive and waste systems all empty into the cloaca. Urine, eggs or sperm, and faeces will all therefore pass out of the cloaca at different times. This is unlike the situation in mammals, where there are separate openings for all these materials.

What do courtship and mating look like?

(See also Chapters 9 and 10 on emotional behaviour and social interactions respectively.)

During courtship, male tortoises will sniff around females and chase them repeatedly to gain their attention. Their intentions are very clear, as they become very stimulated by the prospect of a mating opportunity. The male is trying to get the female to stop walking and allow him to mount the rear of her shell (McArthur et al., 2004; Wegehaupt, 2009a,b; Biedenweg and Schramm, 2019).

Females need male tortoises around for short periods in order to be stimulated to produce eggs. It is thought that male pheromones may play a part in normal egg production but there is little data on this. In addition, the courtship and mating behaviours may play a part in stimulating ovulation, and therefore the production of fully formed eggs. Lack of a male may play a part in the development of follicular stasis, a serious condition of female tortoises (see Chapter 7 on common illnesses and diseases).

Male Mediterranean tortoises, during warm weather, spend much of their time seeking out a female for mating purposes. This drive becomes so strong that males may stop feeding if females are unavailable. Levels of frustration may rise and the tortoise may show frantic walking or pacing behaviours with endless attempts to overcome physical barriers in order to escape in an effort to find a female.

Mating rituals may involve the male head bobbing in front of the female, followed by physical stimulation of the female through repeated ramming the back of her carapace (Spur-thighed and African Spurred/Sulcata tortoises), or biting the back of her legs (Kleinmann's, Hermann's and Horsfield's tortoises). These mating behaviours are to encourage the female to stand still and allow the male to mount her so that copulation can take place. This is quite a precarious position for the male. There is a real possibility that he could fall off, onto his back, if the female keeps moving. The courtship process is designed, therefore, to get her to stand still and allow mating to take place.

Males of some species will also vocalize during copulation. *Testudo kleinmanni* tortoises make a very distinctive sound (see Chapter 17 on Egyptian tortoises). Male Spur-thighed tortoises also make a very strange sound while mating. They are silent at all other times.

Repeated shell-butting or leg-biting can cause physical injury to the female, and being subject to this behaviour repeatedly can cause stress. This is particularly likely if the female is trapped in the corner of an enclosure and cannot get away, if there are too many males compared to females being kept together, or if the males are particularly amorous. For these reasons it is always advisable not to overcrowd enclosures, or to have more males than females if the tortoises are in a multi-sex group. Individual enclosures should also be available so that males and females can be separated if the sexual attraction of the males towards the females becomes too much.

What controls breeding in the wild?

The reproductive cycle of tortoises is dependent upon the seasons in temperate regions, or where the year has wet/dry seasonal variation (Highfield, 1996; Wegehaupt, 2009a,b; Biedenweg and Schramm, 2019). Climatic conditions will determine the optimum conditions for mating, egg-laying and incubation, and ensure that enough food is readily available for both adults and hatchlings. For some species, such as Hermann's tortoises (Wegehaupt, 2009a) it is apparent that a hibernation (brumation) period is required prior to the breeding season. Without this hibernation/brumation period these

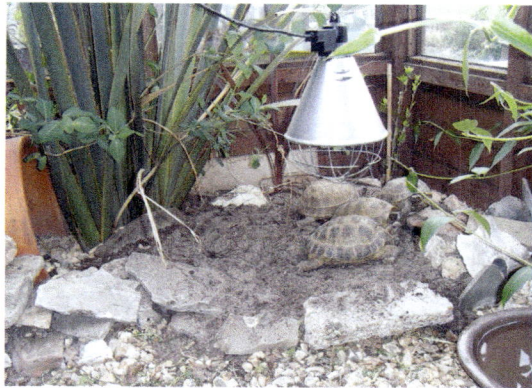

Fig. 11.15. Using a greenhouse with overhead lights to provide warm surfaces for egg-laying (Eleanor Lien-Hua Tirtasana Chubb).

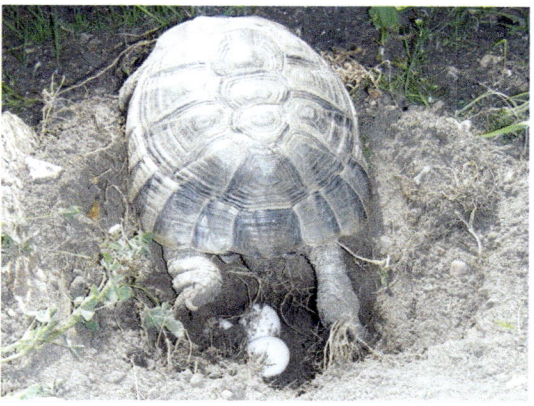

Fig. 11.16. Female Spur-thighed tortoise laying outdoors (Eleanor Lien-Hua Tirtasana Chubb).

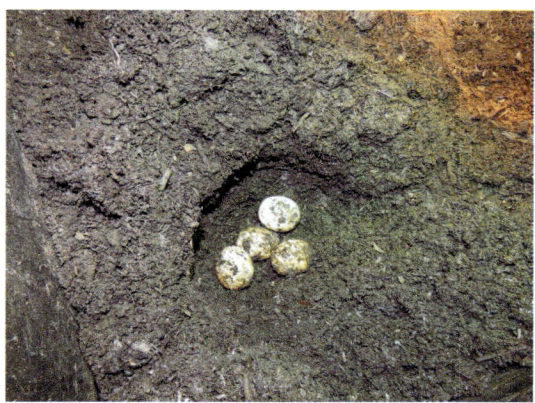

Fig. 11.17. The eggs uncovered in the nest.

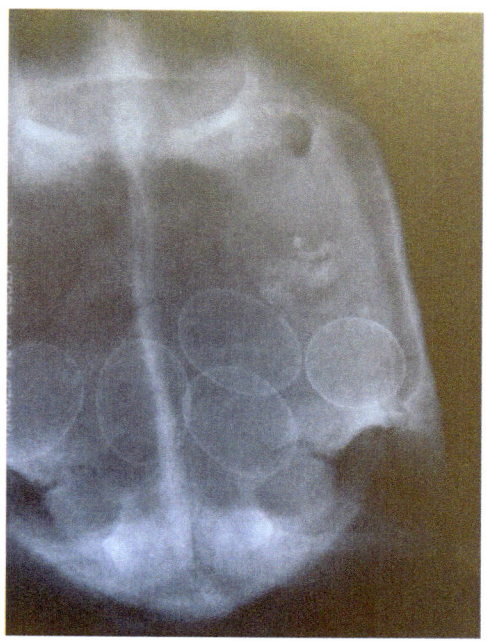

Fig. 11.18. X-ray of female tortoise containing eggs.

species of tortoise do not breed (Wright and Raiti, 2019).

Where the climatic conditions remain constant throughout the year (as in tropical rainforests, for example), breeding can occur at any time, and may occur several times during the year (McArthur *et al.*, 2004; Wright and Raiti, 2019).

For species subject to seasonal changes (Mediterranean and Horsfield's tortoises), females start to produce eggs within follicles as temperatures rise in the spring. These will continue to grow in size until the end of spring. In the wild, ovulation should then take place and the eggs are laid. During the summer when temperatures are high, the female's ovaries become inactive. In the autumn, falling temperatures may again cause the ovaries to reactivate, leading to further production of smaller follicles. If eggs are not laid the female may hibernate (brumate) with these retained follicles.

In more northerly climates, in captivity, this pattern is not well defined enough for the normal cycles to take place. There are rarely extended periods of consistently warm weather in Northern Europe, for example, to replicate the spring and summer of the warmer natural climates where tortoises originate. This means that while follicle

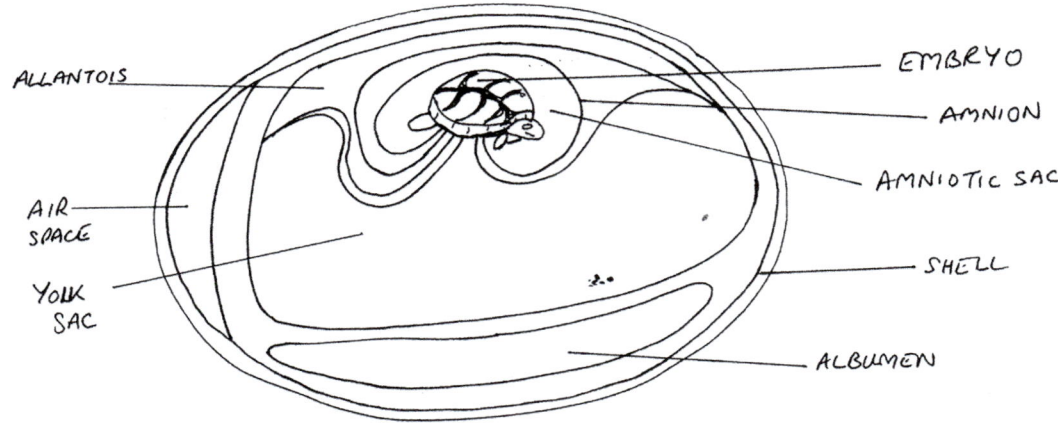

Fig. 11.19. Diagram of tortoise egg.

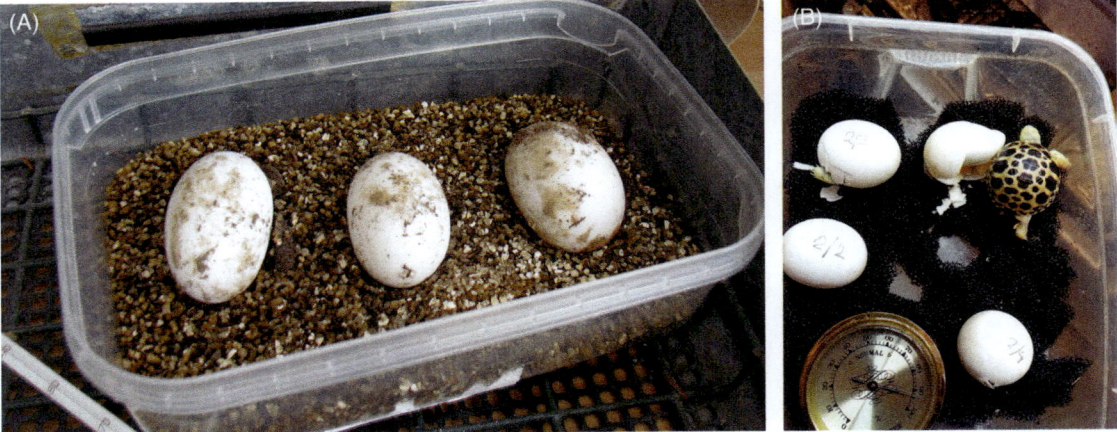

Fig. 11.20. (A) Eggs in a tray of vermiculite as they would be kept in an incubator. (B) Eggs of *Geochelone platynota* hatching (Andy Lewis).

production is stimulated by small temperature rises, the sustained warm temperatures needed for ovulation and egg-laying are much less common. Sometimes a warm autumn can have the effect of stimulating ovulation but rarely is there sustained warm weather at this time of year. This makes egg-laying less likely and leads to female tortoises hibernating with fully formed eggs (McArthur, 1996; McArthur *et al.*, 2004; McArthur, 2012).

Where females are thought to have retained eggs, they can be X-rayed in the autumn prior to hibernation/brumation as shown in Fig. 11.18. Female tortoises do hibernate successfully with eggs, but there may be complications that require veterinary attention, which means that a veterinary check before hibernation is a good idea.

Egg-laying in the wild – when does it take place?

Egg-laying in the wild is synchronized to seasonal changes. For example, where there are wet and dry seasons, hatching starts with the onset of the wet season, as is seen in Radiated, Sulcata and Leopard tortoises (Doody *et al.*, 2021). As the seasons vary in length, the incubation period is long, and hatching may be delayed to coincide with the most favourable environmental conditions for hatchlings. Thus, in these species, hatching of eggs does not occur during the dry season, when there is most likely to be a lack of available food.

In Mediterranean tortoises, hatching takes place in the spring when, once again, food is most abundant and most accessible even to very small tortoises (Wegehaupt, 2009a,b).

In tropical regions conditions are relatively constant throughout the year with regard to temperature, daylength and food availability. Because of this, tortoises such as Red-foots and Hingebacks are able to mate all year round. As food is always available for hatchlings and the climate always equitable, eggs can hatch at any time and this is not restricted by changing seasonal patterns.

How do I prepare mature adult tortoises for breeding in captivity?

It is essential to provide optimal conditions for adult tortoises if you intend to breed from them. They must be healthy and well enough to reproduce without harm to themselves (Biedenweg and Schramm, 2019). The captive environment must provide the females with nesting and egg-laying opportunities, as shown in Fig. 11.16, and suitable arrangements must be made for incubation of any eggs produced (Wright and Raiti, 2019).

The adult tortoises should be provided with plenty of calcium in their diet. This applies particularly to the females, as large amounts of calcium are needed to form the calcified eggshells properly.

Freely accessible water should always be plentiful in order to ensure full hydration of the adults.

The environmental conditions should be optimal to ensure the health of adult tortoises. Any that have been unwell or injured should not be mated, as this process makes significant demands on their physiology and metabolism. An unhealthy tortoise is likely to suffer a significant decline in health if it tries to breed when in poor condition.

What is important for nest-building and egg-laying in captivity?

Females carrying eggs will often bask more frequently than usual as they try to remain warm in preparation for the nest-building and laying processes. They will also be actively looking for nesting sites where the soil is warm enough for the incubation of their eggs (Wegehaupt, 2009a,b; Biedenweg and Schramm, 2019; Wright and Raiti, 2019).

Highfield (1996) identified temperatures of 30–41°C as the most likely to be chosen at nest sites by Spur-thighed (*Testudo graeca*) females. These temperatures are very unlikely to be achieved for any length of time in most captive situations in temperate climates. Providing suitable opportunities for egg-laying outside can therefore be challenging, as the temperatures are simply not warm enough. On the other hand, creating the depth of substrate needed indoors, where correct temperatures can be maintained for egg-laying and incubation, can also be challenging, particularly if the bigger species of tortoises are being kept.

South-facing slopes seem to provide females with the most likely conditions needed for nesting outdoors (Fig. 11.16). Provision of soft loose soil/sand substrates for digging into is essential. These may need to be recreated artificially, using overhead lights to further increase the temperature around potential nest-building sites. This can be done most easily within a greenhouse (Fig. 11.15). It is important to keep cats away from these sites, as these are very tempting as toileting areas for them.

Once the female is satisfied that she has found a suitable location, she will begin digging the hole in which to lay her eggs. This may take some hours and involves a great deal of energy expenditure. The female will have very exact requirements (Highfield, 1996). Once started, this process will continue until the nest is completed (unless the female is prevented from finishing by environmental conditions, for example she becomes too cold to continue).

Sulcata females will initially dig with the front legs until the hole is about 30 cm deep, and then turn around and use their back legs to complete the nest building. This process could take up to 6 hours (Wilson and Wilson, 1997).

Having observed nest-building in Horsfield's, Spur-thighed and Hermann's tortoises, I have noticed that as the female digs with her back legs, she will continue to do so until her legs are no longer in contact with the substrate. Digging is carried out by a circular motion as the back legs move down, back and outwards. Digging only stops when the leg-circling can be completed without the legs coming into contact with the substrate at all. The female's legs simply appear to be waving around in mid-air.

The depth of substrate needed for a nest should be approximately twice the carapace length. For a

Red-footed tortoise or a large Spur-thighed tortoise therefore, with a carapace length of 300 mm, the depth of nest dug could also be 300 mm. For large species such as Sulcatas, the depth of nest-digging will be much greater.

The female will sometimes urinate in the hole to increase humidity levels if the substrate is very dry. This is another reason for ensuring full hydration of adult females during breeding seasons.

Once the eggs have been deposited, the female will fill in the hole with all the loose soil previously dug out. The eggs will be completely covered. Once the tortoise walks away from the nesting site there will be virtually no indication that she has ever been there. If you do not see the female digging the site and then leaving, you are unlikely to know that a clutch of eggs has been laid. Figure 11.17 shows eggs in the nest which have been uncovered after laying.

Occasionally a female who is desperate to lay but who has not been provided with suitable nest-building sites will drop her eggs in the enclosure or the floor of the terrarium or tortoise table, where they will be broken as she walks over them. You cannot be certain that she has laid all the eggs that she is carrying, however, and veterinary advice should be sought in this event.

Incubation of eggs – how can this be done?

The eggs must be removed carefully from the nest site, immediately after the female has laid them, covered them over and walked away. They should then the placed in an incubator and kept in the same position on the incubator substrate. Once in place they should not be moved, or turned as you would do with birds' eggs. This is because tortoise eggs lack the chalazae, or twisted spiral membranes a seen in bird eggs, that hold the embryo in position if the egg is moved. It is therefore relatively easy for the tortoise embryo to be dislodged from the yolk sac. Figure 11.19 shows the egg structure. Tortoise eggs should never be disturbed whilst they are in the incubator.

The embryo will take its nutrition from the yolk held within a sac on which the embryo sits. As the embryo grows and increases in size and mass, the egg yolk will shrink. The embryo is contained within a sac of fluid – the amnion, which protects it against damage and allows gas exchange through the chorio-allantois. Uric acid as a waste product is able to precipitate out, as a solid paste, into the allantois. This means that this toxic waste is no longer a problem for the developing embryo (Highfield, 1996). The position of these membranes and other structures is shown in Fig 11.19.

The incubation substrate on which the eggs are placed will vary with species but vermiculite, sphagnum moss or perlite are commonly used, as all are soft enough to hold the eggs in position. These substrates can also accommodate different humidity requirements, as they absorb and hold water (Wright and Raiti, 2019). Generally, the eggs should be half-buried in the substrate (Fig. 11.20).

The use of commercially available incubators for tortoise eggs is now common (Fig. 11.21). For example, Exo Terra® has a reptile incubator for sale, as does VEVOR®. Zoo Med® sells a Reptibator for this purpose. Grumbach Company sells high-quality incubators (Kune, 2019). It is also possible to build an incubator. This would need to be well-insulated and well-ventilated (Fig. 11.22).

The incubator maintains the correct temperature for the development of the eggs. It should be well-insulated and located in an area where the external temperature is fairly constant. Heat sources such as incubators need to be safe in terms of fire hazard and of course thermostatically controlled. There also needs to be an opportunity to ensure that humidity levels can be maintained at 50–80% within the incubator, depending upon species.

Air flow should be controlled during incubation to ensure that the embryos can absorb sufficient oxygen through their shells, and to avoid the build-up of carbon dioxide (Highfield, 1996).

Incubation temperatures are important for normal development and sex determination. Tortoises show environmental sex determination, with higher temperatures producing female offspring while lower temperatures produce males (Wright and Raiti, 2019).

Monitoring of the temperature and its maintenance within narrow ranges is essential for the development of the embryos and to know the sex of the hatchlings (Wright and Raiti, 2019). An accurate thermometer should be used within the incubator and digital thermometers with alarms can be set so that any change in temperature outside the range set triggers a warning sound. The thermometer sensor needs to accurately detect the temperature as closely as possible to that within the eggs themselves, so should be positioned very close to the eggs. Table 11.1 shows examples of the numbers of eggs laid and incubabtion parameters for several species.

Table 11.1. Incubation temperatures and incubations lengths for different species of tortoise (based on Highfield, 1996; Wright and Raiti, 2019).

Species	Clutch size (number of eggs)	Length of incubation (days)	Incubation temperatures (°C)
Horsfield's tortoise *Testudo horsfieldi*	4–7	60–75	28–32
Spur-thighed tortoise *Testudo graeca*	4–7	60–80	28–32
Hermann's tortoise *Testudo hermanni*	5–12	85–100	28–32
Radiated tortoise *Geochelone radiata*	6–14	95–120	30–33
Leopard tortoise *Geochelone pardalis*	10–20	140–155	28–32
African Spurred tortoise *Geochelone sulcata*	15–30	120–170	28–32
Egyptian tortoise *Testudo kleinmanni*	3	70–140	30–34
Red-footed tortoise *Geochelone carbonaria*	3–6	90–175	28–32

What happens if the eggs fail to hatch?

Having provided a suitable environment for hatching and the maximum length of incubation having passed, there comes a point when the eggs are no longer likely to hatch. This is always disappointing and the reasons for the failure are many and varied. The eggs may not have been fertile (even though a male and female were present during the process). The eggs may not have been properly formed and may have shells that are too thick or too thin (Fig. 11.23). Eggs with these problems would usually show signs of being collapsed or dented and this may have been seen during the incubation period.

If the hatchlings are found to be dead within the shell, the breeding by the adults is likely to be taking place normally but there is a problem with the incubation set-up. This is possibility due to temperature or humidity variations outside the required range. Infections from fungi or bacteria can cause a problem (Highfield, 1996). If the set-up repeatedly fails to produce hatchlings, of course the whole incubation process should be reviewed.

What should I do when the eggs are hatching?

Once the baby tortoises start to break out of the shell, the process can take many hours. The babies or neonates will open the shell with the beak to allow access to air but may remain within the shell for many hours while gathering their strength to break free from the shell (Fig. 11.24A) (Highfield, 1996). The hatching process will normally take place at the same time for any given egg clutch. Keeping the humidity levels high so that the membranes and the hatchling do not dry out is achieved using a water-spray bottle to gently introduce water into the air space around the eggs (Wright and Raiti, 2019). Generally, the hatchling is best left to get out of the egg unaided unless clearly in distress, or exhausted, after a prolonged hatching period. The shell and membranes can be gently separated from the hatching in this situation to help the baby emerge.

The egg yolk should have been reabsorbed by the hatchling before birth but there may be a small amount remaining attached to the underside of the shell (Fig. 11.24B). It is important that this is not

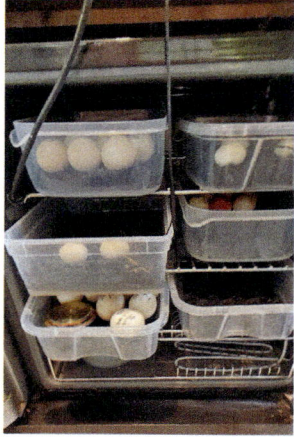

Fig. 11.21. Home-made incubator (Andy Lewis) converted from fridge.

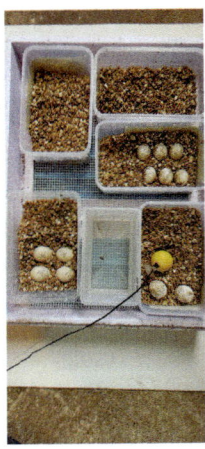

Fig. 11.22. Tortoise incubator showing thermostat (commercially produced by Bruja) with eggs (Andy Lewis).

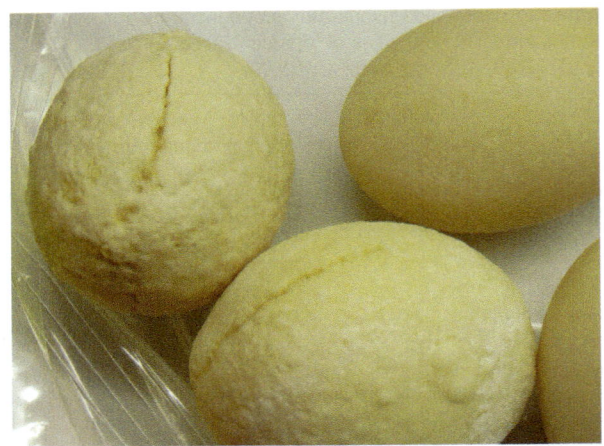

Fig. 11.23. Eggs that are abnormal with thick shells and not likely to hatch.

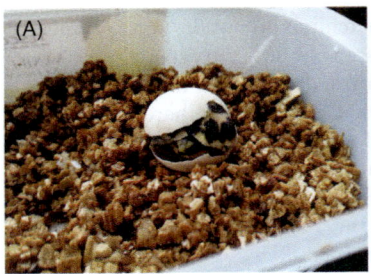 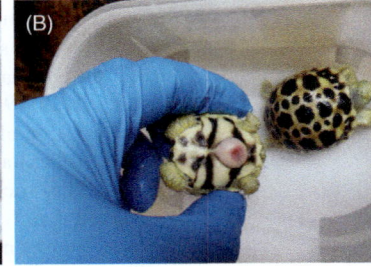 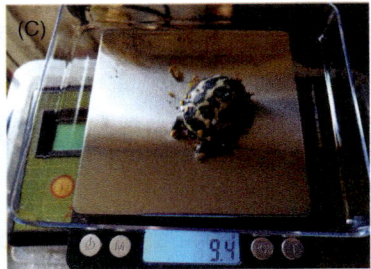

Fig. 11.24. (A) *Pyxis arachnoides* egg hatching (Andy Lewis). (B) *Geochelone platynota* hatchling with egg yolk attached (Andy Lewis). (C) Weighing hatchlings (Andy Lewis).

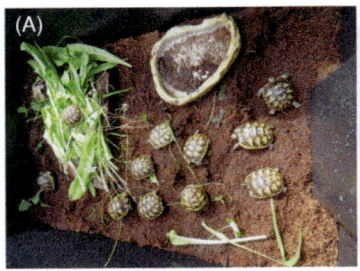 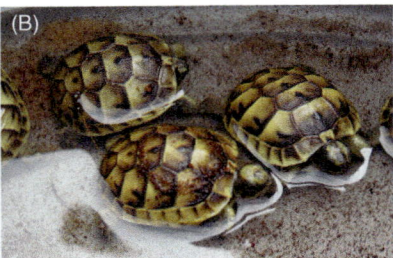 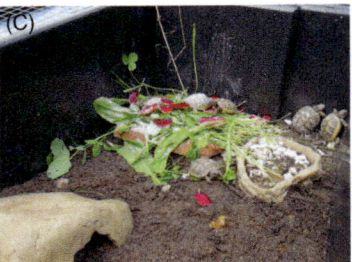

Fig. 11.25. Hatchlings and young Mediterranean tortoises in suitable accommodation to provide food, access to water (in a bath as well as in the enclosure) and plenty of calcium availability.

damaged while it is reabsorbed by the baby. The surface and environment should be clean and soft for the few days this may take.

As the hatchling emerges you will see that it is rounded in shape and folded in half across the middle of the plastron. This takes some time to flatten, possibly up to 2 days. Once this happens the plastron will be flat, and the baby tortoise can move around normally (Highfield, 1996). The shell will be relatively soft initially to allow these

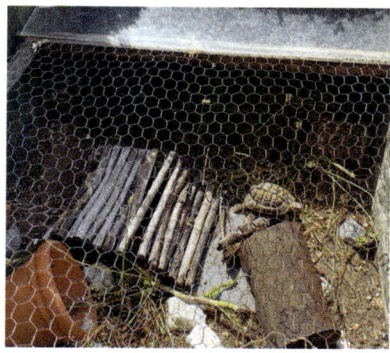

Fig. 11.26. Young tortoises in protected enclosures with wire cover.

changes, but the carapace and plastron will soon harden into their normal shape.

Once a clutch of eggs has hatched, the young tortoises can be moved into their accommodation. The hatching weight being measured in Fig. 11.24C is shown. This should provide access to suitable temperatures and humidity levels, and access to food, water and additional calcium (Fig. 11.25). The calcium can be offered as chalk, eggshells or powder as a supplement on the food. Healthy hatchlings will start to feed within a few hours. The diet should be that of the healthy adult right from the start. Herbivorous tortoises will eat wild plants and weeds immediately.

The enclosures should provide protection from predators, as young tortoises are particularly vulnerable to attacks. Enclosures often have wire coverings, for example, when the hatchlings and juveniles are outdoors (Fig. 11.26).

Conclusion

Consideration of the ethical aspects of breeding captive tortoises will lead each of us to come to a conclusion as to whether it is an appropriate course of action for our own tortoises. The species of tortoise, its age, health, and the suitability of individuals to go through the courtship, mating and breeding processes should all be taken into account when making decisions. Of course, only healthy individuals should be used for breeding.

Considerations of the Five Domains (Five Freedoms) should be part of our decision making. These important welfare considerations identify the ability to carry out normal behaviours as being one of the five welfare requirements. Lack of opportunity to meet and potentially mate with other tortoises can have negative effects on health and well-being. Conversely, if not managed effectively, keeping individuals together for breeding purposes can also be detrimental to health and welfare. Putting individuals together for breeding purposes carries the risk of spreading disease, for example, as well as potentially causing stress, particularly to the females.

Some species of tortoise are much easier to breed than others. Sulcata tortoises, for example, are very fertile, lay large numbers of eggs (up to 30 in each clutch), and can lay up to six clutches per year in the right conditions. Yet they are a challenge to keep as pets. Given that they can weigh 100 kg as adults, while the size of enclosure needed to provide sufficient grazing is measured in acres, they do not make suitable pets in most domestic situations, not least because of the enormous cost of paying for heat and light all year round.

The question arises, therefore: just because we can breed tortoises, does that mean we should? In the case of some tortoise species, their demands are so difficult to meet that there are sound arguments for not breeding them and indeed limiting the numbers kept in captivity. Identifying the suitability, or otherwise, of species to be traded as part of the pet trade would seem to be a logical step in moving forwards with improving the welfare of captive tortoises (Warwick *et al.*, 2018).

It is a tempting and attractive prospect to breed our own captive tortoises, but we must all think very carefully before taking that first step – is it really the right thing to do?

References and Further Reading

Biedenweg, F. and Schramm, R. (2019) *The Egyptian Tortoise* Testudo kleinmanni *Lortet 1883. A Fascinating Little Beauty*. Tartaruga-Verlag Ricarda Schramm, Grebenhain, Germany

Chitty, J. (2015) *Latest methods in chelonian treatment: improving standards for captive Chelonia in the UK*. In: Proceedings of Tortoise Welfare UK Conference, 8 November 2015

Chitty, J. and Raftery, A. (2013) *Essentials of Tortoise Medicine and Surgery*. Wiley Blackwell, Chichester, UK.

CITES: Convention on International Trade in Endangered Species of Wild Flora and Fauna, Geneva. Website: www.cites.org

Doody, J.S., Dinets, V. and Burghardt, G.M. (2021) *The Secret Social Life of Reptiles*. John Hopkins University Press, Baltimore, Maryland.

EAZA and EEP: EAZA = European Association of Zoos and Aquaria. EEP = EAZA Ex-situ Programmes (population management programmes). Reptile EEPs include *Testudo kleinmanni*, *Emys orbicularis*, *Chelonoidis nigra* species complex, *Uroplatus henkeli*, *Mauremys annamensis*, *M. mutica*, *M. nigricans* and *M. sinensis*, *Astrochleys yniphora* and *Chelodina mccordi*. EAZA website: www.eaza.net

ESF: European Studbook Foundation. Private non-profit organization in Europe, headquarters Sneek, Netherlands, with country coordinators elsewhere. Conservation of reptiles and amphibians through captive breeding, especially endangered species. Website: https:/studbooks.eu

Highfield, A. (1996) *Practical Encyclopaedia of Keeping and Breeding Tortoises and Freshwater Turtles*. Carapace Press, London.

Highfield, A.C. and Martin, J. (1995) *Captive breeding of the Egyptian tortoise Testudo kleinmanni*. Tortoise Trust. Available at https://www.tortoisetrust.org/articles/kleinmanni.html

IUCN: International Union for Conservation of Nature, Gland, Switzerland. Maintains IUCN Red List of Threatened Species. Website: https://iucn.org

Jepson, L. (2006) *Mediterranean Tortoises*. Interpet, Dorking, UK.

Johnson, J.D. (2019) Ch 20 Urogenital System. In: Girling, S.J. and Raiti, P. (eds) *BSAVA Manual or Reptiles*, 3rd edn. BSAVA, Quedgeley, UK, pp. 342–353.

Kune, U. (2019) Astrochelys radiata – keeping and breeding in South Spain. *RADIATA* 28(2).

Lumbis, R. and White, C. (2022) Ch 5 Nutritional welfare. In: Rendle, M. and Hinde-Megarity, J. (eds) *BSAVA Manual of Practical Veterinary Welfare*. BSAVA, Quedgeley, UK, pp.124–146.

McArthur, S. (1996) *Veterinary Management of Tortoises and Turtles*. Blackwell, Oxford, UK.

McArthur, S. (2012) Chelonian Medicine: Improving Standards for Captive Chelonia in the UK. In: Proceedings of Tortoise Welfare UK Conference, 17 November 2012

McArthur, S., Wilkinson, R. and Meyer, J. (2004) *Medicine and Surgery of Tortoises and Turtles*. Blackwell, Oxford, UK.

Mellor, D.J. (2016) Updating animal welfare thinking: moving beyond the 'Five Freedoms' towards a 'Life worth Living'. *Animals* 6, 21.

Warwick, C., Steedman C., Jessop C., Arena P., Pilny A. and Nicholas, E. (2018) Exotic pet suitability: Understanding some problems and using a labelling system to aid animal welfare, environment, and consumer protection. *Journal of Veterinary Behavior* 26, 17–26.

Wegehaupt, W. (2009a) *Mediterranean Tortoises, Where and how they live in the wild*. Kressbronn, Germany

Wegehaupt, W. (2009b) *Naturalistic Keeping and Breeding of Hermann's Tortoises*. Kressbronn, Germany

Wilson, R. and Wilson, R. (1997) *The Care and Breeding of the African Spurred Tortoise* Geochelone sulcata. Carapace Press, London.

Wright, K. and Raiti, P. (2019) Ch 5 Breeding and neonatal care. In: Girling, S.J. and Raiti, P. (eds) *BSAVA Manual of Reptiles*, 3rd edn. BSAVA, Quedgeley, UK, pp. 70–89.

Yeates, J. (2022) Ch 1 Animal ethics and welfare. In: Rendle, M. and Hinde-Megarity, J. (eds) *BSAVA Manual of Practical Veterinary Welfare*. BSAVA, Quedgeley, UK, pp. 1–18.

12 Tortoise Hibernation/Brumation

Abstract
Not all species of tortoises hibernate (or brumate, as is the more correct term in reptiles). Tropical tortoises are non-hibernating species. They will die if placed in hibernation. Hibernation takes place naturally in species where the winter climate is too cold and there is insufficient food available for the tortoise to remain active. The hibernation process involves preparation for hibernation, the hibernation or brumation itself, and then the process of waking up and becoming active afterwards.

During hibernation, metabolic processes slow to the minimum needed to sustain life. During hibernation, there is a very low demand for calories or oxygen. The process is temperature-dependent and is stimulated by decreasing daylength. It is a way of surviving periods that would otherwise lead to high levels of mortality. Hibernation also allows some species to extend their range away from the warm tropical areas around the equator. This chapter discusses preparation for hibernation in captivity. Suitable locations for hibernation are described, together with the need to check the tortoise's condition throughout the period of dormancy. Bringing the tortoise out of hibernation safely and back to a period of activity is also described. The chapter examines what can go wrong and why. Ways to deal with hibernation difficulties are also discussed.

What is hibernation/brumation?

Hibernation/brumation is a period of dormancy, or sleep, during which the animal is inactive. Hibernation as a strategy is not restricted to tortoises but is seen in a number of species, including mammals, where the period of inactivity can last several months. Examples of mammals that hibernate include bears, hedgehogs, bats and dormice. During the period of torpor, the animal will rely on stored body fat to sustain life.

In reptiles the inactive period is more correctly called brumation, as this is the appropriate term for ectotherms (Wright and Raiti, 2019) but the effects are similar – the reptile does not feed, drink, produce wastes or show activity during this period of dormancy. Reptiles can react to touch, however, which is different from hibernation in mammals where they are completely unable to respond. **For the sake of familiarity, the term hibernation is used here.**

Tortoises will still respond to light or touch with a small degree of limb or head movement but otherwise appear to be 'lifeless'. The low metabolic level means that breathing and heart rate are very slow. Heart rate may be reduced to one beat per minute.

The process is similar across hibernating species in that there is a period of preparation triggered by environmental changes. Most significant are a reduction in daylength and temperature. Once daylength is short and the temperature stays below the trigger level, the animal will remain hidden in a natural retreat, such as a burrow, crevice, den or cave. This offers protection from the worst of the cold weather and from any precipitation (Biedenweg and Schramm, 2019; Wegehaupt, 2009a).

Hibernation has few biological advantages to a species – it extends the range of habitat that is available, but otherwise it is a survival mechanism only. During hibernation, the animal is unable to function normally. Reproduction is not possible. This is biologically a disadvantage, as the overriding drive for all living species is the production of young, to ensure continuation of the species. Hibernation is therefore an interim period allowing life to continue during adverse conditions, ready for the next season of activity and breeding.

In tortoises, the hibernation period in the wild is likely to be around 8 weeks maximum. We should be aware of this when hibernating captive tortoises. As we try to mimic the natural environment in our environmental provision, so too should we mimic the length of natural hibernation. Horsfield's tortoises may hibernate for longer, as they live at the extreme most northerly range for tortoises. Not only may they hibernate for longer periods; they may also hibernate several times during the year.

Not all tortoises hibernate, in fact only a few species do so. Tropical species living near the equator in a climate that remains warm all year round do not need to hibernate, so their bodies are not equipped for hibernation. Any attempt to hibernate them is likely to lead to severe health problems (Scheelings, 2019) and ultimately their death. These tortoises must have access to warm temperatures and food all year round. Their bodies have not adapted to a period of torpor and inactivity. It is a survival mechanism they do not need, and they are not in any way set up to achieve this.

Why do tortoises hibernate?

Some species of tortoise hibernate in order to survive cold conditions or when there is not enough food available to sustain them. During hibernation the tortoise has a very low demand for calories and oxygen, as metabolic processes slow to the minimum necessary to sustain life.

The critical temperature triggering hibernation is 10°C. Above this temperature the tortoise will start to wake up. The temperature should be maintained at about 5°C throughout hibernation. Below 2°C the tortoise will start to freeze. The most important factor for maintaining a safe hibernation is the temperature.

Hibernating species commonly seen in captivity are listed in Box 12.1. Non-hibernating species are also listed in Box 12.2. However, these lists are not exhaustive. In all cases you must be aware of the particular species you are caring for and its natural environment, in order to determine whether or not it is a hibernating species. Tropical species do not hibernate, and hibernation is likely to lead to their death as they are not adapted for periods of cold, or of inactivity.

In the wild the triggers that start the hibernation process are as follows (McArthur *et al.*, 2004; Highfield and Highfield, 2008; Wegehaupt, 2009a):

- Reduced photoperiod – shortening daylength is the first change to which the tortoise responds
- Reduced light intensity – the sun is not as strong as the angle of the earth tilts away from the sun. This happens in autumn and the result is a slightly reduced light intensity
- Reduced food supply – plant species die off and dry out. This makes it more difficult to find food and reduces the water content available in the food
- Fall in temperatures – once temperatures fall the tortoise will respond with reduced activity, until activity stops when the temperature is continuously below 10°C.

Which species hibernate?

If in doubt as to the species – do not hibernate until proper identification can be carried out.

How do I hibernate my tortoise safely?

Hibernation is a difficult process for tortoises and holds many potential pitfalls. We have to do everything we can to support tortoises as they prepare for hibernation, during the hibernation itself and then post-hibernation.

With increases in global temperatures, it is becoming more difficult to be sure that temperatures during the winter will not rise above the critical 10°C. Thus, it is even more important to monitor temperatures on a daily basis using a maximum–minimum thermometer (Fig. 12.14) to check the changes in any 24-hour period. The thermometer should be placed in a location as close as possible to where the tortoises actually are in the hibernation set-up.

It is absolutely vital to ensure that the tortoise is well-prepared for hibernation. It is essential that only suitable species and healthy individuals of suitable weight are hibernated.

Keeping the hibernation short will reduce the risks and make the hibernation as safe as possible. Regular checking of the tortoise during hibernation will ensure that any problems are spotted quickly. If the tortoise wakes up, this can be seen and suitable action taken.

When waking the tortoise up after hibernation, the optimal conditions necessary to get the tortoise feeding again immediately must be provided. The tortoise must also be given plenty of opportunity to rehydrate.

When not to hibernate:

Tortoises should not be placed into hibernation:

- When the tortoise is not a hibernating species
- If the tortoise is underweight or dehydrated
- When the tortoise is unwell (or has been unwell) or has any injuries
- If the tortoise has not been properly prepared for hibernation (for example by fasting before going into hibernation)

Box 12.1. Hibernating species commonly kept in captivity.

Hermann's tortoise – *Testudo hermanni*
Marginated tortoise – *Testudo marginata*
Spur-thighed tortoise – *Testudo graeca*
Horsfield's tortoise – *Agrionemys horsfieldi*

Note that there are some small North African subspecies of *Testudo graeca* which do not hibernate. These include *T. g. nabeulensis* (Tunisian) and *T. g. soussensis* (Moroccan), (see Chapter 15) and there are other smaller species that also do not hibernate.

The **Horsfield's tortoise** (*Testudo horsfieldi*) hibernates for extended periods compared with other species, due to the range it inhabits, which has prolonged periods of cold. In between, however. there are also periods of extreme heat during which this tortoise may aestivate (see Table 12.1). This makes the Horsfield's tortoise much more of a challenge to keep in captivity than most keepers understand (see Chapter 16 on Horsfield's tortoises). In captivity it is safer to keep to the principles set out here for hibernation of this small species.

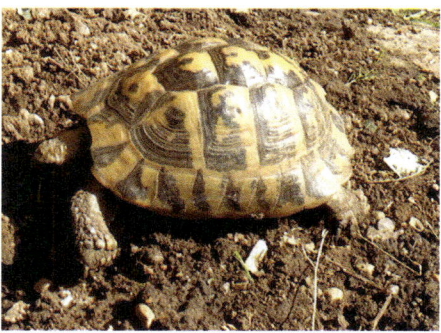

Fig. 12.1. Hermann's tortoise – *Testudo hermanni*.

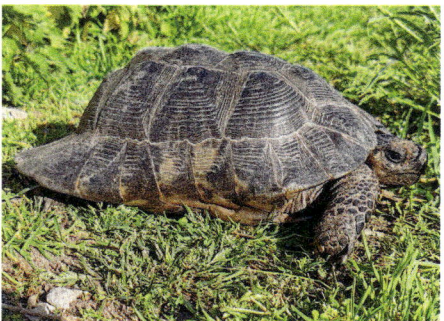

Fig. 12.2. Marginated tortoise – *Testudo marginata* (Dillon Prest).

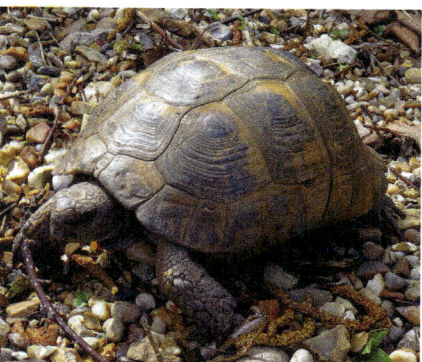

Fig. 12.3. Spur-thighed tortoise – *Testudo graeca ibera*.

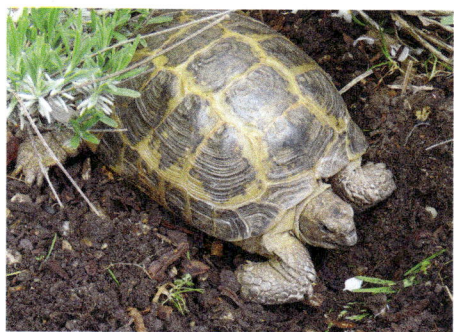

Fig. 12.4. Horsfield's tortoise – *Agrionemys/Testudo horsfieldi*.

Table 12.1. Hibernation (brumation) and aestivation.

Hibernation (Brumation)	Aestivation
Period of dormancy or inactivity	Period of dormancy or inactivity
Allows survival in adverse conditions	Allows survival in adverse conditions
Takes place when temperatures fall and daylength shortens	Takes place at the height of summer
Conditions are too cold for normal metabolism	Conditions are too hot for normal metabolism
There is little food available due to the coldness of the climate	There is little food available due to the dryness of the climate

Box 12.2. Non-hibernating species – tropical.

These tortoises should never be hibernated

Leopard tortoise – *Centrochelys pardalis*
Sulcata (African Spurred tortoise) *Centrochelys sulcata*
Radiated tortoise – *Geochelone/Astrochelys radiata*
Indian Star tortoise – *Geochelone elegans*
Burmese Brown tortoise – *Manouria emys*
Red-footed tortoise – *Geochelone/Chelonoidis carbonaria*
Yellow-footed tortoise – *Geochelone/Chelonoidis denticulatis*
Hingeback tortoises – *Kinixys* spp.:
  Kinixys belliana – Bell's hingeback
  Kinixys erosa – serrated or forest hingeback
  Kinixys homeana – Home's hingeback

Egyptian tortoise – *Testudo kleinmanni*
Aldabran tortoise – *Aldabrachelys gigantea*
Galapagos tortoise – *Chelonoidis niger*

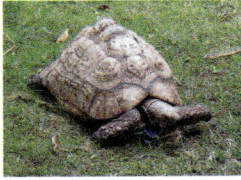

Fig. 12.5. Leopard tortoise.

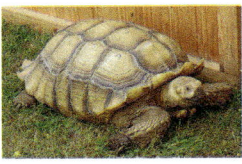

Fig 12.6. Sulcata tortoise.

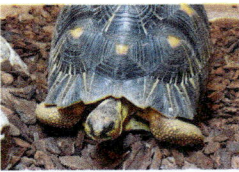

Fig 12.7. Radiated tortoise.

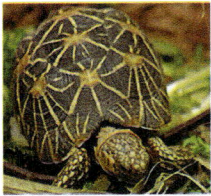

Fig 12.8. Indian Star tortoise (Eleanor Lien-Hua Tirtasana Chubb).

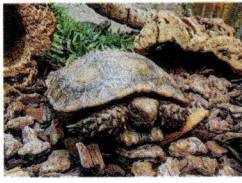

Fig 12.9. Burmese Brown tortoise (Dillon Prest).

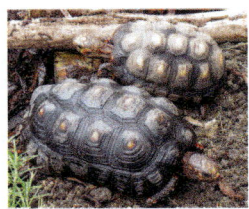

Fig 12.10. Red-footed tortoise.

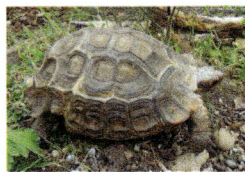

Fig 12.11. Serrated or forest hingeback tortoise.

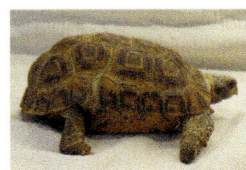

Fig 12.12. Bell's Hingeback tortoise.

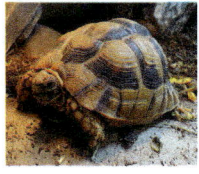

Fig 12.13. Egyptian tortoise.

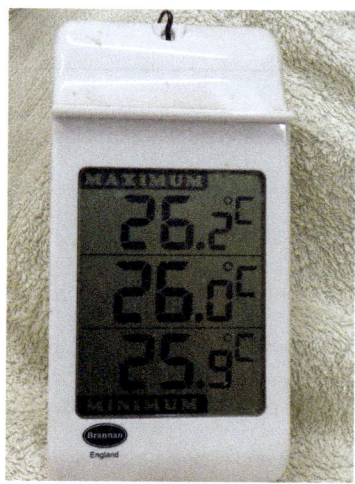

Fig. 12.14. Maximum–minimum thermometer showing the maximum recorded temperature as 26.2°C, the current temperature as 26.0°C and the lowest temperature as 25.9°C in a shed for tropical tortoises.

- For safety, very young tortoises such as current hatchlings should not be hibernated
- Once they have reached the age of 2–3 years a short hibernation of 2–3 weeks could be introduced, bearing in mind that there is always a risk involved.

Planning for hibernation

Hibernation must be planned. You should not be caught by surprise. Many people have contacted me over the years because they have 'lost' their tortoise in September. If the weather has been cold in the early autumn in northerly climes, the tortoises may take it upon themselves to find a suitable location to burrow down into the soil in readiness for an early hibernation. Tortoises are very good at finding sheltered hiding places for this and, once dug-in and under the soil surface, they can be very hard to find and may be lost in the garden for the entire winter. This is to be avoided, as you cannot then support the tortoise, which will end up hibernating for far longer than is advisable and in colder and wetter conditions than are safe.

When should your tortoise hibernate?

This is the description of the process in northern climates, which are colder and wetter than the natural habitat. When the weather starts to cool and the days shorten, you need to keep a careful eye on your tortoise to avoid the situation above. You will need to start to bring the tortoise in, or put it into its overnight area, with heat and light to extend the days and keep the tortoise warmer to slow down the preparation for hibernation.

As Table 12.2 shows, in the UK and northern Europe this begins in August. If the weather is cold and rainy, the tortoise will slow down more quickly. You will want to hibernate your tortoise in the coldest months, so you may have to delay the onset of the process if the tortoise is to sleep in December and January. Thinking ahead is important so that the tortoise does not simply dig in outside. Planning ahead to ensure that the slow-down and preparation are under control, rather than simply haphazard, will increase the likely survival of your tortoise. Even if you opt for an outdoor location (see below) for hibernation, in a covered greenhouse or similar, the tortoise will still have some protection that you have provided and a degree of supervision, which can be the difference between surviving hibernation or not. The example timescale in Table 12.2 is an outline, with details of all the stages shown in subsequent sections.

The four stages of hibernation

Stage 1: Preparation

Before considering a period of hibernation for your tortoise it is vital to ensure that the tortoise is healthy. The tortoise should have been behaving normally during the warmer months:

- Basking – as part of temperature regulation.
- Walking – exploring the environment and seeking out food.
- Urinating – normal urates should be seen.
- Defecating – faeces should be solid, very dark and not smelling unpleasant.
- Reproductive behaviours – if kept with other tortoises, courtship, mating and breeding behaviours should be normal in the season before hibernation.

You should have observed such regular daily activities before the cooling-down period begins. Behaviour in tortoises is the most important indicator of good health (see Chapter 8 on behaviour)

As the weather gets cooler, tortoises start to become torpid. Close observation is needed to ensure that

Table 12.2. Example timescale for hibernation preparation and hibernation itself in Northern Europe (McArthur *et al.*, 2004; Wright and Raiti, 2019).

Months	Actions
Late August–September Daylength shortens and weather cools	• Supplement outside living with indoor heat and light to extend the day and delay hibernation. • Monitor behaviour/feeding. • Carry out pre-hibernation checks. • Weigh and measure. • Make a decision about whether to hibernate and how. • Start hibernation planning. • Prepare the hibernation location and check the temperatures there with a max–min thermometer. • Check you have suitable accommodation for overwintering if hibernation is not possible.
October–November	• Inside accommodation for much of the time (weather dependent). • With artificial heat and light provided but for shorter periods each day, gradually reduced over the next 1–2 months. • Continue pre-hibernation checks and monitor health and behaviour closely.
November–December	• Month of continued slow-down with lots of bathing/drinking opportunities and temperatures allowed to come down to 12–15°C. • Stop feeding and allow fasting for 4 weeks before hibernation, to allow the gut to empty. • Continue pre-hibernation checks and monitor health and behaviour closely.
December–February	• Hibernation for up to 8 weeks. • Check regularly for any problems and weigh every 2 weeks.
February–March	• Wake up and provide plenty of water. • Support inside accommodation with heat, and with light for around 12–14 hours daily to regain normal activity. • Ensure feeding starts and observe behaviours daily. • Keep temperatures above 15°C at night.
March–summer	• Increasing amounts of time outdoors as weather improves and temperatures rise. • Give maximum access to outdoor enclosures throughout the summer. • Monitor for normal feeding and behaviour.

there are no other significant changes in behaviour (other than those associated with becoming cooler and preparing for hibernation). The tortoise will become slower and less active, feeding less as the daylength shortens and the temperature falls.

Pre-hibernation health check

(See also Chapter 6 on health checks)
Check the following:

- Eyes – should be open and bright. Any swelling, discharge or closing of the eyes should be investigated before proceeding with the hibernation, with veterinary advice as appropriate.
- Ears – any swelling, discharge or damage should be investigated before proceeding, with veterinary advice as appropriate.
- Nose – there should be no discharge from the nares, which may indicate a respiratory infection.
- Mouth – should be opened to check for a pink healthy colour (some tortoises with a naturally yellow coloration may be more yellow). There should be no damage to the tongue or tissues. Any sign of stomatitis or mouth-rot (seen as yellow deposits) or any bleeding or purple coloration of the tongue should be investigated before proceeding, with veterinary advice as appropriate.
- Limbs – should not be damaged or swollen. Excess fluid build-up leads to swelling. Any lumps and bumps or injuries should be investigated before proceeding, with veterinary advice as appropriate.
- Tail – there should be no discharge, signs of diarrhoea or nasty smell from this area. If any of these are present, they should be investigated before proceeding, with veterinary advice as appropriate.
- Shell – should be complete with no soft areas, damage, bleeding or fluid loss.

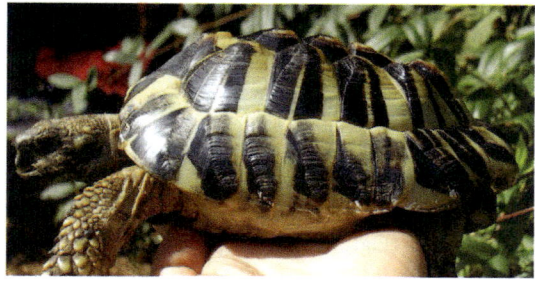

Fig. 12.15. Tortoise with collapsed vertebral column and flattened carapace with restricted space for internal organs, including lungs, due to excessive growth.

Many tortoise keepers get their tortoise checked by a veterinarian before hibernation, especially if they are inexperienced, or if the tortoise has not hibernated before. This is always a good idea and should definitely be carried out if any doubts exist about the suitability of a tortoise to hibernate.

Checking the tortoise is of a suitable weight to hibernate

These calculations should be used as a guide only. Each tortoise is an individual case and the decision as to whether to hibernate should be a holistic one. Information should be gathered on all aspects of the tortoise's history, general health, pre-hibernation behaviour and results of regular checks. Any veterinary advice given should be followed. The more familiar you are with your own tortoise and its normal behaviour and habits, the better the position you will be in to determine whether hibernation should take place and, if so, for how long.

In order to decide if the tortoise is of a suitable weight to hibernate its weight should be compared with its length. Two measurements are needed:

1. Weight in grams – the tortoise should be put onto the scales so that the legs are not in contact with the surface. Using a large stable tub, such as a vitamin tub, to raise the body and legs off the scales may be needed for large tortoises. Accurately measure the weight of the animal in grams. The tortoise should be kept the right way up (hence use of the tub) to avoid undue stress.

2. Straight carapace length (**SCL**) in millimetres – when the tortoise is measured its head should be withdrawn so that the straight shell length can be measured (rather than the length over the dome of its shell).

Comparing the weight to the length can be done in the following ways: (1) the Jackson ratio; or (2) the bone density ratio.

THE JACKSON RATIO (see Chapter 6, on health checks) For Spur-thighed and Hermann's tortoises the Jackson ratio can be used as a scale to compare weight with length. **The Jackson ratio must not be used for any other species.** The graph is more accurate the bigger the tortoise is in length and weight. The steep parts of the curve give the most accurate readings. Lower down the graph, where juvenile and small tortoise measurements would be taken, the readings are less accurate.

THE BONE DENSITY RATIO The bone density ratio can be used (see also Chapter 6 on health checks) as a general guide, but it is not species-specific. The guidance is helpful, but the best approach is to keep monthly records of weight over time so that you can see what a 'normal' weight is for your tortoise, as explained in Chapter 6.

The bone density ratio involves a mathematical calculation to compare length with weight. In the formula below:

L = Straight carapace length in centimetres (cm) (convert millimetres to centimetres by dividing by 10; for example: 1 mm = 0.1 cm; 25 mm = 2.5 cm; 10 mm = 1 cm; 100 mm = 10 cm)

W = Weight in grams (g)

Formula for bone ratio (called N):

$N = W(g) \div L(cm)^3$

Bone ratio (N) = Weight in grams/ (Length in centimetres)^3

This means that having measured the weight (W) in grams (g) and having identified the length (L) in centimetres (cm), you need to find the cube of the length in cm. To do this:

Multiply the length in cm × the length in cm × the length in cm

If a tortoise has a length of 10 cm:

L = 10 cm × 10 cm × 10 cm = 1000 cm^3

If the tortoise weighs 1000 g:

W = 1000

The bone ratio $N = W(g) \div L(cm)^3$

In this case $N = 1000 \div 1000 = 1$

Tables 12.3 and 12.4 show the results from calculations that are used as a guide as to whether the tortoise is of a suitable weight to hibernate. Table 12.5 gives two examples of tortoise calculations using this method.

Note also that Marginated tortoises, in particular, represent a challenge when comparing weight to length because of the large flare they have on the carapace. This can distort the ratio of length to weight, making the tortoise seem underweight. Hibernation of Marginated tortoises should always be undertaken with care for this reason and caution should be taken when deciding on the length of hibernation for this species.

Hibernation of very young tortoises (e.g. hatchlings) is something that many owners find daunting. Generally, in my experience owners feel more confident to hibernate a juvenile tortoise once it is around 3 years of age. The hibernation should be very short to start with, say 2–3 weeks, and gradually increased with age and increase in size (see details below).

Tortoises with significant shell deformities that have very pronounced pyramiding or very flattened shells may be so compromised that hibernation is best avoided (Fig. 12.15). In these cases, the tortoise is likely to have other health issues that may reduce the probability of survival; for example, if lung capacity is greatly reduced.

Keep a record of your tortoise's hibernation events each year (Box 12.3) for comparison over time and as part of the pre-hibernation checks to be sure there are no significant changes from previous years.

Stage 2: Slow-down period

Tortoises cannot simply be placed into hibernation without them first undergoing a slow-down process. They need this to make themselves ready for hibernation.

The slow-down process takes approximately 4 weeks for an adult tortoise of 2 kg or more – this is the time needed for them to completely empty their gut of any remaining food. For smaller or juvenile tortoises this can be around 3 weeks if the weight is around 1.5 kg; for tortoises less than 1 kg in weight this is around 2 weeks.

You should stop feeding the tortoise during the slow-down period so that the tortoise can fast. This is one reason why you should not leave the tortoise in the garden, where it might continue to feed on grass, weeds and plants unsupervised, for the last 4 weeks before hibernation. It is these last 4 weeks (2–3 weeks in very small tortoises) that are for fasting. Fasting allows all the food in the gut to move through and be passed as faeces. This is important,

Table 12.3. Safe hibernation ratio ranges.

Tortoise size	Safe hibernation ratio ranges
Healthy tortoise less than 15 cm length	Bone value (N) is between 0.22 and 0.25
Healthy tortoise greater than 15 cm length	Bone value (N) is between 0.21 and 0.23

Table 12.4. Bone ratio results and hibernation advice.

Bone value (N)	Hibernation
If N ≥ 0.25 (greater than or equal to 0.25)	Tortoise is obese but could be hibernated if there are no other conditions
If N ≤ 0.17 (less than or equal to 0.17)	Tortoise is underweight and should not hibernate

Table 12.5. Two examples of actual tortoise measurements and hibernation recommendations.

Tortoise details	Cube of length in cm	Bone ratio N	Recommendation
Spur-thighed adult male weighing 1920 g and 20.4 cm long	$(20.4)^3 = 20.4 \times 20.4 \times 20.4 = 8489.66$	N = 1920 ÷ 8489.66 = 0.23	Tortoise is longer than 15 cm and is within safe range for hibernation N = 023. Hibernation for 8 weeks could take place
Hermann's, adult female weighing 4500 g and 29.8 cm long	$(29.8)^3 = 29.8 \times 29.8 \times 29.8 = 26463.6$	N = 4500 ÷ 26463.6 = 0.17	Tortoise is longer than 15 cm and is at the limit of the safe range for hibernation N = 0.17. Short hibernation would be recommended or no hibernation

> **Box 12.3.** Hibernation records for each tortoise.
>
> | Tortoise Name | **Hibernation 2021–22** |
> |---|---|
> | | Weight in grams = |
> | | SCL in cm = |
> | | Bone ratio = Weight in grams ÷ SCL in cm^3 = |
> | Species | Length of hibernation in weeks = |
> | | Fasting period dates (4 weeks) = |
> | | Hibernation period dates = |
> | Gender | **Hibernation 2022–23** |
> | | Weight in grams = |
> | | SCL in cm = |
> | Age | Bone ratio = Weight in grams ÷ SCL in cm^3 = |
> | | Length of hibernation in weeks = |
> | | Fasting period dates (4 weeks) = |
> | | Hibernation period dates = |
> | | **Hibernation 2023–24** |
> | | Weight in grams = |
> | | SCL in cm = |
> | | Bone ratio = Weight in grams ÷ SCL in cm^3 = |
> | | Length of hibernation in weeks = |
> | | Fasting period dates (4 weeks) = |
> | | Hibernation period dates = |

because undigested food left in the gut can ferment and give off gases such as carbon dioxide, which can build up and cause damage to the gut as there is nowhere for them to escape.

Putting the tortoise into a tepid bath for around 15 minutes stimulates defecation. This helps move food through the gut. The tortoise needs to be at a temperature of around 13–15°C. Bathing also allows full hydration of the body tissues and ensures that the tortoise has a full bladder. This is needed to allow urate production and to remove toxins from the blood.

To achieve the reduced temperatures needed to prepare the tortoise for hibernation, outdoor accommodation can be used during the daytime if temperatures are suitable, and the weather is dry (see below). Alternatively, a cold room indoors can be used, or a rodent-free outbuilding as long as temperatures are monitored using a maximum–minimum thermometer. The tortoise must be checked every day and be bathed regularly (see below), but the location must be safe and secure from predators. Indoor enclosures can be used with lights and heat being gradually turned down and then turned off while monitoring temperatures.

In summary, for an adult tortoise, temperature reduction during slow-down period should be as follows (McArthur *et al.*, 2004; Wright and Raith, 2019):

First two weeks:

- Reduce daytime temperatures to 20–15°C
- Reduce night-time temperatures to 15–8°C
- Bathe daily – allowing the tortoise to dry off before temperature falls below 10°C

Third week:

- Reduce daytime temperatures to 15–10°C
- Reduce night-time temperatures to 13–8°C
- Bathe three times weekly – allowing the tortoise to dry off before temperature falls below 10°C

Fourth week:

- Temperatures to remain around or just below 10°C
- The tortoise will be very inactive – no bathing is required
- Hibernate if all has gone to plan

Juveniles (young developing tortoises aged up to 10 years) and small adult tortoises

Follow the same principles as for adult tortoises above but shorten the total slow-down period to 2–3 weeks, depending upon size and weight. The smaller the tortoise, the more quickly everything will happen. The first stage will take 5–9 days; the second stage will take 5–8 days; the third stage will take 4 days. My experience is based on hibernating tortoises of 3 years or older.

Fasting

During the slow-down period the digestive system must be emptied of food. It is essential that you keep the tortoise in a location that does not provide any food items. To be sure that fasting is complete, no

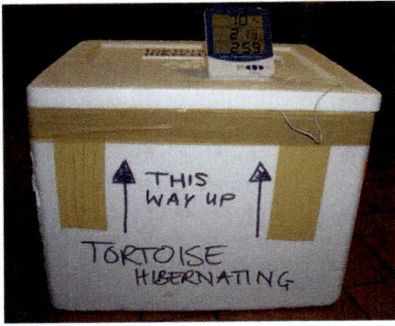

Fig. 12.16. Hibernation box with two layers, insulating material of polystyrene and air holes (Eleanor Lien-Hua Tirtasana Chubb).

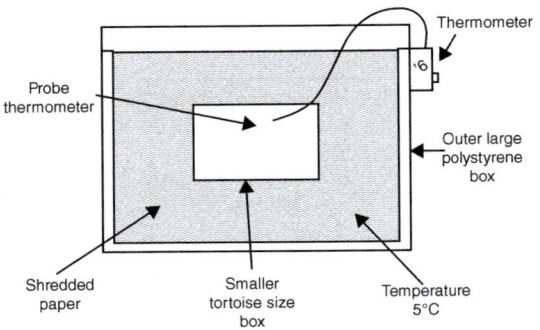

Fig. 12.17. Diagram of hibernation box (Tortoise Trust).

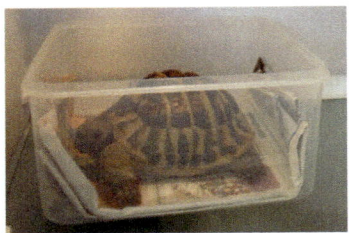

Fig. 12.18. Tortoise in suitable box in fridge.

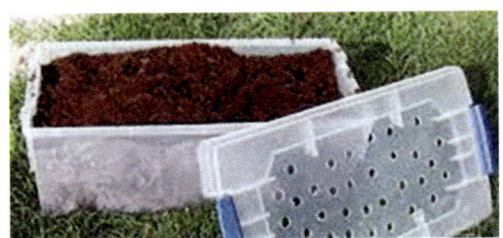

Fig. 12.19. Hibernation box that can be used in soil, with air holes.

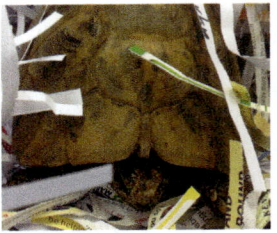

Fig. 12.20. Tortoise in hibernation box of shredded paper.

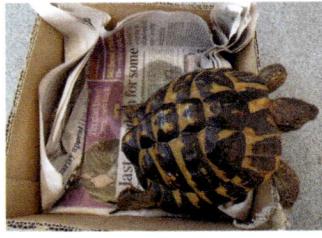

Fig. 12.21. Tortoise in fridge hibernation box being woken up because urination has occurred.

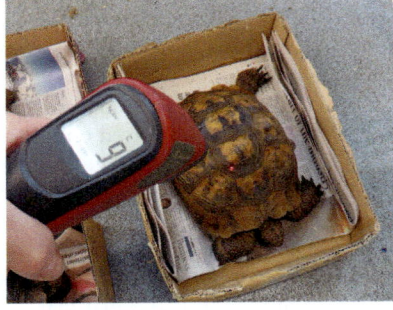

Fig. 12.22. Infrared thermometer showing post-hibernation temperatures on waking as temperatures slowly increase to room temperature before the tortoise is put under heat or light.

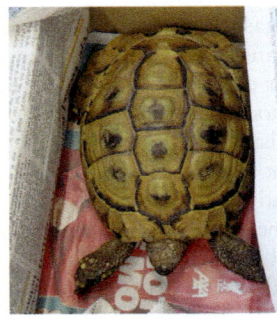

Fig. 12.23. Tortoise waking up in small hibernation box as used in fridge.

Chapter 12

defecation should be seen for the final 7–10 days of preparation for an adult; 5–8 days for juvenile and small tortoises. As stated, this prevents build-up of gases such as carbon dioxide due to gut flora activity during hibernation. As the tortoise cools down, the appetite will reduce naturally. The need for food is also reduced, as less energy is needed for movement.

Stage 3: Hibernation

Where should I hibernate my tortoise?

Your choice will depend on your own circumstances and location. If you live in a very cold northern climate you may struggle to keep temperatures above 2°C in an outbuilding and you may decide to use an unheated room in your home. In more temperate climates you may struggle to keep the temperatures cold enough to maintain hibernation. In recent years winter temperatures have regularly risen above 10°C in the UK and in parts of Europe for several days at a time during December, for example.

The loft space of a house should not be chosen as a safe location for hibernation, because there will be significant fluctuations in temperature there. On a sunny day the space may warm above 10°C; when there is frost or snow the temperature is very likely to be below 2°C, the temperature at which the tortoise will begin to freeze.

When making your decision the two absolutely vital factors are:

- Temperature
- Safety

There are several options.

OPTION 1 (Figs 12.16 and 12.17) An insulated box in a safe location – such as a cold garage or outhouse. The building should be brick or concrete rather than wood so that there are smaller fluctuations in temperature. This also reduces the opportunities for predators and rodents to get in. The box should be on a secure shelf raised off the ground.

You will need to place the tortoise inside a box packed with shredded paper, which should be large enough for the tortoise to turn around inside and move up and down. Holes about 1 cm across should be placed in the box to allow air flow. Then a second box, preferably wood, is needed, into which the first can fit, with about 6–10 cm gap between the two boxes. Another layer of shredded paper should be added between the two boxes (both beneath and at the sides of the interior box). This provides double insulation. Again, air holes are needed. The tortoise is then inside a box, inside a box. This reduces any fluctuations in temperature.

OPTION 2 (Fig. 12.18) A fridge that is working well – not an old machine and not one with a freezer compartment. This should be a separate fridge just for this purpose, not the one you keep all your food in! This protects you from any disease from the tortoise being near your food and protects the tortoise from being near food products that might have a strong odour or contain chemicals that may affect breathing. There will also be too much disturbance to the tortoise if you are opening the fridge throughout the day.

The fridge should be running well. The door should be opened each day to refresh the air – to allow fresh oxygen in and remove any carbon dioxide build-up. When you open the door to refresh the air you should also check the condition of your tortoise. You will need a box into which the tortoise will just fit, to place the tortoise in so that it cannot fall off the fridge shelf when the door is opened. The box can contain compost or just contain the tortoise (Fig. 12.19). The box should be open to the air.

OPTION 3 Hibernaculum – this is a container (usually a plastic box) used to house the tortoise. It contains dry compost or leaves, and should be located in a covered position. The tortoise must not be exposed to wet or damp conditions. Sinking the box into the soil and covering with a cold frame could be one solution, or digging it into a greenhouse that has a soil (rather than concrete) base. The container should not be open to the weather, or it is likely to fill with water. Monitoring of the temperature is essential, as sunshine can significantly raise the temperature under glass, even on cold winter days. The container should be buried in loose earth to reduce temperature changes and to provide higher humidity.

As mentioned in the planning and preparation sections above, allowing a tortoise to hibernate 'naturally' by simply letting it dig itself in wherever and whenever it feels ready, is not recommended in a climate that is colder and/or wetter than the natural habitat. Once the tortoise is in captivity, living in an environment outside the natural range, the hibernation process cannot be natural. The conditions are already not ideal in most captive situations, or indeed may be wholly unsuitable for a hibernation without support. Just as we try to mimic the natural conditions when creating tortoise enclosures, we have to try to mimic the conditions and the duration of a natural hibernation. In a cold climate a tortoise will hibernate for far longer than in the wild, which is very damaging in the long term (see Chapter 7 on common illnesses and diseases). Hence all the preparation and planning discussed here.

Whichever option is chosen, an alarm with a maximum–minimum thermometer should also be fitted (Highfield, 1996). This will alert you to temperatures rising above 10°C or falling below 2°C.

How long should you hibernate your tortoise for?

Keep the hibernation short – 8 weeks is a sensible maximum for healthy adults (McArthur, 2003). This is how long they would hibernate in the wild. For juveniles over 2 years, start the first hibernation with 2–3 weeks only, then wake the tortoise. As the tortoise increases in size, this can gradually be increased by adding a week every 2 years, up to the 8 weeks maximum.

Should you check your tortoise during hibernation?

If your chosen hibernation option allows, you should check your tortoise for movement and response to light touch every day. Even though the tortoise is hibernating, it will remain responsive when you touch a limb gently. There will be a small limb movement in response to touch. As long as you do not take your tortoise into a warm room to carry out this check, it should not wake up (Fig. 12.20). If you open the tortoise's box and its eyes are open, however, you must get the tortoise up. It has woken up and cannot be placed back in hibernation without risk of damage to health (see section below on difficulties in hibernation). Hibernation must be abandoned, the tortoise woken up and supported with warmth and light (see Stage 4: Waking up).

Regular inspection is essential for monitoring progress. A tortoise in a large box may make limited movements up and down, in response to temperature variation. You may find the tortoise in a different place in the box from one day to the next. This is normal and does not necessarily mean that the tortoise has woken up. In a fridge or small space, such movements will not take place. If the temperature remains constant and below 10°C, at around 5°C, the tortoise will not move significantly during hibernation. Excessive movement indicates that the temperature is too high. This should not happen with proper placement and monitoring.

Wake the tortoise immediately if urination or defecation occurs (Fig. 12.21). These are both signs that the tortoise is in significant difficulty and needs support straight away. Hibernation must be abandoned, the tortoise woken up and supported with warmth and light (see Stage 4: Waking up).

Check the tortoise's weight weekly to ensure that weight loss does not exceed 1–2% of body weight each month. As the tortoise sleeps, the heart rate slows greatly to around 1 beat/minute. Breathing rate is also very low, with a correspondingly low demand for oxygen. Toxins produced slowly and passed into the blood are reabsorbed into the bladder. This is only possible if the bladder is full of water, hence the need for full hydration during the slow-down period.

The tortoise can be weighed without problem. Make sure you do this in the cold rather than moving it into a warm part of the house. Place the tortoise gently on the scales, record the weight and then return it immediately to the hibernation location. If the tortoise has lost more weight than is acceptable, it should be woken up and hibernation abandoned. The total weight loss during the whole hibernation period should be less than 5% of the starting weight, given that the monthly weight loss should not be more than 2%. The tortoise must be supported with warmth and light (see Stage 4: Waking up).

Monitor the temperature every day using the maximum–minimum thermometer so that you can check the temperature throughout each 24-hour period. The temperature must remain as constant as possible between 4°C and 8°C and ideally stay at around 5°C throughout.

Stage 4: Waking up after hibernation

Having decided on a suitable length of time for hibernation, you will most likely be deliberately waking your tortoise up, rather than allowing it to wake up naturally. You must have suitable indoor accommodation already in place. The tortoise will need to be supported in this accommodation until the outside temperatures improve and the tortoise can go outside for short periods. Allowing your tortoise to simply wander around on the floor is not suitable, even if your house is well heated. Even in a well-heated home, the temperature at floor level is much lower than the air temperature that you will be aware of. The floor temperature in a centrally heated house will be about 16–20°C, which, without access to basking lights, will not allow most species to reach anything like their preferred optimum temperature, which will be around 28–32°C.

It is important not to shock the tortoise by warming up too quickly. Take the tortoise out of the cold space or fridge and place it on the floor in the box, in a heated room. Open the boxes if you have used Option 1, or dig up the tortoise and bring it in if you have used Option 3. Over the next 2–3 hours, allow the tortoise to come up to around 20°C, which can be checked with an infrared thermometer (Fig. 12.22).

The tortoise should start to move around as it reaches 10–12°C and then warms up further. The eyes should open as temperature rises or, if not, they should open once the tortoise is bathed. Once at room temperature around 20°C, the tortoise can be put into a lukewarm bath at about 20–25°C. This will aid further warming and start the process of rehydration.

Once the tortoise has been at 20–25°C for 2–3 hours, the opportunity can be given for further warming in the normal indoor enclosure. Do not place the tortoise directly under the basking lights but allow the tortoise to move into this warmer area as it wishes. The tortoise will gradually warm up to the preferred optimum temperature of around 28°C, depending upon species.

Daily baths should be given for 5–7 days before returning to the normal twice-weekly regime. Fresh water should be available within the enclosure in addition to the regular bathing. The tortoise should feed within 24 hours of waking – offering some soft succulent food may be helpful to start feeding.

Cucumber can be a useful appetite stimulant. Easy-to-digest foods such as lamb's lettuce or salad leaves can also be used initially. It may be helpful to add Criticare (energy + protein) and/or Reptoboost (electrolytes, energy, probiotic) (both Vetark® products) to the bath if the tortoise is slow to feed. If the tortoise is not feeding after 5 days, veterinary advice should be sought.

In northern climates, the tortoise will then remain in the indoor accommodation until the spring weather improves sufficiently for it to start going outside for part of the day (see Chapter 3 on the captive environment). This will be temperature- and weather-dependent. The tortoise must be protected from any extremes of temperature, especially at this time, as the immune system needs time to recover and work efficiently again after hibernation. Optimal conditions are needed post-hibernation for the tortoise to regain normal function and behaviour. Hibernation is always a stressful process for the tortoise, regardless of how well it has been prepared.

Dos and Don'ts of Hibernation

Table 12.6 is a summary of what to do and what not to do in managing a tortoise's hibernation.

What can go wrong during hibernation?

Freezing

One of the most distressing outcomes of a poorly managed hibernation is that the tortoise is exposed to very cold temperatures for an extended period. The result will be that the tortoise starts to freeze. Like all living things, the tortoise has a high percentage of water in its body. Some tissues (such as the eye) have very high concentrations of water. One of the first effects of freezing is that the eyes become damaged as the water in them freezes. This can lead to blindness which in turn can reduce appetite and willingness to feed (McArthur *et al.*, 2004).

A maximum–minimum thermometer or use of an alarm is essential monitoring equipment during hibernation so that you know if there has been exposure to temperatures below 2°C for any length of time. The tortoise must be moved to a location where the temperature remains at around 5°C.

Dehydration

Without sufficient water in the tissues (and in the bladder as a storage location), the levels of toxins formed in the blood as a result of slow metabolic processes will gradually rise. These toxins pass into the bladder, diffusing into the water there, and are therefore removed from the blood. This stops them building up. This process will continue until hibernation is over. The tortoise can then expel its bladder contents (including the toxins) and take in a fresh water supply. If the tortoise enters hibernation in a dehydrated state, the toxins cannot be removed from the blood effectively as there is no water in the bladder into which they can dissolve. This is why giving daily baths is so important before hibernation and again after the tortoise

Table 12.6. Dos and don'ts of hibernation.

DO	DON'T
Hibernate healthy tortoise if the right species.	Hibernate sick or underweight tortoise.
Ensure good hydration and fasting for 4 weeks before hibernation.	Hibernate tortoise until all food has been emptied from the gut.
Hibernate for up to 8 weeks only – shorter for juveniles.	Hibernate too long – 8 weeks maximum for healthy adults.
Choose a safe place: • a frost-free garage or shed • no rodents • off the floor.	Use the loft/roof-space of your home: • the temperature will fluctuate and the tortoise may well freeze • there is a possibility of rodents being in the space without you being aware of this.
Option 1: Put the tortoise inside a strong cardboard box, large enough for it to turn around. Put this box inside another wooden box, for extra insulation and protection. Do not seal the box to ensure an air flow. Use safe insulation material around the tortoise such as shredded paper. The location must be dry on a stable bench or shelf. Choose a place with suitable temperatures: • between 2°C and 10°C • ideal temperature is 5°C. Use a maximum–minimum thermometer to check the temperature. Use an alarm to monitor temperature and alert you to temperatures below 2°C.	Use a wooden shed where the temperature will fluctuate too much and where access by rodents is easier. Use hay or straw as the insulation material around the tortoise. Allow the tortoise to become damp or wet. Allow temperature fluctuations – a steady 5°C is ideal. If temperatures rise above 10°C the tortoise will wake and must be taken out of hibernation immediately. If temperatures fall below 2°C the tortoise will start to freeze.
Option 2: Use a fridge to maintain suitable temperatures of 4–8°C. This can be very safe if a maximum–minimum thermometer is used to check the temperature.	Put the tortoise back into hibernation after it wakes up.
For both Options 1 and 2: Check your tortoise daily for any signs of distress, or if any urination or defecation takes place. Check your tortoise's weight each month. You can do this without waking the tortoise. The tortoise should not lose more than 1% of its weight in one month. A 1000 g tortoise should not lose more than 10 g in one month. A 1000 g tortoise should not lose more than 20 g in total over a 2-month (8-week) hibernation.	Leave your tortoise in hibernation if urination or defecation takes place. Leave your tortoise longer than 8 weeks or if the tortoise loses too much weight.
Option 3: Make sure the hibernaculum location is secure from rodents and does not fluctuate in temperature outside the desired range (4–8°C).	Allow the tortoise to hibernate outside without some protection from the weather.
For all options: Control the length of hibernation to a maximum of 8 weeks. Control the temperature to keep within the desired range (4–8°C). Ensure that you check the tortoise regularly.	Put the tortoise back into hibernation after it wakes up. The tortoise can only hibernate once before going through the whole cycle again. Leave your tortoise in hibernation if urination or defecation takes place. Leave your tortoise longer than 8 weeks or if the tortoise loses too much weight.

wakes up. If the tortoise urinates during hibernation, this is always a signal that it is in significant difficulties – the tortoise should be woken up immediately.

Breathing difficulties

If the tortoise has a respiratory infection that has been dormant, the pathogen may start to cause signs and symptoms during hibernation, as the tortoise is in a weakened state. The bacteria or virus may start to multiply and accelerate the disease, as the tortoise's immune system is less efficient during hibernation. This could include organisms causing URTD/RNS/rhinitis (see Chapter 7 on common illnesses and diseases). Any overproduction of mucus that blocks the nares may create a life-threatening situation for the tortoise while in hibernation. If a nasal discharge is observed, the tortoise should be woken up immediately.

Metabolic bone disorder can lead to a collapse of the carapace and so internal space for all the organs is reduced. One of the organs affected may be the lungs. They may be too small to allow adequate gas exchange. In hibernation the effects of this may be exacerbated and may lead to breathing difficulties. Great care should be taken when hibernating tortoises with significant shell deformities, and a decision not to hibernate may be the best one. If hibernation does take place, it should be kept short to reduce even further the potential stress on the body.

Injuries or infections

Other signs of infection, or any injuries arising during hibernation (e.g. rodent bites), should be taken as an emergency situation. The tortoise should be woken immediately. Any changes in the tortoise, such as swelling, leakage of fluids, or failure to respond when touched, may indicate an underlying disease. The tortoise should be woken from hibernation immediately and veterinary attention sought.

Tortoise defecates

This implies that the tortoise was not fully empty of food at the start of hibernation. One effect of this can be a build-up of gas as the undigested food material continues to be broken down very slowly, causing fermentation, which can produce waste gases such as carbon dioxide. This builds up in the gut with no means of escape. The tortoise should be woken up immediately if faeces are produced during hibernation.

Tortoise urinates

As stated above, urination during hibernation is a sure sign that the tortoise is in trouble. Wake the tortoise immediately, warm it up and provide opportunities to rehydrate at least three times daily in a warm bath. Seek veterinary advice as necessary if the tortoise continues to lose water repeatedly.

Tortoise loses more than 1% of body weight in a month

The tortoise may have been too light in weight when the hibernation started or there may be another underlying health issue. Once excess weight loss, greater than 1–2% of body weight in a month, is detected the tortoise should be woken up and supported to start feeding. If the tortoise does not start eating within 5 days, veterinary attention should be sought.

Excessively long hibernation

Hibernation of more than 8 weeks for a healthy adult may result in the tortoise being unable to get started again when woken up. For juveniles and small tortoises, the hibernation period should be shorter. During hibernation, fat stores release energy slowly to allow metabolism to continue very slowly. An immediately available store of carbohydrate (to provide energy quickly as the tortoise wakes up) is in the liver in the form of glycogen. If the tortoise has used up this store during a very long hibernation, there is no easily available food to increase blood glucose levels and help the tortoise get feeding again. Post-hibernation anorexia may be the result (see Chapter 7 on common illnesses and diseases) and the tortoise may need extensive support and recuperation to be able to feed again.

Conclusion

Hibernation is a natural part of the annual cycle in some species of tortoise. These are temperate species adapted to cope with colder conditions. Tropical tortoises are not adapted to hibernate, as their natural environment remains warm enough throughout the year for this not to be necessary. They are not biologically adapted to hibernate and this is a dangerous process for which they are not equipped to survive.

Safe hibernation requires good planning and preparation to ensure that the tortoise is likely to survive this period of deep sleep and inactivity. In captivity the hibernation period must be controlled by us, in terms of checking the tortoise regularly and in terms of length. Restricting the length of hibernation to around 8 weeks maximum ensures that the tortoise is not too stressed by the process and does not get into the difficulties associated with very long hibernations.

Whether the hibernation takes place in a very controlled environment, such as a fridge, or a more natural hibernation is attempted in a controlled outdoor environment, our intervention is required. Being in captivity means that the conditions are never going to be exactly those found in the wild. The tortoise will always need our support.

It is thought that in the UK over 6 million Mediterranean tortoises may have been imported between the 1940s and the introduction of the 1984 ban controlling the trade in these species (Highfield, 1996). It is sobering to note that the vast majority of these tortoises died within a few years of coming to the UK, many during hibernation. We know so much more about the process now, and can make hibernation much safer for our tortoises as a result.

References and Further Reading

Biedenweg, F. and Schramm, R. (2019) *The Egyptian Tortoise* Testudo kleinmanni *Lortet 1883. A Fascinating Little Beauty*. Tartaruga-Verlag Ricarda Schramm, Grebenhain, Germany.

Chitty, J. and Raftery, A. (2013) *Essentials of Tortoise Medicine and Surgery*. Wiley Blackwell, Chichester, UK.

Highfield, A. (1996) *Practical Encyclopaedia of Keeping and Breeding Tortoises and Freshwater Turtles*. Carapace Press, London.

Highfield, A. and Highfield, N. (2008) *Taking Care of Pet Tortoises*. The Tortoise Trust Jill Martin Fund. Available from www.tortoisetrust.org

Highfield, A. and Highfield, N. (2009) *Keeping a Pet Tortoise*. Interpet, Dorking, UK.

McArthur, S. (1996) *Veterinary Management of Tortoises and Turtles*. Blackwell, Oxford, UK.

McArthur, S. (2003) Post hibernation anorexia (PHA) Testudo species. *BCG Symposium,* 29 March 2003.

McArthur, S., Wilkinson, R. and Meyer, J. (2004) *Medicine and Surgery of Tortoises and Turtles*. Blackwell, Oxford, UK

Scheelings, T.F. (2019) Ch 1 Anatomy and physiology. In: Girling, S.J. and Raiti, P. (eds) *BSAVA Manual of Reptiles*, 3rd edn. BSAVA, Quedgeley, UK, pp. 1–25.

Varga, M. (2019) Ch 3 Captive maintenance. In: Girling, S.J. and Raiti, P. (eds) *BSAVA Manual of Reptiles*, 3rd edn. BSAVA, Quedgeley, UK, pp. 36–48.

Wegehaupt, W. (2009a) *Mediterranean Tortoises, Where and how they live in the wild*. Kressbronn, Germany.

Wegehaupt, W. (2009b) *Naturalistic Keeping and Breeding of Hermann's Tortoises*. Kressbronn, Germany.

Wright, K. and Raiti, P. (2019) Ch 5 Breeding and neonatal care. In: Girling, S.J. and Raiti, P. (eds) *BSAVA Manual of Reptiles*, 3rd edn. BSAVA, Quedgeley, UK, pp. 70–88.

13 Mediterranean Tortoises

Abstract
This chapter discusses the three species of temperate tortoises, collectively described as Mediterranean tortoises because they naturally live in the countries that surround the Mediterranean Sea in Central Europe. This range of countries includes areas of Southern and Eastern Europe, together with coastal regions of North Africa. The tortoises are commonly called Spur-thighed, Hermann's and Marginated tortoises.

The chapter describes the three species and their subspecies although there is no consensus on the nomenclature as the field studies and research are patchy. There is some work taking place to identify different populations and subspecies using DNA testing, but this is in its infancy. These species have been collected for the pet trade from early days and all are CITES-listed as endangered or threatened with extinction. They are collectively the most commonly kept species in captivity and have been in captivity for longer than other species.

The chapter looks at their natural habitat, much of which is now degraded due to human activities, as the basis for creating captive environments that mimic conditions found in the wild. As temperate species these tortoises can hibernate/brumate, but large numbers have been subjected to very poor conditions in captivity for many years, including excessively long hibernations, which have been responsible for high mortality rates in wild-caught and captive-bred animals.

What are Mediterranean tortoises?

Mediterranean tortoises were the first tortoises to be imported from the wild to supply the rapidly expanding pet trade. Importation of these animals in huge numbers skyrocketed in the 1960s. So many tortoises were taken from the wild during this period that native populations crashed. In 1984, the UK prohibited the importation of wild-caught Mediterranean tortoises. Subsequently trade in Mediterranean tortoises has been controlled through the Convention on International Trade in Endangered Species (CITES). Because of their endangered status in the wild, legal trade is confined largely to captive-bred animals only. Unfortunately, a thriving illegal trade in tortoises still exists, as shown in Fig. 13.2 which was taken in 2024.

As the sale and importation of all Mediterranean tortoises is controlled by CITES, there may well be requirements for certification or registration of these species in your country. As wild populations in many species are considered to be endangered, only captive-bred tortoises should be bought. You are advised to check your own government's legislation on the selling and buying of Mediterranean tortoises.

Mediterranean tortoises come from countries around the Mediterranean Sea. These include the northern-shore countries – Spain, France, Italy, Slovenia, Croatia, Bosnia Herzegovina, Montenegro, Albania, Greece and Turkey (plus their associated islands), together with the southern-shore countries of Africa and the Middle East – Morocco, Algeria, Tunisia, Libya, Egypt, Israel, Jordan, Lebanon and Syria.

Tortoises that come from the northern shores of the Mediterranean live in temperate climates. The land is usually covered with a blanket of thick vegetation, which often includes shrubs and wooded areas.

Whilst tortoises found in North African and Middle Eastern countries experience a higher year-round temperature, their habitat is usually more arid and desert-like, with less vegetation coverage than that found on the European side of the Mediterranean.

The geographical area in which Mediterranean tortoises can be found is relatively small. A wide range of environments are encompassed, as shown in the map in Fig. 13.1. If a captive tortoise is to thrive it is important that the specifics of its original natural environment are reflected in the conditions under which it is kept.

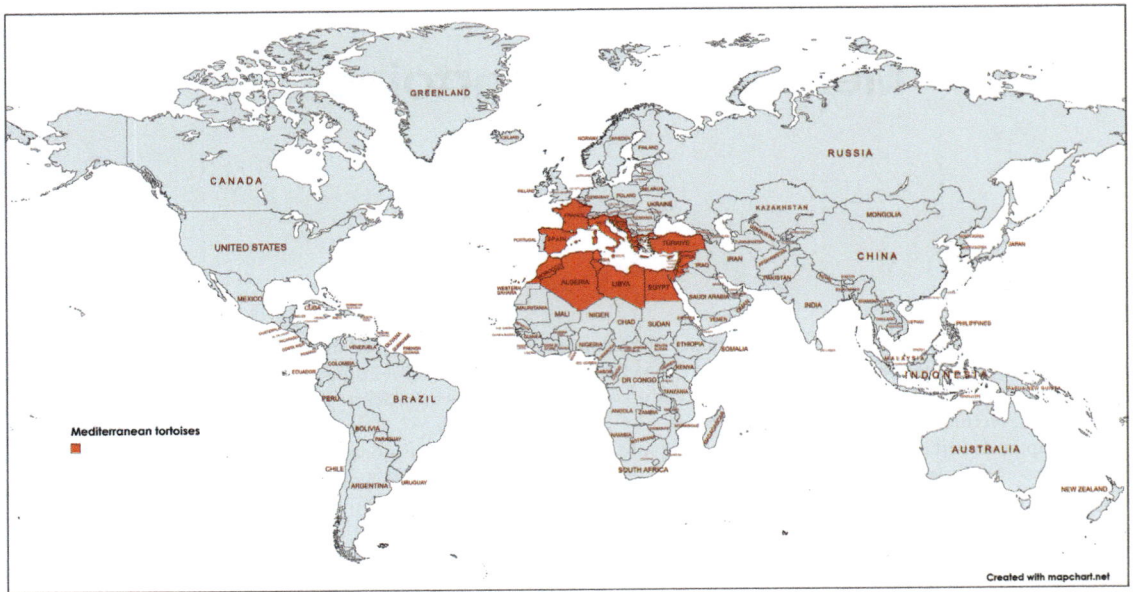

Fig. 13.1. Map of countries where Mediterranean tortoises are found around the Mediterranean Sea and into the Middle East. (https://www.mapchart.net/world.html)

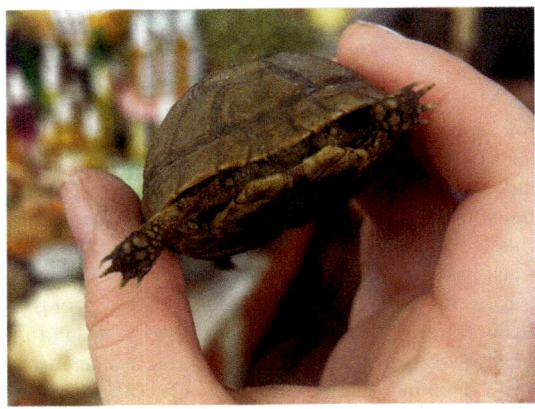

Fig. 13.2. This tiny juvenile in a Moroccan market clearly has the spurs on the thighs indicating that it is a Spur-thighed tortoise (Corinne Wayends).

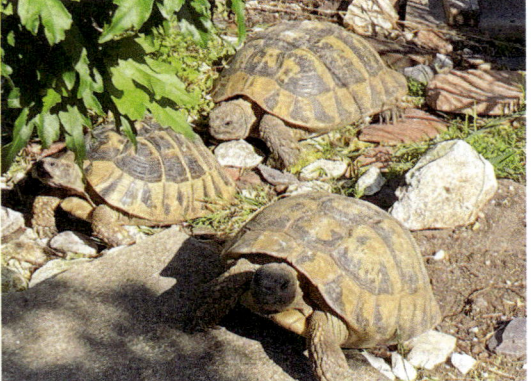

Fig. 13.3. Hermann's tortoises.

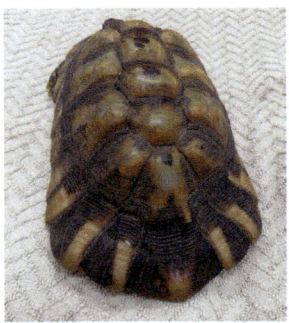

Fig. 13.4. Marginated tortoise.

What are the different types of Mediterranean tortoises?

Mediterranean tortoises have been divided into three main species:

- Spur-thighed tortoises (*Testudo graeca*) (Figs 13.5–13.8)
- Hermann's tortoises (*Testudo hermanni*) (Fig. 13.3)
- Marginated tortoises (*Testudo marginata*) (Fig. 13.4)

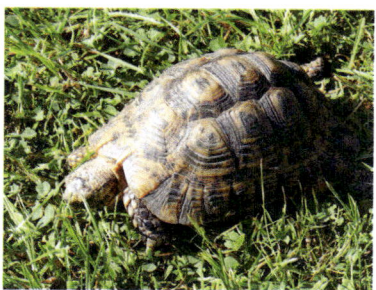

Fig. 13.5. North African Spur-thighed tortoise.

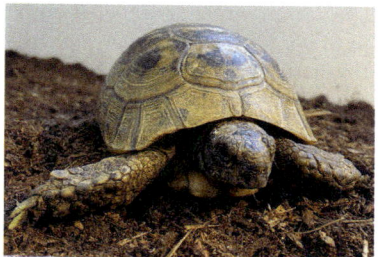

Fig. 13.7. North African Spur-thighed tortoise.

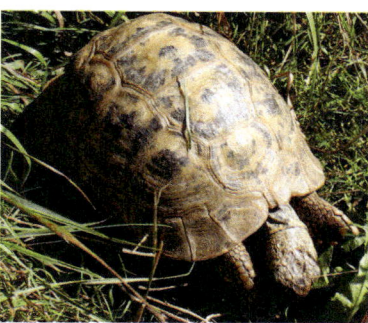

Fig. 13.6. North African Spur-thighed tortoise.

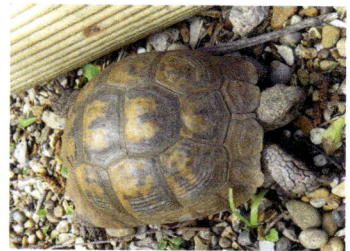

Fig. 13.8. Turkish Spur-thighed tortoise.

While Mediterranean tortoises have been divided into these three named species, classification may not be as straightforward as was initially thought. Subspecies of Spur-thighed and Hermann's tortoises exist, while the many local variations found within each species and subspecies confuse the picture further (Highfield, 1996; Vetter, 2002).

What are Spur-thighed tortoises (*Testudo graeca*)?

Testudo graeca is sometimes called the Greek tortoise, which is unhelpful as they are found in many countries in addition to Greece. The shell pattern and colour vary significantly (Figs 13.5–13.8).

As the name suggests, the defining feature of this widely varied group is a pair of 'spurs' on the upper thighs of the back legs (see Chapter 11, on breeding). Although seen in both males and females, the purpose of the spurs is to help the male hold onto the female during mating. As with many other species, the female is generally larger than the male, by up to a third, to allow sufficient capacity within the body for egg production (Highfield, 1996; Jepson, 2010).

There are many subspecies and types of *Testudo graeca* but the most commonly encountered are from two subspecies: *Testudo graeca graeca* (Figs 13.5 and 13.6) and *Testudo graeca ibera* (Fig. 13.8).

The classification of the species is complex, with many unknowns regarding subspecies. There may well be separate species in some cases, and there are populations that are genetically very similar but that look remarkably different. Conversely, similar-looking tortoises may be from different areas with different genetic make-ups (Vetter, 2002).

Which parts of the Mediterranean do *Testudo graeca* come from?

Testudo graeca graeca are found in on northern Mediterranean shores in southern Spain, and in the Balearic Islands and Sardinia. They are also found in North Africa, in Morocco, Tunisia, Algeria, Libya and Egypt, and into the Middle East in Iran and Jordan (Fig. 13.9).

Testudo graeca ibera are found in the southern European countries of Spain, Greece and Italy, and also in Turkey (Europe and Asia) and in Asiatic countries including Georgia, Armenia, Bulgaria and

Romania, with overlapping regions of both subspecies also in Syria, Iran and Jordan (Fig. 13.10).

While the natural habitats of these two subspecies of tortoise do vary, both groups have broadly similar environmental needs in captivity (McArthur et al., 2004). These include:

- A preferred temperature range of 15–34°C (days up to 34°C and night-time minimum 15°C).
- The correct humidity level. This will depend on whether they originate in wooded areas (more humid), open scrubby areas, or desert-like regions (least humid).
- A substrate that combines some vegetation, possibly some scrub, together with either loamy soil, or rocky, sandy soil (again determined by what they would be used to in their original habitats).

Spur-thighed tortoises (*Testudo graeca* spp.) are all herbivorous and tend to be very active, usually spending their days walking great distances in search of vegetation to eat. They need a high-fibre, high-calcium, low-protein, low-fat diet. We can best provide this by feeding a wide variety of leafy flowering plants and succulents.

These tortoises need basking opportunities and a well-drained substrate. Water to drink and bathe in should be provided at all times.

It should be noted that some (not all) *Testudo graeca* hibernate in the wild. While some only hibernate during the winter, others aestivate during very hot summers. Aestivation is a period of dormancy in very hot conditions, usually above 38°C, in the summer, such as those seen in North African and Middle Eastern countries. Where temperatures can also be cold in the winter, for example in higher mountainous regions, tortoises will both hibernate and aestivate in the same year. Both hibernation (dormancy in cold weather) and aestivation (dormancy in hot weather) are strategies for coping with extreme weather, or with the lack of available food at certain times of the year (see Chapter 12 on hibernation/brumation).

Are the two subspecies of *Testudo graeca* very similar?

1. *Testudo graeca graeca*

This is a very complex group and individuals show considerable variation in size, shape and shell coloration across the range of countries in which the species is found (shown in Fig. 13.9). Figure 13.11 shows one sub-species from Morocco.

Some *Testudo graeca graeca* individuals are very small indeed and because of this can be extremely fragile and delicate, requiring extra special care. *Testudo graeca graeca* tortoises from North Africa do not hibernate, as the temperature there never falls low enough for them to need to do so. These tortoises do not tolerate very cold conditions and need support in the form of artificial heat and lighting throughout the autumn, winter and early spring if kept in cold climates. They are particularly susceptible to disease such as runny nose syndrome (upper respiratory tract disease, URTD), which can be passed to them from other Spur-thighed tortoises, including *Testudo graeca ibera* (see Chapter 7 on common illnesses and diseases).

An example of a very small *T. graeca graeca* is Ursa, a tiny male tortoise originally bought in a Tunisian market, then smuggled back to Britain illegally in his purchaser's pocket. When I first saw him, he was close to death. As an impulse buy his purchaser did not have a suitable set-up for him at home, and very little knowledge of how to care for him correctly. He was put into a UK garden in temperatures that were nothing like those of Northern Africa and he would not eat the salad food that he was offered. Thinking that he was a baby (and not a fully grown adult) his purchaser attempted to tube-feed him on milk, not appreciating that, as reptiles, tortoises do not produce or drink milk. Milk is a damaging food source for herbivorous tortoises, being high in protein and fat content. When it was explained that Ursa needed specialist care if he was to survive, he was handed over to me.

Ursa was, by this time, so dehydrated that he was blind. His head and limbs hung out limply. He needed life-saving fluid therapy urgently. A specialist tortoise veterinarian injected fluid directly into his body cavity as an emergency measure. After that came the long process of intensive care (which went on for over a year), and gradually, with the right conditions and diet, he began to recover and feed himself. Over the next 18 months he became much more alert and active. He remains fit and healthy 33 years later.

While some North African *T. graeca graeca* (like Ursa) are small, others are much larger. Penny, a large female *T. graeca*, weighs 3.7 kg. Her coloration and size are typical of a *T. graeca graeca/whitei* tortoise from Algeria (not yet formally named as a subspecies but used here for distinction). Interestingly, female tortoises like this large *T. graeca whitei* were relatively common among

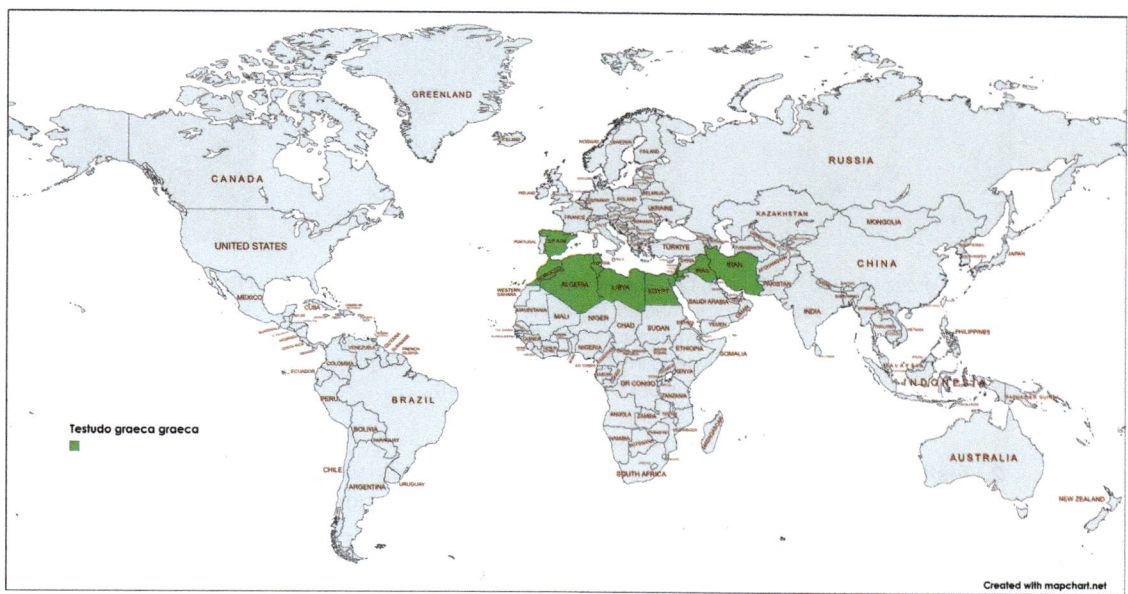

Fig. 13.9. Map of the countries where *Testudo graeca graeca* are found. (https://www.mapchart.net/world.html)

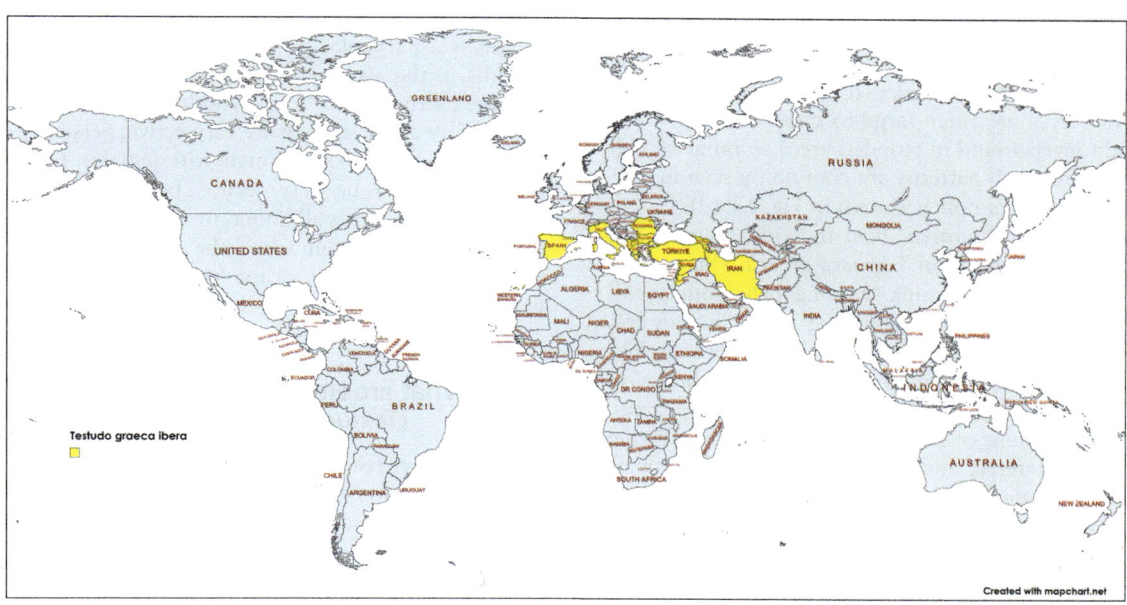

Fig. 13.10. Map of the countries where *Testudo graeca ibera* are found. (https://www.mapchart.net/world.html)

those wild-caught and imported for the pet trade before the UK ban in 1984. Males were much rarer. It may be that the larger females were seen and captured more easily or that the males were less hardy and so rarer in the wild, or were less able to cope with conditions in captivity. Figure 13.12 shows a male and female *T. graeca whitei*. Unfortunately, many *T. graeca whitei* have now passed away and so these tortoises are becoming increasingly rare in captivity.

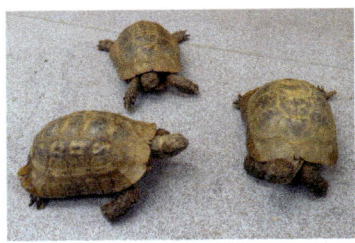
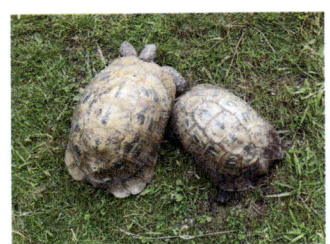
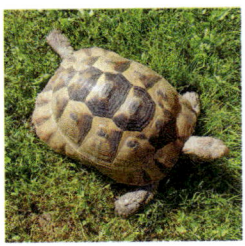

Fig. 13.11. *T. graeca graeca* (more recently *soussensis*) from the Souss Valley in Morocco.

Fig. 13.12. *T. graeca graeca* from Algeria (likely to be a subspecies *T. graeca whitei*, also known as Gilbert White's tortoise after the famous naturalist who owned Timothy, whose shell is on display at the Natural History Museum in London).

Fig. 13.13. Captive-bred *T. graeca ibera*.

2. *Testudo graeca ibera*

This subspecies of Spur-thighed tortoise is another complex group. *Testudo graeca ibera* originates from the southern European countries, and Asiatic countries bordering the Mediterranean, as shown on the map in Fig. 13.10.

The habitat in which they live is more scrubby and wooded than that found in North Africa. This affects their coloration. Tortoises from Turkey, for example, tend to be darker, with shells that look more mottled, in order to provide camouflage. Their eyes are often large to cope with the lower light levels found in wooded areas. A range of colours and shell patterns are commonly seen in captivity (one example is shown in Fig. 13.13).

Typically, *T. graeca ibera* individuals are much more aggressive than *T. graeca graeca*. This is most obvious during mating. Mating behaviour in all tortoises can appear disturbing to the human eye, involving as it does the male chasing and circling the female, and ramming the back of her shell with the front of his, a process repeated many times. This ramming of the shell is an attempt gain the female's interest and stop her from walking away. If the female is stationary the male can mount her shell from the rear, allowing the eggs to be fertilized internally (see Chapter 11 on breeding). The ramming behaviour is far more violent and persistent in *T. graeca ibera* than in *T. graeca graeca* and is often accompanied by biting the skin and flesh of the hind legs, sometimes drawing blood. If no females are present, male *T. graeca ibera* will chase, ram and bite the legs of other males, and attempt to mate with them.

Males will also attempt to mate with any tortoise-like object such as shoes or boots, or stone or wooden tortoise sculptures. This behaviour can be problematic in captivity, causing increased stress and serious physical damage to all parties. If the enclosure is too small, and a number of tortoises are kept together, the opportunities for animals to escape from each other is limited, which can lead to damage to both males and female, and significant health risks related to stress (see Chapter 9 on emotional states).

This is a particular problem during the summer months, as the warmer weather causes the males to become more sexually active. Adult males generally have to live alone, as they are very active, persistent and aggressive in trying to mate with females. Their enclosures must be very secure, because lots of male tortoises go walkabout in the spring after hibernation/brumation when the drive to find a mate is strongest; they escape from enclosures and gardens and may be lost to their original owner.

What are Hermann's tortoises (*Testudo hermanni*)?

There are three recognized subspecies of Hermann's tortoise: *Testudo hermanni hermanni*, *Testudo hermanni boetgeri* and *Testudo hermanni hercegovinensis*. Other subgroups may exist, but DNA analysis and data are limited. As with all tortoise species, precise classification can be tricky (Vetter, 2002).

Hermann's tortoises come from France, Spain, Italy, Croatia, Serbia, Bulgaria, Romania and Greece and may also be found in North Africa, as shown in Fig. 13.14 (Wegehaupt, 2009b). As with other Mediterranean species, much of the original habitat and range is now lost, with a few isolated populations being all that are left in the wild.

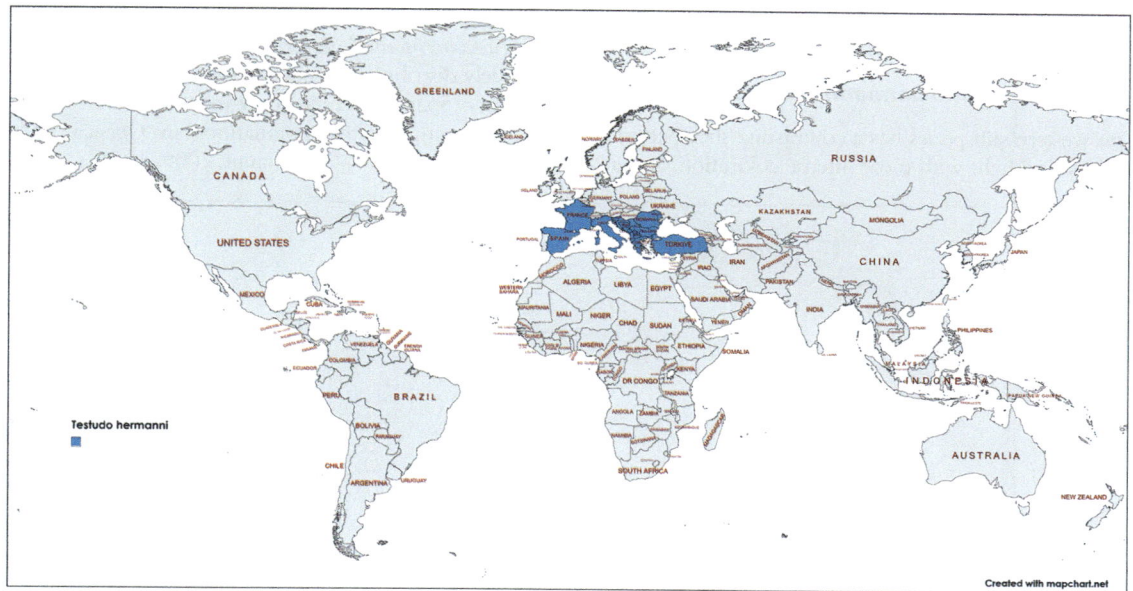

Fig. 13.14. Countries where *Testudo hermanni* are found. (https://www.mapchart.net/world.html)

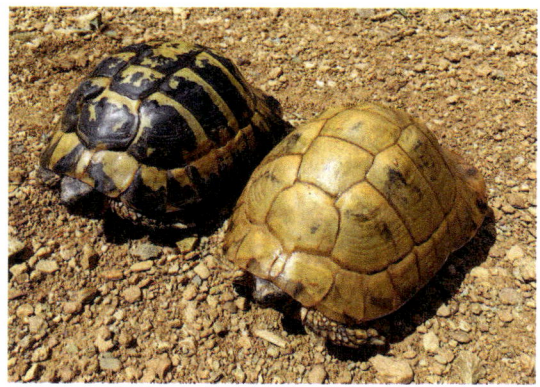

Fig. 13.15. *Testudo hermanni* tortoises are seen in a range of colours and patterns.

Hermann's tortoises look similar to Spur-thighed tortoises, although the shell is slightly less domed, and the males may appear almost triangular in appearance. Again, there is great colour variation in Hermann's tortoises – some are much lighter in colour, others have a distinct pattern of black and pale areas (Fig. 13.15).

Hermann's tortoises can be identified by possession of a single tail spur, rather than spurs on the thighs as seen in Spur-thighed tortoises. This spur is very long in Hermann's males and again is used by the male to hold onto the female for long enough to mate. As with Spur-thighed tortoises, the mating ritual can be seen as rather alarming but this time it is focused on biting the rear legs of the female, rather than shell ramming.

Hermann's tortoises are often voracious feeders in captivity. When seen in captive hatchlings, this gluttonous behaviour can result in the youngster growing too fast and exhibiting subsequent deformities of shell, limbs and body (see Chapter 7 on common illnesses and diseases).

One of my female Hermann's tortoises, Matilda, managed to damage her lower jaw, which dislocated and parted despite veterinary efforts to repair it. This injury had no impact whatsoever on her ability to eat, and certainly did not put her off her food. Despite her injury, she continued to eat well and thrive as a healthy adult tortoise for over 20 years.

Are the three sub-species of *Testudo hermanni* very similar?

1. *Testudo hermanni hermanni*

This western subspecies has a contrasting shell pattern of dark and light with more intense coloration, and a more domed carapace than the eastern subspecies (*Testudo hermanni boetgeri*). *T. hermanni hermanni* is a widely distributed subspecies found across southern regions of Spain and France, Italy and the Mediterranean Islands, with healthy populations in Corsica and Sardinia (Fig. 13.16) (Wegehaupt, 2009a,b).

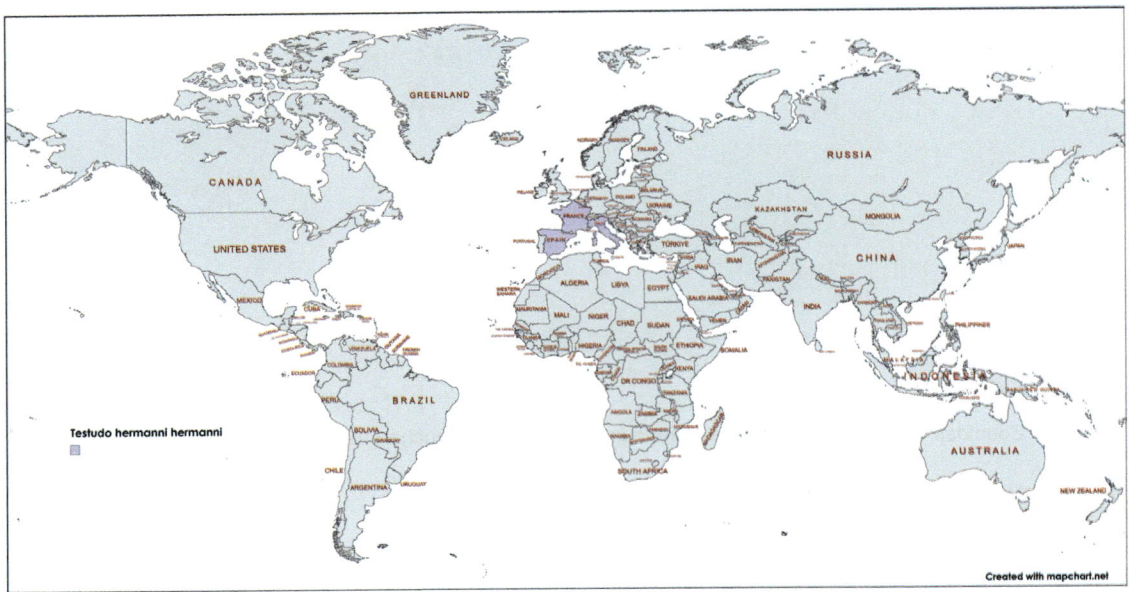

Fig. 13.16. Countries where *Testudo hermanni hermanni* may be found. (https://www.mapchart.net/world.html)

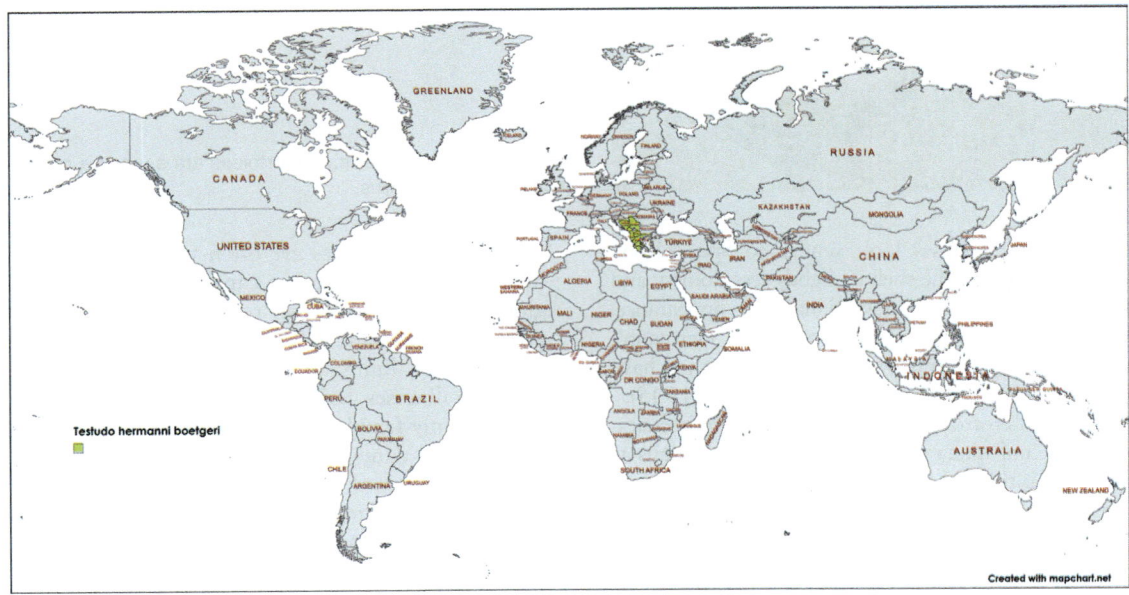

Fig. 13.17. Countries where *Testudo hermanni boetgeri* may be found. (https://www.mapchart.net/world.html)

2. *Testudo hermanni boetgeri*

This eastern subspecies also has a patterned shell, but the colour tends to be lighter and paler. *T. hermanni boetgeri* populations are found in Montenegro, Serbia, Kosovo, Macedonia, Greece and Albania (Fig. 13.17).

3. Testudo hermanni hercegovinensis

T. hermanni hercegovinensis tortoises are found only in Dalmatia, a coastal region of southern Croatia (Fig. 13.18). This tortoise has not been universally agreed as a separate subspecies. It is very similar to *T. hermanni hermanni*, with a domed carapace.

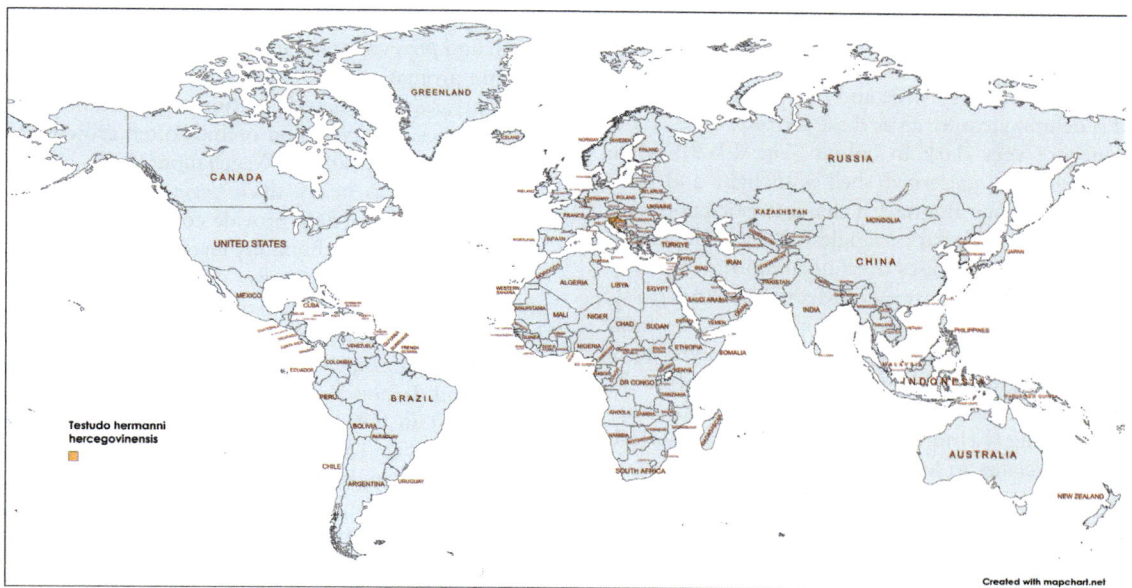

Fig. 13.18. Countries where *Testudo hermanni hercegovinensis* may be found. (https://www.mapchart.net/world.html)

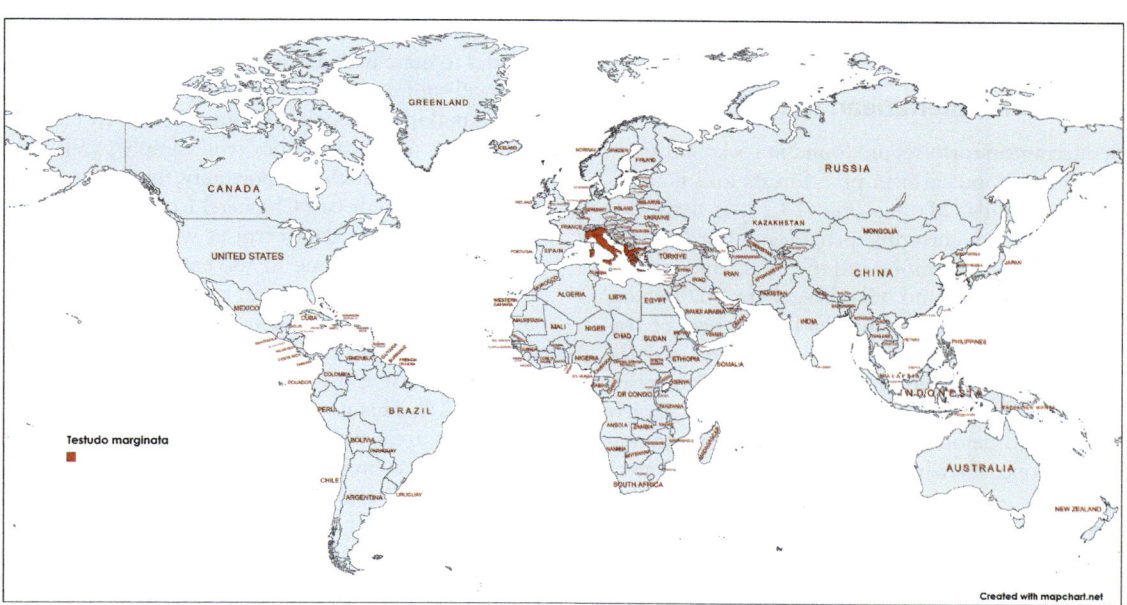

Fig. 13.19. Countries where *Testudo marginata* may be found. (https://www.mapchart.net/world.html)

Mediterranean Tortoises

What are Marginated tortoises (*Testudo marginata*)?

Marginated tortoises can be found in Greece (the Peloponnese Peninsula), Sardinia, Albania and Italy (Fig. 13.19) (Vetter, 2002).

Marginated tortoises are larger than other species of Mediterranean tortoise, with a characteristic flared shell at the rear margin (or edges) of the carapace. They can be identified by the fact that the back of their shell is very wide and flared out at its edges. This defining feature gives these tortoises their name. Some are very dark in colour (Fig. 13.20) while others have a patterned shell with light and dark coloration. They also have a characteristic pattern on the plastron, with dark triangles on the shell plates.

Marginated tortoises are uncommon in captivity compared with other types of Mediterranean tortoise, as far fewer of them were imported (mainly from Greece). The most commonly imported species were the Spur-thighed and Hermann's tortoises before the 1984 ban in the European countries. Now that captive breeding is a more significant source, some breeders do specialize in Marginated tortoises. This species comes from hot dry areas generally, and does not tolerate cold wet conditions. It may be that mortality of wild-caught animals, prior to the 1984 European importation ban, of this species has been higher in captivity than in other Mediterranean species – hence their limited numbers.

What is the natural environment of Mediterranean tortoises?

Mediterranean tortoises are found in rocky terrain in coastal areas, but also in pine forests and maquis-overgrown hills. Maquis (Fig. 13.21) is a type of vegetation that currently provides a border zone between forested regions and the coast, and is often situated on slopes and hills (Wegehaupt, 2009a,b).

Originally maquis contained a huge variety of vegetation, with trees, shrubs and bushes. This was the original primary habitat for Mediterranean tortoises. Unfortunately, this primary habitat is now largely gone, due to deforestation, and a secondary maquis has developed in what remains. In deforested areas the topsoil was often washed away, leaving only impoverished, often rocky, soil, as seen in Fig. 13.22 with a Spur-thighed tortoise in view. Luckily poor soil is ideal for the growth of wild-flower species.

Secondary vegetation often contains coniferous trees, such as pines, and other evergreens such as the ubiquitous mastic tree (*Pistacia lentiscus*), together with oaks, common box and carob plus wild olive and fig trees. Shrubs include junipers, broom, rock roses and tamarinds.

In some areas where there is erosion and a sandy soil, dense thickets of low shrubs form what is termed garrigue. This is most commonly seen near the coast. The garrigue is also called *tomillares* in Spain and *phyrgana* in Greece. Garrigue areas often contain aromatic herbs and spices such as lavender, rosemary, sage, thyme and marjoram. Bright flowers such as lilies, amaryllis and orchids often grow here too (Wegehaupt, 2009a,b; Wegehaupt, 2021).

Where there is heavy thick vegetation, microclimates are created. These provide cooler, shady areas and areas with higher humidity levels. As water is not readily available (especially during the summer months), such areas with their higher humidity and heavy morning dews become important sources of water for tortoises, who lick it from plants and from the ground. Tortoises will seek out puddles after rainfall and sit in the water drinking with their heads submerged (Fig. 13.23). They will also empty their bladders in the puddles, excreting nitrogenous wastes (mainly uric acid and urates) as a milky white liquid.

As they are often inaccessible to humans, these areas of thick vegetation remain a stronghold for tortoises. Although largely solitary, Mediterranean tortoises do use common tracks and come across other tortoises frequently in their home territories (Fig. 13.24).

In spring, males are very active, looking for females to mate with. Generally, when tortoises meet, they will sniff each other (especially around the face) before making a decision about whether to engage further. In most cases they will simply walk on. Where there is a mating opportunity, they will engage in courtship rituals (see Chapter 11 on breeding).

For much of the day tortoises will seek shelter – unless they are basking in the early morning sun. They do not like to be out in the open, as they feel vulnerable, especially when young. Each tortoise will have a retreat, often under bushes, or a scrape where they rest and sleep, slightly buried in the soil (Fig. 13.25). This is one of the ways in which they can access areas of higher humidity (see Chapter 3 on the captive environment).

The original habitat for all Mediterranean tortoises is now largely lost because of human activities and development (Fig. 13.26). While a few isolated areas of primary habitat remain, generally these tortoises are now only found in secondary habitats of maquis and garrigue.

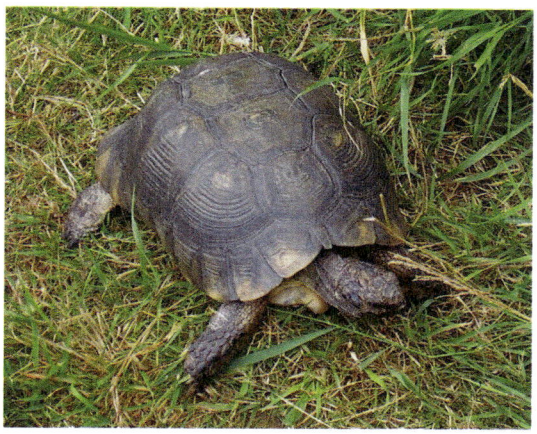

Fig. 13.20. Marginated tortoise with very dark carapace.

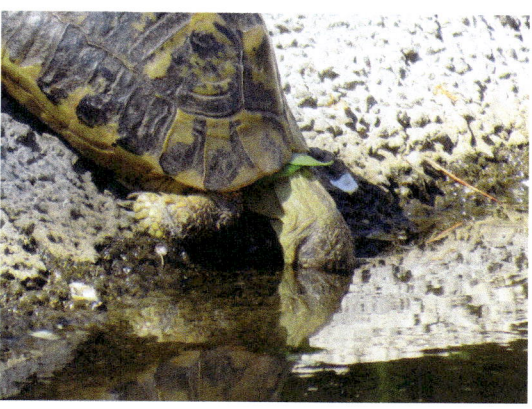

Fig. 13.23. Hermann's tortoise in Majorca drinking.

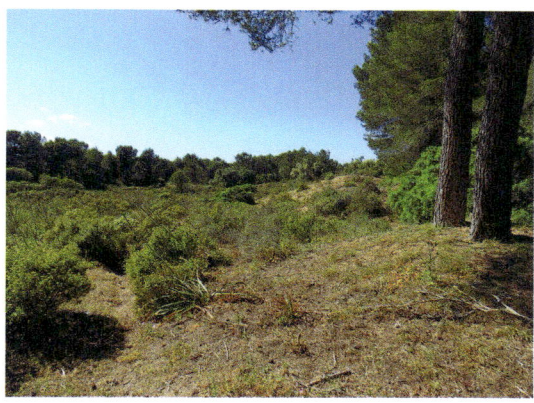

Fig. 13.21. Primary maquis, of which there is relatively little left.

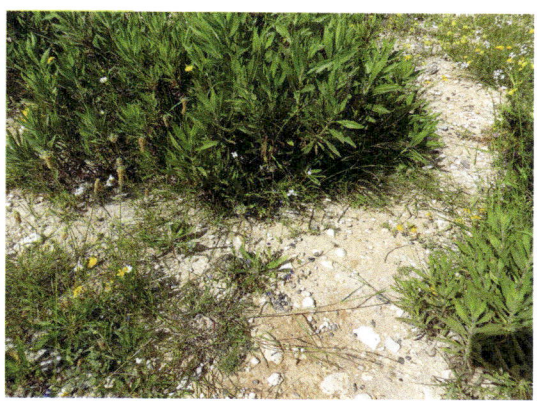

Fig. 13.24. Paths and tracks through vegetation.

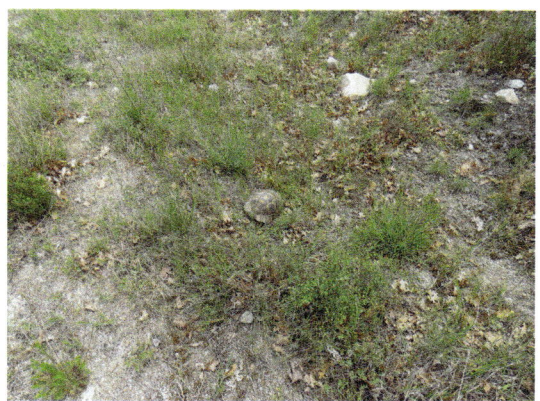

Fig. 13.22. Closer view of Mediterranean habitat (with Spur-thighed tortoise) in northern Greece.

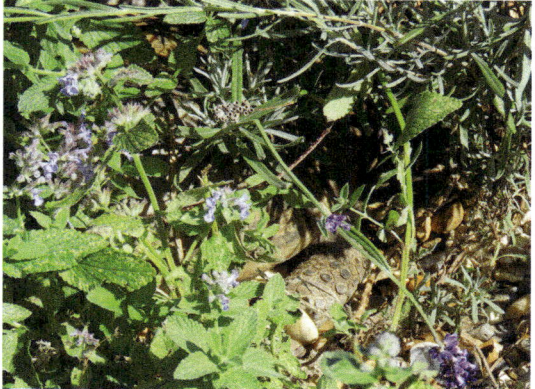

Fig. 13.25. Tortoise using vegetation to hide under for shade and shelter.

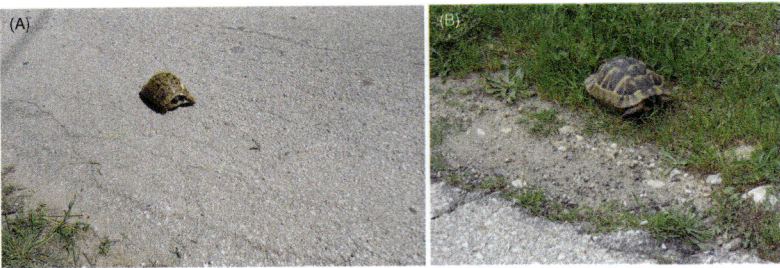

Fig. 13.26. Human activities often spell disaster for tortoises through tourism, building developments, roads and loss of habitat. (A) Elderly Hermann's female crossing the road. (B) Male Spur-thighed in northern Greece.

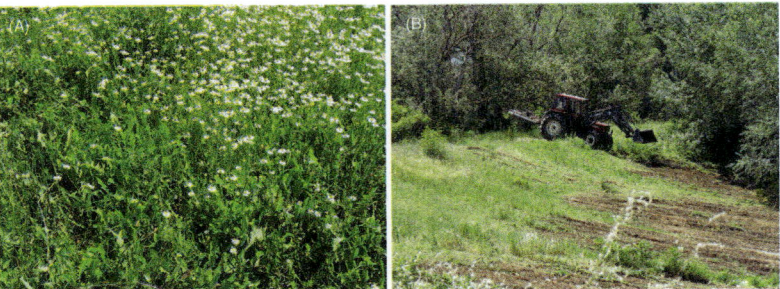

Fig. 13.27. Farming methods often leave no space for tortoises. The habitat is devastated, changing from (A) lush vegetation, much of which is a food source, to (B) bare earth or a monoculture for human food.

The impact of agriculture has been to reduce tortoise populations and to isolate them. Often only small pockets of suitable habitat remain, populated by tiny groups of tortoises with limited genetic diversity. Farming has created barriers, such as rock/stone walls and fences, which tortoises cannot cross. Loss of forest and woodland because of clearance has also decimated tortoise populations (Fig. 13.27). Grazing by goats and sheep has resulted in soil erosion in some areas. The landscape is reduced to a moon-like desert, or fields of rubble where no plant life (and therefore no tortoises) can exist (Wegehaupt, 2009a,b).

Roads are also a major hazard, not simply because of the risk of tortoises being run over, but also because they present obstacles on hillsides with sides too steep to climb or have concrete kerbs. These are often too high to climb, leaving the tortoise trapped and unable to get back into the cover of vegetation. This makes it easier for predators, or human collectors, to see tortoises, making roads a significant factor in the decline of populations.

Predators like wild boar will take not only eggs, hatchlings and juveniles but also adult tortoises. Foxes and dogs will gnaw on their shells or eat their limbs.

Smaller tortoises are also prey to birds of the corvid family or eagles, as well as rodents, badgers, martens and snakes. Younger tortoises tend to be less well camouflaged, and less cautious than adults. This makes them easier prey both to spot and to eat. Young tortoises often live in small colonies, which reduces an individual's chances of being eaten. Juveniles will often stay in their hatching area for several years, provided that there is adequate food (Wegehaupt, 2009a,b).

In captivity careful husbandry may well remove the danger from predation, but the challenge is to provide an environment that allows our tortoises to make choices and gives opportunities which enable them to maintain homeostasis. They require opportunities to achieve a suitable body temperature, access to sufficient daily light levels, and to eat food that will keep them healthy and well (see Chapter 3 on the captive environment).

What types of accommodation do Mediterranean tortoises need in captivity?

Many owners of captive tortoises put a great deal of thought and effort into providing large enclosures (both inside and outside) that replicate (as far as is possible) the types of environment that their tortoises would be used to in the wild (Fig. 13.28). There are many examples of captive tortoises from this group that are surviving but not thriving. In some cases they are coping with extreme examples of poor husbandry, and have done so for many years (see Chapter 7 on common illnesses and diseases). They are not called the 'Great Survivors' for nothing (Gerlach, 2012).

The amount of time a tortoise spends outside in its enclosure will depend upon the climate in which the tortoise is being kept (Fig. 13.29). If the climate is like that of the Mediterranean, conditions will be very like those of the natural habitat. It is important to realize, however, that as soon as a tortoise is taken out of its natural environment and confined, its choices are immediately, and necessarily, limited. It is an owner's responsibility to compensate for this and to provide suitable living conditions (Fig. 13.30) (Highfield, 1996).

If the climate is colder than that of the Mediterranean, additional support in the form of artificial heat and light will be needed for all or parts of the year (see Chapter 4 on artificial light and heat). This is ideally provided by setting up basking lights in an insulated shed or greenhouse which is attached to, and therefore accessible from, the outdoor garden (Fig. 13.31). This allows the tortoise to access both outside and indoor spaces whenever required (see Chapter 3 on the captive environment).

If the tortoise is living in captivity in a climate that is hotter than the Mediterranean, plenty of shade provision will be needed. If the temperature exceeds 38°C these tortoises may aestivate, which is a period of dormancy (similar to hibernation) in a cool, shady location to avoid excess daytime temperatures. Tortoises become dormant, resting in the coolest possible spots until the temperature is reduced, as they cannot remain active in these temperatures. Artificial cooling may be required if this situation continues for extended periods during the warmest months of the year in your location.

As much time as possible should be spent by your tortoise outside, with access to natural sunlight, in order for it to stay healthy. Ultraviolet (UV) and visible wavelengths of light are needed together with infrared radiation. All three wavelengths are provided by natural sunlight. The daily rhythm of tortoise activity is controlled by this natural light – UV and visible light provide stimulation for activity, while infrared light provides the warmth that allows this activity to occur (see Chapter 4 on artificial light and heat).

Outside tortoise gardens should provide:

- Basking areas
- Places to hide, retreat, shelter
- Enclosed areas for additional warming – covered with polycarbonate or Perspex® to retain heat
- Different substrates – soil, rocks, flat areas
- Opportunities to climb and exercise
- Planting of shrubs and edible flowering plants for shade and food
- Accessible source of water.

While indoor accommodation is unlikely to be as extensive as that found outside, it should provide the habitat enrichment detailed above. Ideally both indoor and outdoor accommodation will be connected (Figs 13.31 and 13.32). This gives the tortoise maximum space and allows it to make choices about how it spends its time, as it would in the wild (Fig. 13.33) (Highfield and Highfield, 2008).

In the wild the tortoise is likely to roam over 5 km a day, so whatever we provide will always be a compromise in terms of size of enclosure (see Chapter 3 on the captive environment). Biedenweg and Schramm (2019), in their publication on Egyptian tortoises, suggested that the territories of male tortoises in the Mediterranean may be in the region of 0.65–1.69 ha, and for females 0.74–2.41 ha. These are very large areas for roaming, which we are unlikely to be able to meet fully in captivity.

Where the inside enclosure is not linked to the outside one, indoor accommodation is needed in the form of a tortoise table, or open enclosure with overhead heat and light (see Chapter 3 on the captive environment). Indoor accommodation is likely to be needed for all tortoises in spring and autumn to extend the daylength and provide additional heat. In autumn this is used to delay hibernation and in spring to get the tortoise feeding again after hibernation. Hibernation/brumation length should be similar to that in the wild at around 8 weeks (McArthur *et al.*, 2004), which means additional support is needed. Cold, wet days in summer may also be a circumstance when indoor accommodation is beneficial.

What is a suitable diet for Mediterranean tortoises?

Like all herbivorous tortoises, Mediterranean tortoises in the wild eat a wide range of plants. In captivity they need to be provided with a diet rich in fibre and low in protein. Plenty of calcium needs

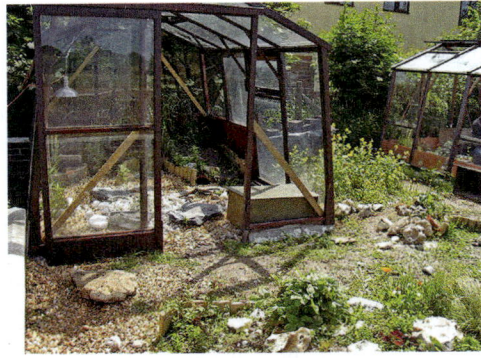

Fig. 13.28. Tortoise enclosure with heat and light in greenhouse and with access to the outside (Eleanor Lien-Hua Tirtasana Chubb).

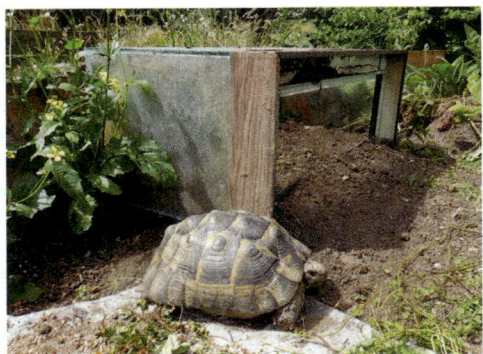

Fig. 13.29. Outdoor garden enclosure for Mediterranean tortoises with shelter providing additional heat from an aquarium on its side (Eleanor Lien-Hua Tirtasana Chubb).

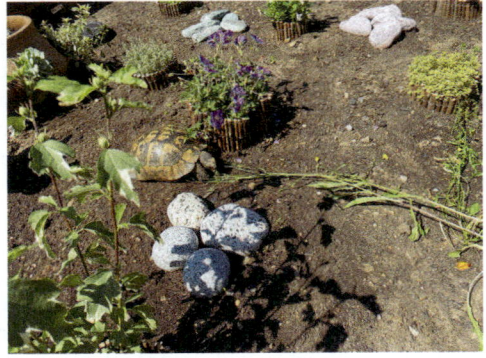

Fig. 13.30. Planting to create shade and to allow natural foraging and browsing.

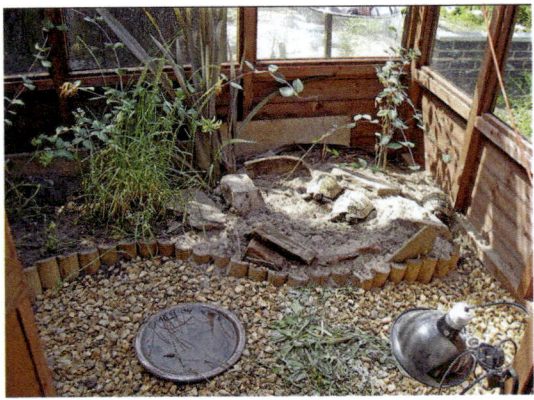

Fig. 13.31. Linked outdoor and indoor accommodation (Eleanor Lien-Hua Tirtasana Chubb).

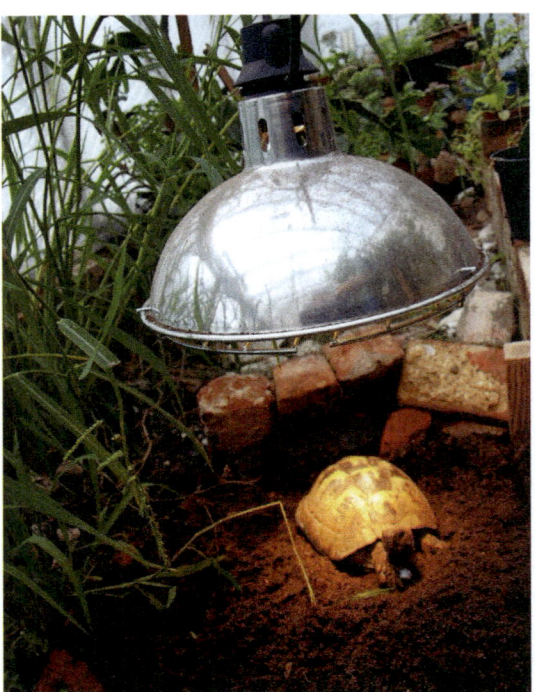

Fig. 13.32. Indoor accommodation substrates.

to be made available. It should be noted, however, that tortoises cannot assimilate this calcium unless they also have access to UV radiation. This is essential for the synthesis of vitamin D3 in the skin, without which calcium cannot be taken up (Highfield and Highfield, 2009).

A comprehensive list of plant species that can be grown as food can be found in Chapter 5 on diets. Some examples of plants that are suitable for regular feeding, as they come into season in northern Europe, can be seen in Table 13.1, taken from *Edible Plants for Tortoises in the UK* (King, 2020).

In my experience, both forms of deadnettle are available in March in the UK, as is garlic mustard and a small amount of dandelion. Geranium in the hardy form remains throughout the winter, as do plantain and bristly oxtongue.

Tortoises start feeding straight away after hibernation. They will gorge on young plants whose spring growth is high in vitamins and minerals. Unfortunately, such plants are often too high in protein to be fed in large quantities. A mixed diet of mature leaves is therefore preferable. Variety in the diet provides a good range of vitamins and minerals, and helps to prevent the tortoise becoming addicted to one or two types of unsuitable food. A mixed, varied diet also reduces the protein content while still ensuring that it remains high in fibre.

Water

It is crucial that water is always available for drinking. After hibernation the tortoise needs to flush out any toxins collected and stored in the bladder during hibernation. Drinking fresh water helps stimulate the tortoise to do this. Suitable humidity levels in the substrate and the air are also needed for good health and for normal growth in hatchlings and juveniles.

What is a typical day for a Mediterranean tortoise in captivity?

Tortoises will typically emerge when the sun comes up and starts warming their enclosure. The tortoise will be aware of the rise, and will want to move outside into the sunshine. This is one of the big advantages of an enclosure that combines indoor and outdoor space. The tortoise can be confined indoors overnight, where additional heat and light may be provided, and the tortoise kept secure from predators and theft (see Chapter 19 on health and safety). The enclosure can then be opened in the morning for the tortoise to go outside as the temperature rises. This is as close to the natural situation as we can create in captivity, in climates where additional heat is needed.

As temperatures start to reach more than 15°C, tortoises become more active. They will typically lie with head and limbs extended on warm slopes to absorb as much sunlight and warmth as possible. Then the search for food begins. Tortoises will eat until mid-morning if food items are available. This will be followed by periods of alternate walking, resting and hiding as they seek the optimum temperature for their metabolism. They may look for water and bathe in the morning or the evening. They may try to find food again in the late afternoon, if it is still warm enough. As the sun starts to fade the tortoise will seek shelter, a retreat or hide. There is likely to be burrowing down into a natural scrape if the substrate, temperature and humidity are suitable. As described, it is safest if these opportunities can be created in an enclosed space, in a secure shed, greenhouse or indoors.

Learning your tortoise's daily rhythms of behaviour and activity, so that you can spot abnormal behaviour and, if necessary, seek attention, is one of the most enjoyable aspects of being a keeper. Observing natural behaviours and gaining a better understanding of your tortoise's needs (see Chapter 8 on behaviour) are key to doing the best job you can as a carer.

Good practice is to check your tortoise a number of times a day, to ensure that it has not escaped, turned upside down or gone missing. In autumn, as the temperature falls and daylength shortens the tortoise may look for a place to dig in, ready to hibernate. Check nightly and first thing in morning, if

Table 13.1. Plants suitable for regular feeding in northern Europe (King, 2020).

Plant	Month in season
Pink deadnettle	March
Goose grass	March
Garlic mustard	April
White deadnettle	April
Alexanders	April
Sow thistles	April
Dandelion	April
Goat's beard	April
Cat's ears	May
Mallow	May
Geranium/Cranesbill	May
Archangel	May
Bristly oxtongue	May
Herb Robert	June
Nipplewort	June
Creeping thistle	July

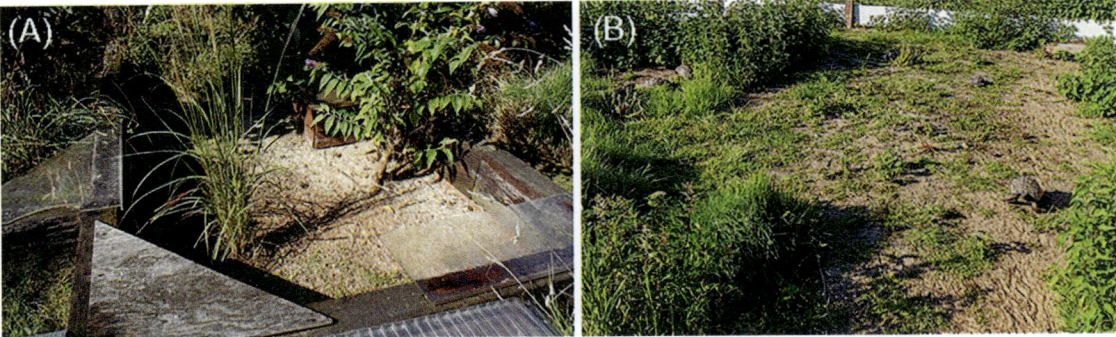

Fig. 13.33. (A) Well-planted small enclosures for enrichment. (B) Large outdoor enclosure (Dillon Prest).

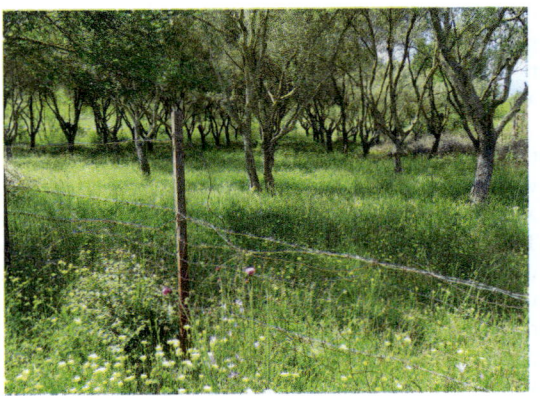

Fig. 13.34. Olive groves can be more usable spaces for tortoises than other farming areas. Note the fencing that they have to contend with, however.

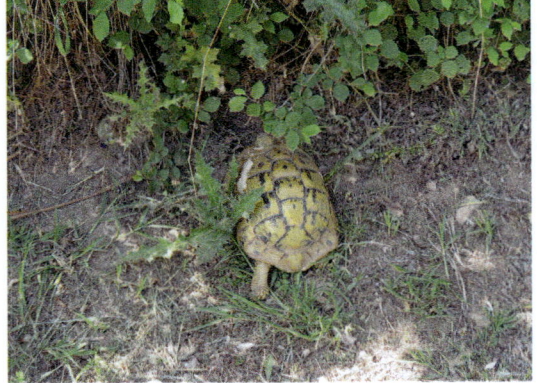

Fig. 13.36. Hermann's tortoise making an escape into vegetation after crossing a road.

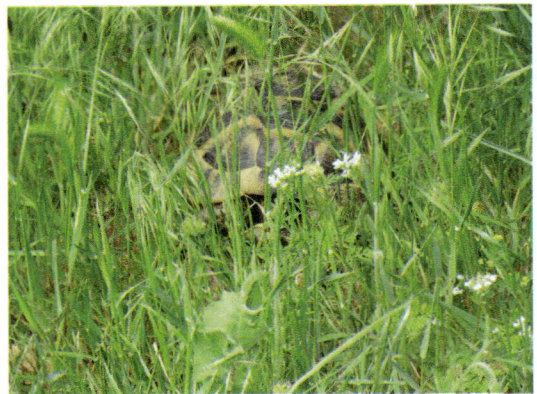

Fig. 13.35. Spur-thighed tortoise in roadside vegetation.

sleeping outside, for predator damage and to ensure that the tortoise is still safely in the enclosure.

Tortoises are strong and persistent. They can easily get themselves into trouble by getting caught up in structures and objects within the enclosure. I once saw a Hermann's tortoise that had been kept in a small enclosure with chicken-wire sides. The tortoise had ripped all the scales from both front legs as he tried to scale the sides in an attempt to get out and find a mate. This is why enclosures should be made of solid materials and why any enrichment and structures must be 'tortoise-proof', bearing in mind that these animals are effective climbers, diggers and very driven to find pastures new if their enclosures are too small.

Mediterranean tortoises in the wild

There is little primary habitat left for these tortoises and what is available is often fragmented due to human activities. Roads are a particular hazard for tortoises to cross. There are cases where their habitat is being destroyed while they still live there (see Chapter 20 on tortoise keeping in the past, present and future). Figures 13.34–13.36 show examples of the remaining natural habitat and some of the situations in which tortoises find themselves trying to survive.

Conclusion

Mediterranean tortoises can make excellent pets provided that they are given the correct care and attention. They are not the 'easy pets' that they may have been advertised as in years gone by. As described here they have particular needs, as all tortoises do. Without those needs being met, they may survive, but not thrive, sometimes for many years. As we now know much more about how to help them to achieve physiological homeostasis, and therefore to stay healthy and well during their expected long lifespan of over 100 years, we have a responsibility to do our best for them.

Spur-thighed tortoises are a very mixed group. Some are fragile and delicate and so may not be able to hibernate. Spur-thighed tortoises can also be more susceptible to diseases such as runny nose syndrome (URTD).

Hermann's tortoises are generally considered to be a hardier species. They often have a voracious appetite and will eat a wide variety of foods.

Marginated tortoises are generally much less common and require a warmer environment than either Spur-thighed tortoises or Hermann's tortoises.

Keeping mixed groups of Mediterranean tortoises is not generally advised unless they naturally cohabit in the wild. Tortoises living in groups in captivity should as a general principle be with others of the same species. Mixing species can be a recipe for disaster in terms of spread of disease (see Chapter 7 on common illnesses and diseases). *Testudo graeca graeca* should not be kept with *Testudo graeca ibera*, as the latter can be a cause of URTD in the former. Runny nose syndrome can be a recurring and problematic respiratory infection in these tortoises. The courtship and mating behaviours are different in different species – another reason for not mixing them. Hybrid matings and egg production, leading to hybrid offspring, are also not helpful in terms of the conservation efforts in Mediterranean tortoises.

Providing suitable homes for Mediterranean tortoises is possible in many parts of the world. As they have been part of the pet trade for over 60 years, we know more about keeping them in captivity than many other species of tortoise. This is an advantage when doing our best to provide suitable accommodation and diets, as the more we know about individual species of tortoise, the better we can do for them in captivity.

References and Further Reading

Biedenweg, F. and Schramm, R. (2019) The Egyptian Tortoise *Testudo kleinmanni* Lortet 1883. A Fascinating Little Beauty, Tartaruga-Verlag Ricarda Schramm, Grebenhain, Germany.

CITES: Convention on International Trade in Endangered Species of Wild Flora and Fauna, Geneva. Website: www.cites.org

Gerlach, J. (2012) *The Great Survivors*. Phelsuma, Cambridge

Highfield, A. (1996) *Practical Encyclopaedia of Keeping and Breeding Tortoises and Freshwater Turtles*. Carapace Press, London.

Highfield, A. and Highfield, N. (2008) *Taking Care of Pet Tortoises*. The Tortoise Trust Jill Martin Fund. Available from: www.tortoisetrust.org

Highfield, A. and Highfield, N. (2009) *Keeping a Pet Tortoise*. Interpet, Dorking, UK.

Jepson, L. (2010) *Mediterranean Tortoises*. Interpet, Dorking, UK.

King, L. (2020) *Edible Plants for Tortoises in the UK* (4th edn). Available from books@tlady.clara.co.uk

McArthur, S., Wilkinson, R. and Meyer, J. (2004) *Medicine and Surgery of Tortoises and Turtles*. Blackwell, Oxford, UK.

Vetter, H. (2002), *Turtles of the World Vol. 1, Africa, Europe and Western Asia*. Chimaira, Frankfurt.

Wegehaupt, W. (2009a) *Mediterranean Tortoises. Where and how they live in the wild*. Kressbronn, Germany.

Wegehaupt, W. (2009b) *Naturalistic Keeping and Breeding of Hermann's Tortoises*. Kressbronn, Germany.

Wegehaupt, W. (2021) *Feeder Plants for Mediterranean Tortoises*. Kressbronn, Germany.

14 Tropical Dry Grassland Tortoises

Abstract

Leopard tortoises, Sulcatas, Radiated, Indian Star and Burmess Star tortoises are included in this chapter. These tropical species from Africa and Asia need warmth and light all year round as they do not hibernate. They are herbivorous and generally grazers, eating a wide variety of grasses, succulents and flowering plants. Their diet needs to be very high in fibre and calcium and low in protein. These species have very attractive shell patterns and are highly sought after as pets.

Keeping them healthy requires sufficient space, warmth and light, which for some species such as Sulcatas is extensive. Some are very large, strong species, making it a challenge to meet their accommodation requirements in captivity. Others are quite delicate and can easily succumb to disease, which makes them a challenge in other ways. They generally require large enclosures with artificial heat and light throughout the year. As tropical species, none of these tortoises hibernate/brumate. From a companion perspective, they can be very rewarding pets throughout the year. Many of them are endangered species in the wild, which raises an ethical dimension to keeping them in captivity. Ethical sourcing of these animals and the role of captive breeding is discussed.

Which species of tortoise?

Tropical dry grassland tortoises come from areas where there are open grasslands, dry scrub and semi-arid conditions. These are found on the continents of Africa and Asia. They come in different sizes, but all are larger tortoises, which means that they need a good deal of space when kept in captivity. As they are tropical, their preferred body temperatures are around 28–32°C. They do not hibernate/brumate. They have also evolved to live in areas with the brightest of sunlight available on our planet, so their demands for UVB and natural sunlight are very high. Accommodation must be provided that allows these tortoises access to suitable temperatures and light sources for the entire year.

A suitable diet, consisting of a variety of plant species, is essential, along with free access to water. Supplementation to ensure sufficient calcium in the diet is recommended. Although the natural environment is largely dry and arid, there will be microclimates created by the vegetation and landscape. These locations, under bushes, shrubs and trees, will have higher levels of humidity, essential for normal growth of juveniles and as part of the natural environment. This gives the tortoises the opportunity to access the environmental choices that they need in order to thrive, rather than just survive.

These tortoises need to bask and seek shade in order to achieve their preferred body temperature. Their environment should be maintained at daytime temperatures above 22°C and at night not below 18°C. In their natural environment it does not get cold for any period of time, so variation in their body temperature from day to night is not great, nor is variation across the months of the year. Because of this they maintain their body temperature from background heat as well as from the sun. As they come from tropical regions, less time is needed for temperature regulation and more time can be spent walking and seeking food. This gives these tortoises an opportunity to feed for more prolonged periods of time, which allows them to grow to a bigger size.

The bigger the tortoise, the larger the enclosure that is needed. Sulcatas need the largest grazing areas, with Leopard tortoises not far behind. For grazing for a large adult Sulcata, 0.2–0.4 hectares would not be unreasonable (i.e. 0.5–1.0 acres). This fact alone makes these animals unsuitable as garden tortoises for most people. Tropical dry grassland tortoises often burrow and dig scrapes, so they need shade as well as open areas and a well-drained loose substrate.

Although the species in this section are all tropical tortoises, with similar environmental and dietary needs, they should not be kept together. Keeping more than one species of tortoise together is generally not advised from a biosecurity perspective, as often there is the possibility of passing on disease. Some are particularly susceptible to catching diseases from other species, as they have no resistance to pathogens they have never previously encountered.

These beautiful tropical tortoises have very specific needs and are not suitable for everyone to keep in captivity, because of the amount of space they need. The costs of keeping them are high also, due to their need for warmth 365 days a year. In the winter, finding suitable food items can be challenging. These are not 'beginner' tortoises and require a great deal of commitment and effort if they are to be kept healthy and well.

It is important to source these species ethically as they are still the subject of illegal trading. Captive-bred animals are available but often at a higher cost. Funding the trade in these endangered species by purchasing wild-caught animals is to be avoided at all costs. They are protected by the Convention on International Trade in Endangered Species (CITES) and there are legal restrictions on their trade in most countries.

Much of what is needed for successful maintenance of these species in captivity is covered in the first section on Leopard tortoises. Subsequent sections focus on the important differences in the species that follow.

Leopard tortoises – *Geochelone pardalis* (more recently *Centrochelys pardalis*)

Leopard tortoises can reach 60 cm in length and females can weigh up to 50 kg (Highfield, 1996). They are called Leopard tortoises because of the coloration of their shells, which is yellowish, splotched with dark blotches, somewhat reminiscent of the fur of a leopard cat (Fig. 14.2). They can easily live for up to 100 years.

Leopard tortoises are herbivorous grazers. They will eat flowering plants, succulents and large amounts of grass species. Their diet must be high in fibre and low in protein. In the wild they will eat the bones of carcasses in order to gain calcium. Growing a large shell and heavy bones means that they have a great need for this mineral. These tortoises burrow into the substrate and can dig quite deep holes. Like all tortoises, they need to drink regularly. Unlike many land tortoises, however, they have the capacity to swim and have been seen swimming across large pools in their natural habitat.

Two subspecies are generally recognized (Vetter, 2002; Highfield, 1996; BCG Caresheet), although as adults they are not easy to differentiate:

- *Centrochelys pardalis babcocki* is the much more common Eastern subspecies ranging in eastern Africa from Ethiopia to South Africa.
- *Centrochelys pardalis pardalis* is the Western subspecies with a much smaller range within South Africa.

What is their natural environment?

These are tortoises of the African Savannah, found across southern and eastern Africa, in Kenya, Tanzania, South Africa and Namibia (Fig. 14.1). They range across the Sahel and Sub-Saharan southern Africa and live sympatrically with African Spurred tortoises (Sulcatas) and some species of Hingeback (see Chapter 15 on tortoises of humid forests).

Here the habitat is semi-arid grassland (Fig. 14.3A), where temperatures range from 15°C to 32°C, the humidity is low, and the substrate is sandy soil, silt and clay for much of their range. There are areas of greater vegetation cover in some countries, such as that shown in Fig. 14.3B, which was taken in the rainy season in Zambia. Figure 14.4 shows just how well camouflaged this species is.

What is a suitable diet for Leopard tortoises in captivity?

In spring and summer grass species, succulents and flowering plants should provide the main source of food as they come into season (see Chapter 5 on diets). Kabigumila (2001) and Milton (1992) both identified large numbers of plant species in the natural diet of this herbivorous species. In Tanzania succulents formed a higher percentage of the diet, although the variety we can provide in captivity is more likely to be achieved through wild-growing weeds and grass species. Succulents can of course be included (Fig. 14.5).

These grazers should never be fed grass clippings, in the same way that clippings are not safe to feed to horses. They are often wet and partially fermented, leading to problems digesting this material.

Having kept this species in captivity for many years, I can confirm that, when they are on the required high-fibre, high-calcium and low-protein diet, their ability to produce large volumes of fibrous faeces is impressive (Fig. 14.6).

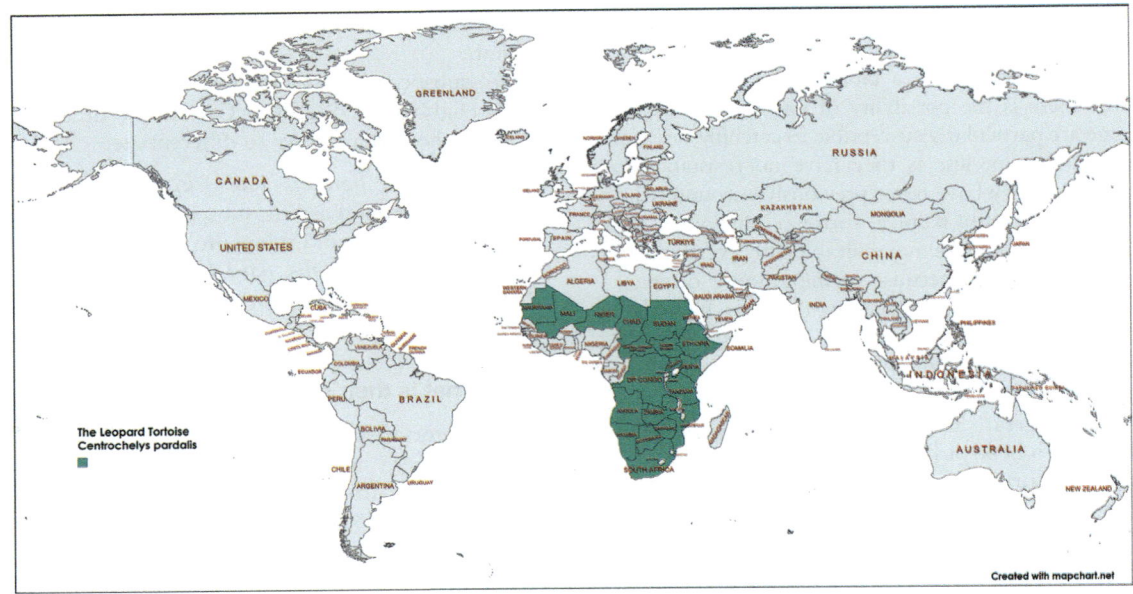

Fig. 14.1. Map of Leopard tortoise distribution. (https://www.mapchart.net/world.html)

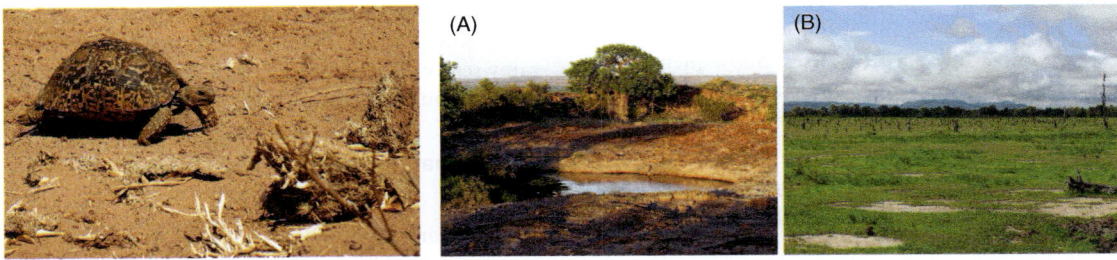

Fig. 14.2. Leopard tortoise in South Africa (Gary Franklin).

Fig. 14.3. The savannah habitat: (A) in South Africa (Gary Franklin) and (B) in Zambia (Sian Bewick).

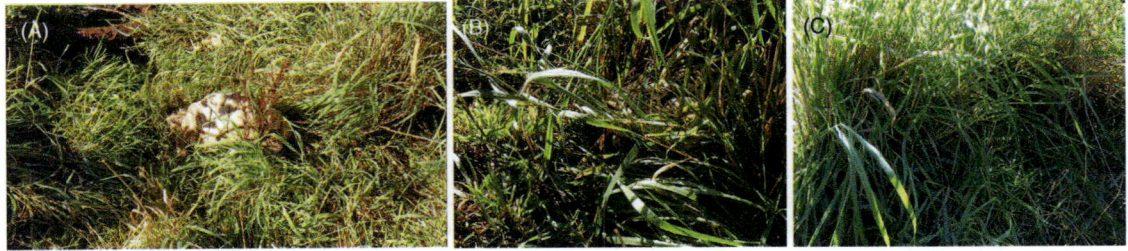

Fig. 14.4. This sequence of photographs shows how superbly well camouflaged Leopard tortoises are in grassland due to their shell patterning.

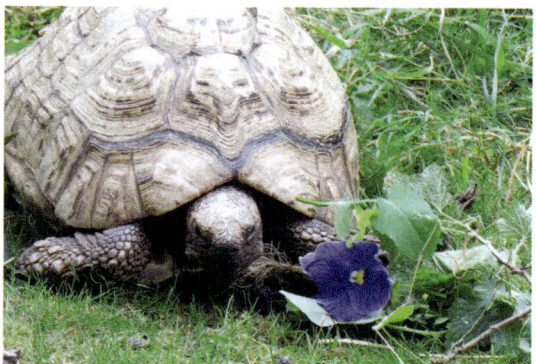

Fig. 14.5. Selection of weeds in the diet provides variety from flowering plants in addition to grass.

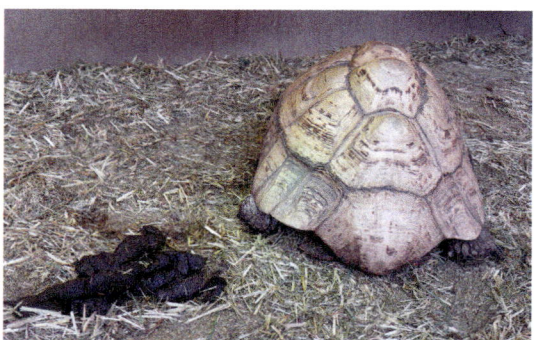

Fig. 14.6. Shaka, my male Leopard tortoise, is a legend here for the huge amounts of poo which he produces on a daily basis throughout the summer. This is very dark, fibrous and does not smell unpleasant – in a similar way to that of mammalian grazers such as cattle and sheep.

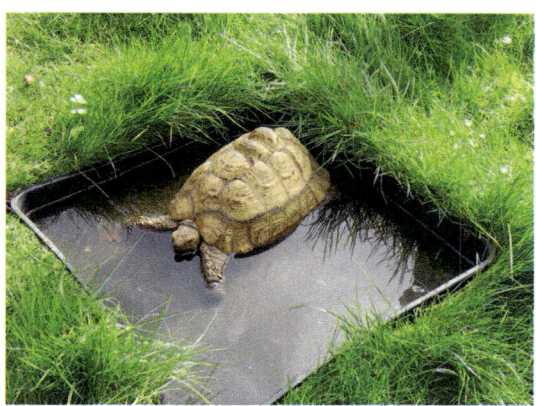

Fig. 14.7. Leopard tortoise in large bath in outdoor enclosure with long grass. This area is unmown, as Shaka grazes the grass short throughout the summer months in the UK.

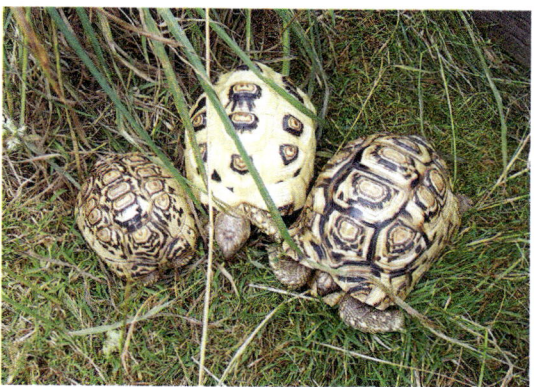

Fig. 14.8. Three juvenile Leopard tortoises. Note that the two individuals on the right and left of the picture have normal shell patterns. The individual in the centre has grown too quickly: it is very pale because the shell growth has not allowed the pigmentation to move, as the scutes have grown so fast. This leaves a pale, unpigmented shell, which may even be soft if this effect has been caused by poor diet and overfeeding is severe.

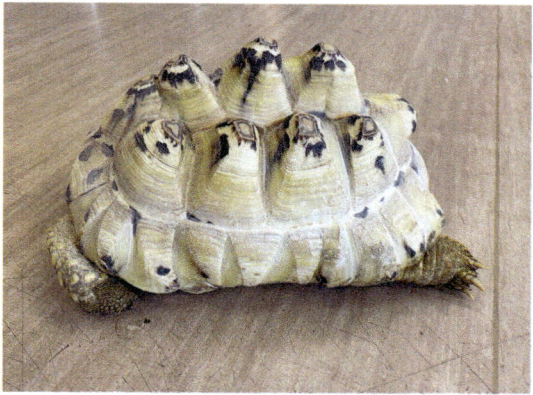

Fig. 14.9. As a relatively fast-growing species, it is easy to overfeed Leopard tortoises. This is an extreme example of shell pyramiding due to poor diet and overfeeding.

In the winter, when weeds and grass are not really growing, it can be a challenge to ensure that Leopard tortoises can continue to eat high-fibre foods like grasses, stems and leaves. Use of hay products (an example would be Readigrass®) is essential to maintain variety in the diet and provide the necessary high fibre. Arcadia® Freshly Pressed Tortoise Food is another good source of high-fibre food for the winter.

Naturally growing species that continue to be available throughout the year may include buddleia, lilac, hardy geraniums and plantain. In the autumn other green shrubs, such as vine, continue to be available as they drop their leaves later in the season. In spring early plants include garlic mustard.

Fruits are not part of the natural diet and so should be avoided. Flowers of edible species can be eaten as part of the mix of leafy plants (Fig. 14.6), along with succulents, such as prickly pear cactus, and grasses. Note that some sources of information continue to refer to the suitability of fruits and vegetables such as kale for this species but, as mentioned above and in Chapter 5 on diets, these foods are to be avoided.

What types of accommodation do Leopard tortoises need in captivity?

Leopard tortoises need large outdoor enclosures as described in Chapter 3 (on the captive environment), ideally at least 600 m² bounded by sturdy fences that they cannot see through. They should have access to this enclosure all year round, even though their time outside may be limited to only an hour in the coldest months of a northern winter. A short period that allows very beneficial grazing on sunny winter days is acceptable as long as they return to their basking lamps indoors before becoming too cold (Highfield, 1996). They walk very large distances in the wild and need the opportunity to exercise in this way in captivity.

They will also need a large insulated shed or outbuilding, ideally at least 15 m², to provide heat and light during the winter months, if they live with you in a temperate or cold climate. These tortoises need to be kept warm and dry, as they can easily get respiratory problems. They do not tolerate the damp or cold draughts of air, for example. Although they may spend much of the winter in their indoor space, the opportunity to graze outdoors should be given whenever possible. It is helpful, therefore, if the indoor and outdoor enclosures are linked. The cost of heating and the need for large indoor and outdoor accommodation means that these tortoises are not suitable for all keepers.

Leopard tortoises also need access to drinking water at all times (Fig. 14.7).

Males when kept together may fight but small colonies can be kept together with greater numbers of females than males present. Facilities are needed to be able to separate males from females if the males' mating and courtship attentions become too much for the females.

To prevent the spread of disease, Leopard tortoises should not be kept with other species of tortoise.

This species breeds well in captivity and there is some variation in the shell pattern of juveniles, in part due to diet and growth rates (Fig. 14.8).

If excessive growth continues there may be a devastating result in a relatively young tortoise, as shown in Fig. 14.9. This poor animal has no possibility at all of a normal life. Due to shell deformities and weak limbs from a diet that is too low in calcium and too high in protein, this tortoise can barely lift its shell off the ground to walk. The future is bleak for this individual, who is unlikely to have anything like a normal lifespan.

African Spurred Tortoises/Sulcatas – *Geochelone sulcata* (more recently *Centrochelys sulcata*)

The Sulcata is the largest continental tortoise, weighing in at around 100 kg when fully grown. It can measure over 80 cm in length (Highfield, 1996). The only larger tortoises are the island species found on the Galapagos and Seychelles (Galapagos and Aldabran tortoises) (Wilson and Wilson, 1997). The lifespan may be as long as 150 years in suitable conditions (Fig. 14.10).

African Spurred tortoises (Fig. 14.11) must not be confused with the much smaller but similarly named Mediterranean Spur-thighed tortoise.

Sulcatas are a very threatened species in their native countries (Petrozzi *et al.*, 2017, 2020). They breed very well in captivity and can grow very quickly. Several clutches of up to 30 eggs can be laid by a female each year in captivity and hatching rates are very high. If not fed a suitable diet, shell deformities and very rapid growth are even more common than in Leopard tortoises. Being so large, the consequences of shell deformities and weak bones in the legs can be even more severe than for smaller tortoises. As they grow and gain weight, their legs may not be strong enough to hold them off the ground. This is likely to lead to difficulties in walking and so to severe welfare issues and a much-shortened life.

I once rescued a young male Sulcata from an owner who could no longer accommodate him because of his size. At that stage he was only

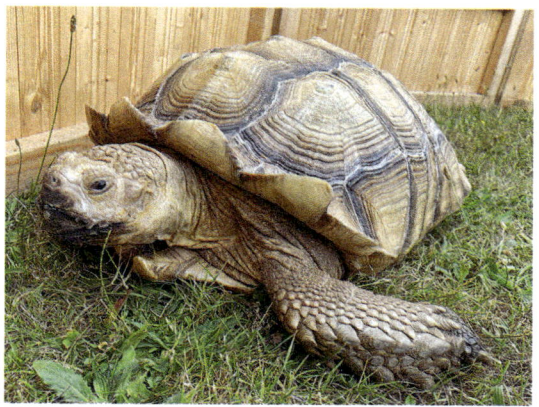
Fig. 14.10. Large male Sulcata.

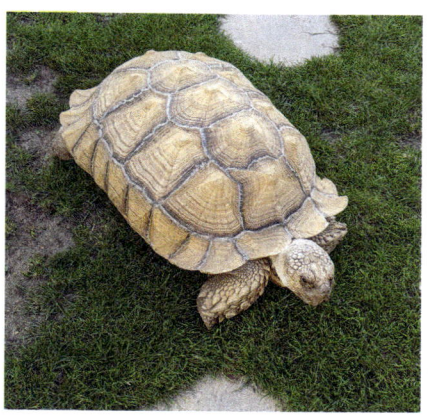
Fig. 14.11. Sulcata Shelly.

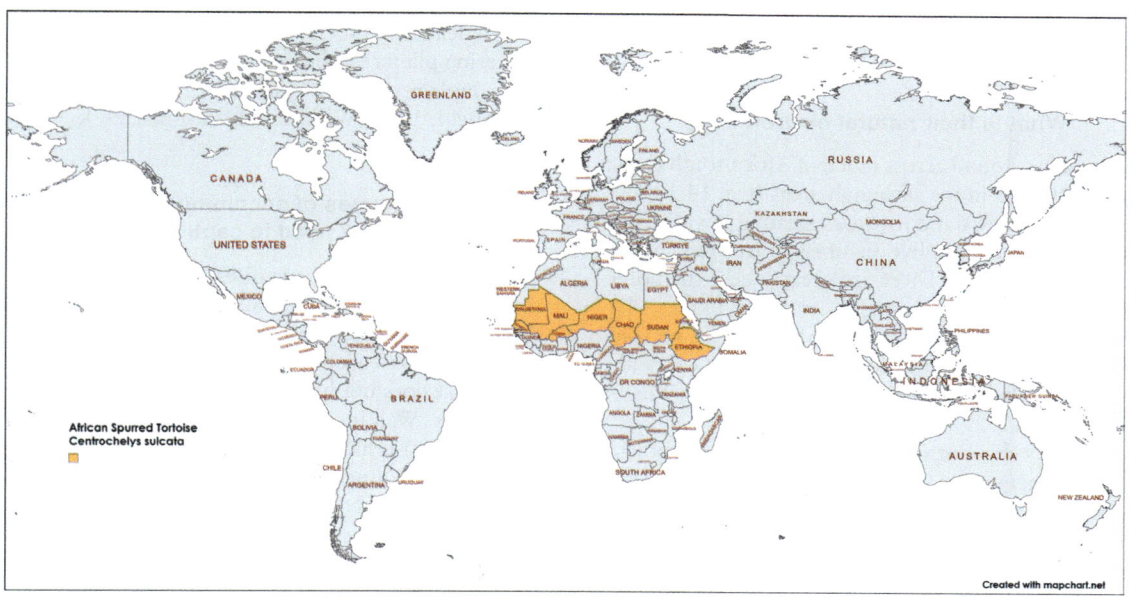
Fig. 14.12. Map of Sulcata tortoise distribution. (https://www.mapchart.net/world.html)

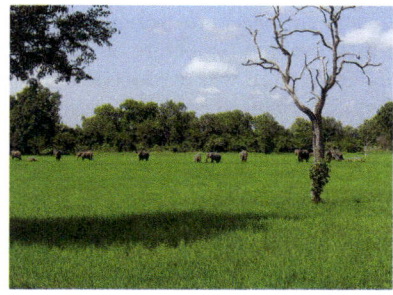
Fig. 14.13. African Savannah in the wet season (Sian Bewick).

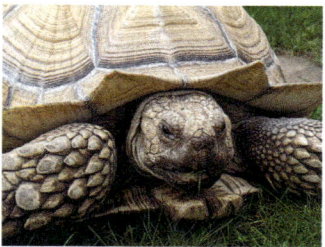
Fig. 14.14. Large gular scutes on the plastron of male Sulcatas are used for fighting and for ramming the female to get her to stand still prior to mating.

8 years old and was already 7 kg in weight and 25 cm in length. As these tortoises are the fastest growing of all tortoise species, many have ended up without a home for this reason. I kept the tortoise for a couple of years knowing that eventually more suitable accommodation would need to be found. As adults, Sulcatas need a large paddock for grazing as well as a well-insulated shed for the winter (if living in a colder climate). When he left me at the age of ten, Smarty was 8.5 kg in weight and 35 cm in length, and thus far too large for the accommodation that I could provide. He now lives in a Dinosaur Park where he has this own huge field together with a large indoor enclosure. He is still growing!

This species is described as charismatic (Petrozzi *et al.*, 2020) and gregarious with high levels of activity and engaging personalities. This has made them a popular pet, especially when young.

What is their natural environment?

Sulcatas are found across much of Africa south of the Sahara Desert in the savannah areas (Fig. 14.12).

They are grassland tortoises needing a warm, dry environment. They live in open grasslands, as do Leopard tortoises. There are areas where the home ranges of both species overlap, as shown in Figs 14.1 and 14.12. The environment has dry, hot seasons when there is limited access to water. Sulcatas are active largely in the wet season (Fig. 14.13) (Wilson and Wilson, 1997).

Sulcatas dig burrows of up to 3 m in depth to provide themselves with shade in the hottest part of the summer. They sometimes aestivate during these hot periods, using the burrow as a shelter. Not many people want 3 m holes in their lawn! This is one of the behaviours that makes keeping these tortoises in domestic settings something of a challenge.

Arguably they are not a suitable pet species, and certainly huge numbers of them have been bred in captivity for the pet trade and then abandoned as they grow large. Around the world many of these tortoises have died due to poor husbandry and lack of suitable accommodation. However, as discussed here, they are threatened in the wild due to habitat destruction and collection for the pet trade (Petrozzi *et al.*, 2020). Captive breeding may therefore play an important role in the continuation of the species in the future, as discussed in Chapter 20 on past, present and future tortoise keeping.

What is a suitable diet for Sulcata tortoises in captivity?

Sulcatas have a similar diet to that of Leopard tortoises as described above (Highfield, 1996). In spring and summer grasses, weeds and succulents should provide the main source of food. Dry foods such as hay and products such as Readigrass® can be used in the winter to increase variety while maintaining the demand for a high-fibre, low-protein diet. Arcadia® Freshly Pressed Tortoise Food is also a good winter feed. Sulcatas are very large, fast-growing tortoises and therefore have a very high demand for calcium and vitamin D3, especially when young. Their diet should always be supplemented two to three times each week with calcium and vitamin D3, using a product such as Nutrobal (Vetark®).

Vine leaves, mulberry leaves, hibiscus leaves and flowering plants can be included in their diet. Fruits and high-protein foods should be avoided (Highfield, 1996; Wilson and Wilson, 1997).

What types of accommodation do they need in captivity?

These are very strong tortoises. Like Leopard tortoises, they will happily walk through any barrier through which they can see. Therefore, it is very unwise to try to accommodate a Sulcata in a glasshouse that does not have insulated wooden or brick solid sides. Walking through glass (or stepping on broken glass) is likely to result in significant injury. All boundaries (including field boundaries) must be very solid and secure, as these tortoises possess immense strength and, once set on a path, will continue undaunted to their destination, particularly if they can see a way out.

Like Leopard tortoises, Sulcatas need a very large, insulated shed or outbuilding provided with heat and light in order to survive the winter months, if they live in a temperate or cold climate. Indoor accommodation will need to be even larger for Sulcatas, as they need to walk every day and travel greater distances. A minimum of 40 m^2 would be recommended indoors; and outdoors 1000 m^2 or 0.5 acres would be suitable.

An additional consideration for this species is that Sulcata males are often aggressive towards each other. This means that they cannot always be kept together in groups. They will fight, as they are territorial and will compete for females. They can cause a great deal of damage to each other because of their strength and size. Males will try to ram each other with the distinctive extensions on their gular scutes of the plastron and will turn each other over (Fig. 14.14). This is dangerous in hot sunny weather because, due to their large size and weight, they cannot easily right themselves (Wilson and Wilson, 1997).

Keeping groups of Sulcatas is potentially problematic due to this aggressive tendency. Females are less aggressive and can often cohabit. Pairs of a male and female can often live together; or in groups with one male and several females. Courtship and mating involve the male stimulating the female to stand still through shell ramming and circling. The male will then mount the female, which is hazardous as it is relatively easy for him to fall off if she moves. This species does not have a deeply concave plastron to help the male stay in position during copulation. As indicated, they are a fertile species and breeding large numbers of juveniles in captivity has taken place over the past 20 years. This has led to over-production and significant welfare issues for adults because suitable long-term accommodation is so hard to find. Rescue organizations have been put under increasing pressure to find these now large tortoises new homes, as their original owners find that they can now longer meet the needs of 70–100 kg animals in their homes.

Radiated tortoises – *Geochelone radiata* (more recently *Astrochelys radiata*)

The Radiated tortoise is another very attractive species with a beautiful shell pattern (Vetter, 2002). The carapace of the shell is highly domed. The shell can be quite smooth but even in wild populations raised scutes are often seen as a normal feature and these small pyramids on the carapace are not considered abnormal. The skin is very pale yellow (Fig. 14.15).

This is a delicate species requiring outdoor and indoor facilities throughout the year. They are susceptible to respiratory disease and should be maintained without contact with other tortoise species. They can live for over 100 years and so are a long-term commitment involving more than one generation of humans, as is the case for most tortoise species.

This species grows to around 40 cm and weighs around 15 kg (Highfield, 1996; BCG care sheets). The lifespan is over 100 years.

What is their natural environment?

Radiated tortoises are listed as critically endangered in their natural habitat in Madagascar by the International Union for Conservation of Nature (IUCN). There is an introduced population on nearby Réunion Island. These are the only locations on the globe where they are found. These tortoises are also listed as Appendix I species by the Convention on International Trade in Endangered Species (CITES) to give the strongest protection to restrict their trade globally.

Radiated tortoises naturally live in the dry forests, scrub areas and woods of southern Madagascar (Fig. 14.16). Unfortunately, much of this habitat has now been lost because of human activity and development. Together with loss of habitat, their numbers have been further reduced by the fact they are a food source for poverty-stricken local people in rural locations. In addition, they have been increasingly caught for the illegal pet trade, where they have a high value. Prices for a Radiated tortoises online can be up to US$5000. Once again ethical sourcing is essential for this endangered species.

They are kept as pets in small numbers, often by specialist keepers. There are captive-breeding programmes in Asia, North America and Europe, mainly in zoos. Some keepers also breed, so some captive-bred individuals are available. If buying one of these, it is very important that you seek out a genuine captive-bred individual and comply with any necessary legislation. As keepers of these lovely tortoises, we do not want to contribute any further to their loss in the wild.

What is a suitable diet for Radiated tortoises in captivity?

Like the other tortoise species here, Radiated tortoises need a high-fibre diet consisting of mixed grasses, flowering plants and coarse leaves and stems (Highfield, 1996; Kuhne, 2019). In the dry season, food consists of dried leaves and only in the wet season would fresh green leaves be available. Keepers often advocate feeding dry food such as dried mulberry leaves and a selection of dried flowers for at least half of each week, and fresh green leaves and stems for the other half (Fig. 14.17) (Kuhne, 2019).

These tortoises also eat succulents such as Opuntia cacti, which can be an important source of water in their naturally arid environment. There are sources suggesting occasional animal protein

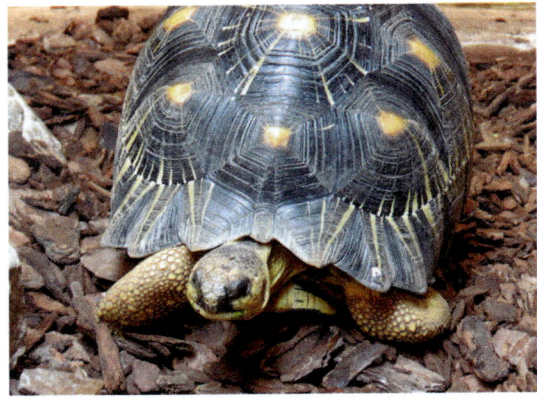

Fig. 14.15. Beautiful shell pattern of Radiated tortoises.

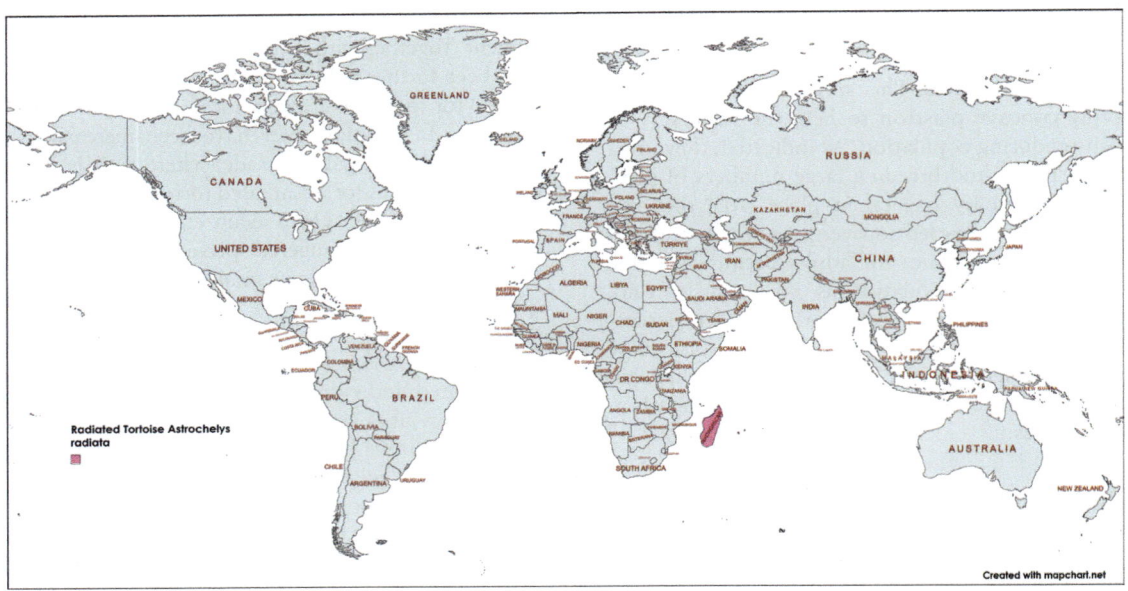

Fig. 14.16. Map of Radiated tortoise locations. (https://www.mapchart.net/world.html)

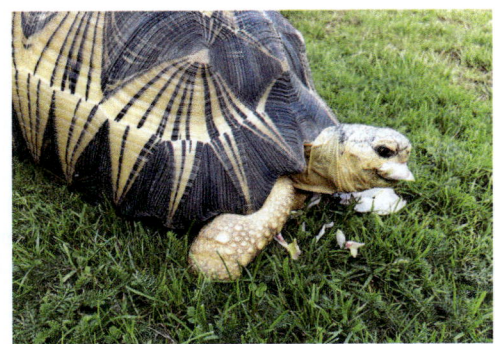

Fig. 14.17. Radiated tortoises will graze on lawns, or in this case select the much more appealing rose petals being offered.

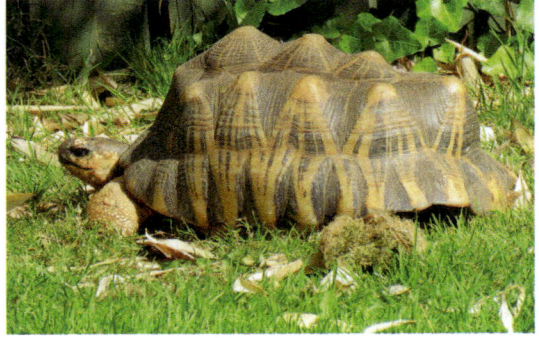

Fig. 14.18. Radiated tortoise with severe pyramiding due to poor diet.

feeds in the diet but there is little evidence for this being a good idea on a very regular basis. Leuteritz (2003) reported that the diet in Madagascar consisted of 29 different plant species, which again emphasizes the need for variety in the diet. The diet consisted of 58% grasses in this study with 7% of the total succulent cacti of Opuntia species. Animal matter, which included bones, shell, hair, carcass, skin and faeces, made up 11% of the diet and was all dried material.

Although all herbivorous tortoises will eat bone and feathers, together with animal faeces, the likely opportunities for any meat in the diet are very limited. This author would not recommend animal protein in the diet for this species in captivity for the reasons below.

Radiated tortoises also require a good source of calcium in the diet and the conditions needed for calcium uptake, including suitable UVB levels, as a source of vitamin D3 as described above. These tortoises require low protein levels in their diet, as for the other species in this section. High-protein diets produce high-nitrogen wastes, which the tortoises are not designed to deal with. Like the other tropical dry grassland tortoises, feeding too much fruit, or vegetables, which may be too high in protein is harmful. Fig. 14.8 shows pyramiding from a poor diet. Fruit is very acidic and may cause digestive problems – in the wild access to berries and fruits is very limited and usually seasonal. A high-fibre diet is essential (Highfield, 1996) to prevent intestinal problems such as diarrhoea, which may result from too much fruit or a diet with too much protein. In the winter, hay and grasses should be included in the diet to increase the variety of plant species fed.

Radiated tortoises in Madagascar were reported as drinking from rainwater puddles (Leuteritz, 2003), which reinforces the need for free access to water for all these species even though they are adapted to live in largely dry arid conditions.

What types of accommodation do they need in captivity?

Radiated tortoises require warm indoor accommodation with artificial light and heat (see Chapter 4 on artificial light and heat) in cold weather. They should not be mixed with other species, for fear of disease transfer. Outdoor grazing together with insulated sheds or outbuildings as indoor accommodation are needed. These tortoises need sufficient space to walk around, whether indoors or outside. Like all the other species in this chapter, they do not hibernate and will need to be kept warm, feeding and active throughout the year. In the wild they walk many kilometres every day, as do all the species in this chapter.

Radiated tortoises can be bred easily in captivity. The males have a longer more pointed tail than females. The females will lay seven clutches a year, each containing six to eight eggs (Highfield, 1996).

Indian Star tortoises – *Geochelone elegans*

This is a very attractive tortoise. Its shell pattern resembles a star configuration, hence the name, making it one of the most recognizable and distinctive land tortoises in the world (Fig. 14.20). These tortoises can be up to 35 cm in length and weigh 12 kg, making them of similar size to the Radiated tortoise.

As with other tropical dry grassland or arid scrub area tortoises discussed in this chapter, this species requires warm indoor accommodation. This can be costly to provide in cold weather. Like all the tropical tortoises discussed here, Indian Star tortoises do not hibernate and they need access to warmth, high light-intensity levels and space to move around, even in the winter.

The shell can be smooth or have raised scutes, as seen in the Radiated tortoise. This species is also delicate and should not be mixed with other species of tortoise. The shell is highly patterned and domed. The Indian Star tortoise is found across India and Sri Lanka and in some locations in Pakistan (Fig. 14. 19) (Highfield, 1996).

These tortoises are in serious decline in their natural habitat largely due to habitat loss, but also for food where people in the locality are very poor, and from poaching for the illegal pet trade. In 2019 the Indian Star was listed as an Appendix I species by CITES, giving it the highest level of protection from trading, as it continues to be over-exploited. It is classed as a vulnerable species, but its numbers are falling so fast, with wild population sizes unknown but decreasing possibly to the point of being endangered. Again, it is important to comply with legislation and source this species responsibly so that you do not contribute to their demise in the wild.

What is their natural environment?

Indian Star tortoises are found across southern India, Pakistan and on the island of Sri Lanka. They live in dry scrub forest and at the edges of arid desert areas (Fig. 14.21) (Highfield, 1996). They have also adapted to live on the edges of farmland and other locations altered by the activities of humans.

Their natural habitat is dry forest, open grass and scrub seen in rural areas of India and Sri Lanka, such as the area shown in Fig. 14.21. Although found in Pakistan, it is not as common there.

The Indian Star tortoise is a grazer and walks considerable distances on a daily basis to find food. The habitat is arid and has high daytime temperatures for much of the year. This leads to crepuscular behaviour, with the greatest activity in the early morning and evenings when the temperature is not too hot. These tortoises burrow and dig scrapes in sandy, loose soils. Indian Star tortoises are adapted to retain water and can withstand periods of drought. In captivity, as with the other species in this chapter, they should have free access to water.

What is a suitable diet for Indian Star tortoises in captivity?

A high-fibre diet is needed, with a mix of grasses and hay species as the basis of the diet, supplemented with flowering plants, coarse stems and leaves from a variety of plants. This tortoise needs a low protein content to the diet, as high-protein diets produce high-nitrogen wastes, which the tortoises are not designed to deal with.

A good source of calcium is also required, together with the conditions needed for calcium uptake, including suitable UVB levels. Adding a supplement to the diet (see Chapter 5 on diet) is a good idea for all tropical tortoises, including the Indian Star tortoise, as they have a high demand for calcium and vitamin D3 for the reasons given above, particularly when they are growing to full size.

Feeding too much fruit, or vegetables high in protein, is to be avoided, as stated above for the species in this chapter. Fruit is very acidic and can cause digestive problems; in the wild, access to berries and fruits is very limited and usually seasonal.

What types of accommodation do they need in captivity?

Indian Star tortoises need a large, insulated shed or outbuilding to provide heat and light during the winter months, if they live in a temperate or cold climate. They need a good deal of space to walk around. This allows them to make the choices needed to ensure that they achieve their preferred body temperature of around 30°C. Their outdoor

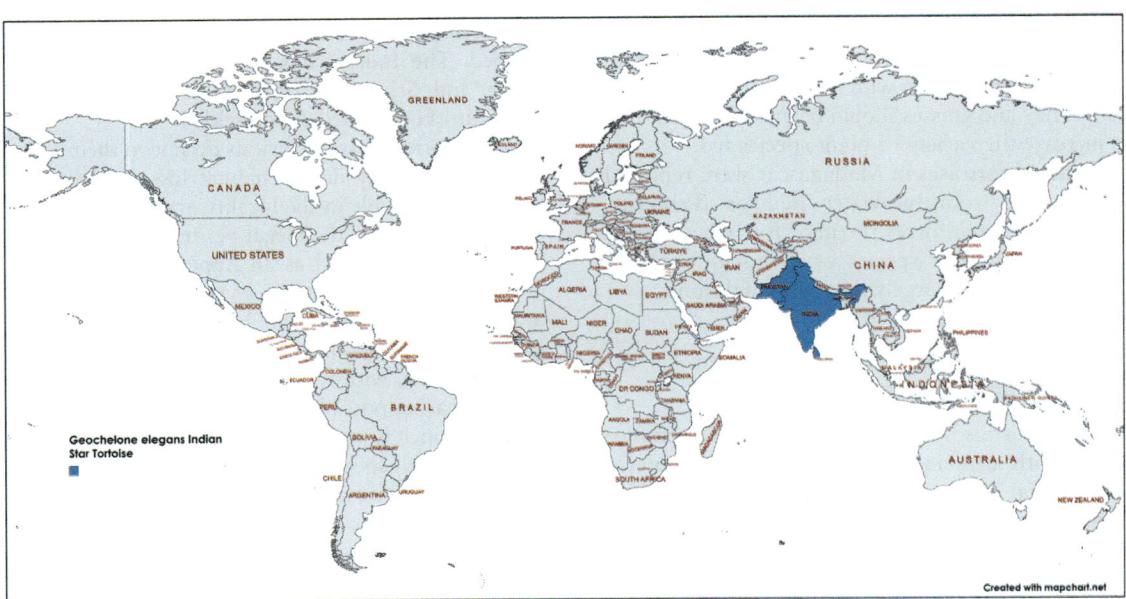

Fig. 14.19. Map of Indian Star tortoise locations. (https://www.mapchart.net/world.html)

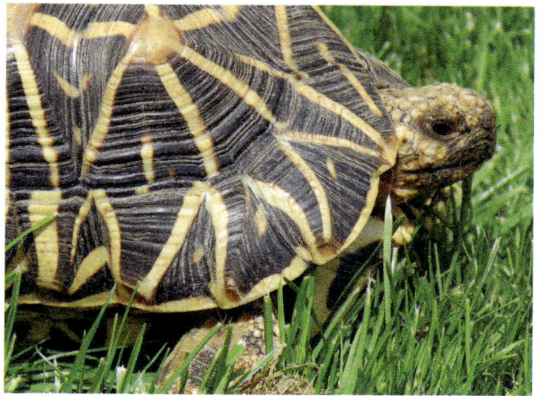

Fig. 14.20. Indian Star *Geochelone elegans*.

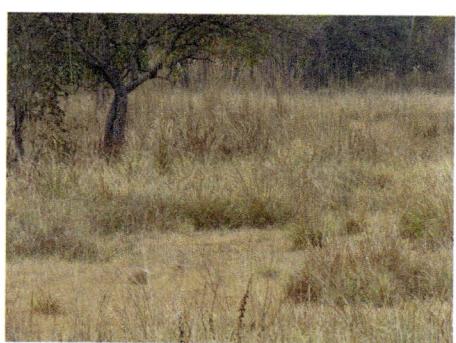

Fig. 14.21. The dry scrub and grasslands of the natural habitat in central India.

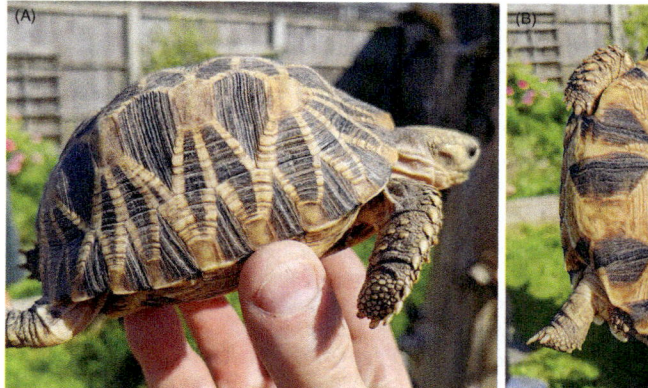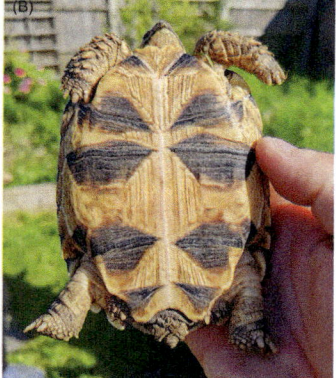

Fig. 14.22. Burmese Star (*Geochelone platynota*) captive-bred in the UK (Dillon Prest and Andy Lewis).

enclosure should also be as large as possible to allow plenty of exercise through walking without becoming stressed in too small a space, which could lead to repetitive behaviours.

Burmese Star tortoises – *Geochelone platynota*

These critically endangered tortoises are not seen commonly in captivity (Fig. 14.22). They are critically endangered in the wild in their home range in Myanmar, where they live in dry forests and scrub areas. They tend to be active in early mornings and late afternoons to avoid the hottest part of the day. They are herbivorous foragers. Virtually extinct in the wild in the 1990s, Turtle Survival Alliance reports that over 20,000 have been bred and 5000 individuals reintroduced into the home range in Myanmar.

Conclusion

These species of dry, open grasslands can be accommodated in captivity. However, the size of some species makes them very difficult to accommodate in captivity, *Centrochelys sulcata* being the largest continental tortoise (only the Galapagos and Aldabran island species are larger). Leopard tortoises are also larger than Mediterranean tortoises, or Horsfield's tortoises, by a significant amount.

They are all tropical species that do not hibernate (brumate). It is essential that, when kept in captivity, there is indoor accommodation as well as outdoor enclosures. If kept in northern Europe or America there will be significant costs in keeping them warm during the winter months. The size of the heated building needs to be considerable to provide sufficient space for walking and a good quality of life while indoors.

Some of these species are critically endangered in the wild, having been collected excessively for the pet trade for a number of years. This added form of exploitation, in addition to the pressures of habitat loss and pollution from human activities, has brought them to the brink of extinction in the wild. It is important to source these animals responsibly, therefore, and not to contribute to the loss of wild populations.

Burmese Star tortoises are rare in the wild and in captivity, and are bred by only a few committed keepers. The species was considered extinct in the wild in the 1990s but this is a success story in terms of captive breeding and the reintroduction of 5000 animals in Myanmar (Turtle Survival Alliance).

Without conservation efforts involving zoos and private keepers, the future looks very bleak. The prospect of reintroducing some of these species is a long way in the future. Conservation efforts will need to include the involvement and cooperation of local people, many of whom live in poor rural areas, where these tortoises command a high value. This has been achieved with Burmese Star tortoises to an extent and shows what can be achieved.

References and Further Reading

Bjorndal, K.A. (1989) Flexibility of digestive responses in two generalist herbivores, the tortoises *Geochelone carbonaria* and *Geochelone denticulata*. *Oecologia* 78, 317–321.

British Chelonia Group (BCG) Caresheets for: Mediterranean (Spur-thighed, Marginated, Hermann's) and non-Mediterranean (Horsfield's, African Hingeback, African Spurred, Radiated, Leopard, Indian Start, Pancake, Egyptian, Red-eared terrapin, Soft-shelled turtles, Box turtles, South American tortoises, Asian turtles and tortoises. British Chelonia Group, Walsham-le-Willows, Suffolk, UK. Website: www.britishcheloniagroup.org.uk

Burmese Star Tortoise (*Geochelone platynota*) Fact Sheet: Summary. San Diego Zoo Wildlife Alliance Library. International Environment Library Consortium.

CITES: Convention on International Trade in Endangered Species of Wild Flora and Fauna, Geneva. Website: www.cites.org

Highfield, A. (1996) *Practical Encyclopaedia of Keeping and Breeding Tortoises and Freshwater Turtles*. Carapace Press, London.

IUCN: International Union for Conservation of Nature, Gland, Switzerland. Maintains IUCN Red List of Threatened Species. Website: https://iucn.org

Kabigumila, J. (2001) Sighting frequency and food habits of the Leopard tortoise *Geochelone pardalis* in Northern Tanzania. East African Wildlife Society. *African Journal of Ecology* 39, 276–285.

Kuhne, U. (2019) Astrochelys radiata – Keeping and Breeding in South Spain. *RADIATA* 28(2).

Leuteritz, T.E.J. (2003) Observations on diet and drinking behaviour of radiated tortoises (Geochelone radiata) in Southwest Madagascar. *African Journal of Herpetology* 52(2), 127–130.

Milton, S.J. (1992) Plants eaten and dispersed by adult leopard tortoises Geochelone pardalis (Reptilia: Chelonii) in the southern Karoo. *South African Journal of Zoology* 27(2).

Petrozzi, F., Hema, E.M., Sirima, D, Douamba, B., Segniagbeto, G.H., Diagne, T., Amadi, N., Amori, G., Akani, G.C., Edem A., Eniang, E.A., Chirio, L. and Luiselli, L. (2017) Habitat determinants of the threatened Sahel tortoise *Centrochelys sulcata* at two spatial scales. *Herpetological Conservation and Biology* 12(2), 402–409.

Petrozzi, F., Hema, E.M., Sirima, D., Segniagbeto, G.H., Akani, G.C., Eniang, E.A., Dendi, D., Fa, J.E. and Luiselli, L. (2020) Tortoise ecology in the West African savannah: Multi-scale habitat selection and activity patterns of a threatened giant species, and its ecological relationships with a smaller-sized species. *Acta Oecologica* 105, 103572.

Tortoise Trust Care Sheet: Indian Star tortoise. Website: www.tortoisetrust.org Turtle Survival Alliance: Burmese Star tortoise. Turtle Survival Alliance, North Charleston, South Carolina. Website: www.turtlesurvival.org

Vetter, H. (2002) *Turtles of the World Vol. 1, Africa, Europe and Western Asia*. Chimaira, Frankfurt.

Vetter, H. (2006) *Turtles of the World Vol. 4, East and South Asia*. Chimaira, Frankfurt.

Wilson, R. and Wilson, R. (1997) *The Care and Breeding of the African Spurred Tortoise Geochelone sulcata*. Carapace Press, London.

15 Tropical Tortoises from Humid Forest Areas

Abstract
Tropical tortoises from humid forest areas require warmth and high humidity levels throughout the year. Tropical areas have a consistently warm temperature throughout the year. This means that the range of temperatures that these tortoises can tolerate is relatively small. These tropical tortoises are omnivores, eating mainly green leaves, flowers and fruits with a very small percentage (5–10%) of animal protein.

The species included in this chapter are Red-footed and Yellow-footed tortoises and Hingeback tortoises which are those more commonly kept in captivity. These tortoises live in areas with other tortoise species. As with all tropical species, none of these tortoises hibernate so must be provided with warm accommodation throughout the entire year. They also require high humidity, particularly the Yellow-footed species, which is not always easy to provide, especially in outdoor accommodation.

These tortoises are more specialist in their requirements as discussed in relation to their natural habitat, which requires significant effort to recreate in northern Europe or North America. The requirement for warmth all year round creates economic implications as the costs of energy continue to rise. These are not for a beginner tortoise keeper, although they are very attractive and can be engaging and active pets. The Red-footed tortoises are generally good eaters and will take anything as food, but, as described in this chapter, the need to provide a miniature tropical rainforest, or cloud forest, in a domestic setting is a challenge. Hingebacks are generally shy and retiring, living a more solitary life, but again are very attractive tortoises.

Red-footed tortoises (*Geochelone carbonaria*, more recently *Chelonoidis carbonaria*) and Yellow-footed tortoises (*Geochelone denticulata*, more recently *Chelonoidis denticulatus*) (Vetter, 2005)

In captivity the Red-footed tortoise is relatively common. Yellow-footed tortoises are kept but less so. This may be because Red-foots live in drier forest and shrub, or even savannah-type areas, with less of a need for very high humidity. Yellow-foots are found in tropical rainforests and have an even higher need for a humid environment (Fig. 15.2) (Highfield, 1996).

The Red-foots are found across South America and into Panama, and on Caribbean islands (although these may be from introduced animals) (Highfield, 1996) as shown in Fig. 15.1. When I lived on the main island of St Vincent & The Grenadines in the mid-1980s, I rented a home that had a resident Red-foot as a pet in the garden. Dottie was a healthy adult female, with a great appetite and a particular attraction to mangoes. There being a tree in the garden, she gorged on them seasonally when given the opportunity. Part of the rental arrangement was to care for Dottie and I was sad to leave her at the end of my tenure.

The Red-footed and Yellow-footed tortoises are considered together here, as their environmental and dietary demands are similar, apart from humidity levels mentioned above. The two species live sympatrically in similar regions, as outlined above, but within different habitats. Generally, in captivity Red-foots are more commonly seen in the UK and Europe Figures 15.3 amd 15.4 show these two species.

Males have very concave plastrons, which gives them the opportunity to remain in position when mounting the female, and the body of these tortoises is both elongate and domed. Adult male tortoises have a narrowing at the waist, which is distinctive. They also have an obviously longer tail than the females, as is the case in most tortoise species (see Chapter 11 on breeding for images).

They have large eyes to be able to see in low light intensities. This is an adaption to life on the forest floor, where the sun is largely blocked out by tall trees. Their eyes and the area around the eyes are continually moistened by tears and the soft skin of their legs is always damp to the touch or is actually wet. This is due to living in areas of high humidity,

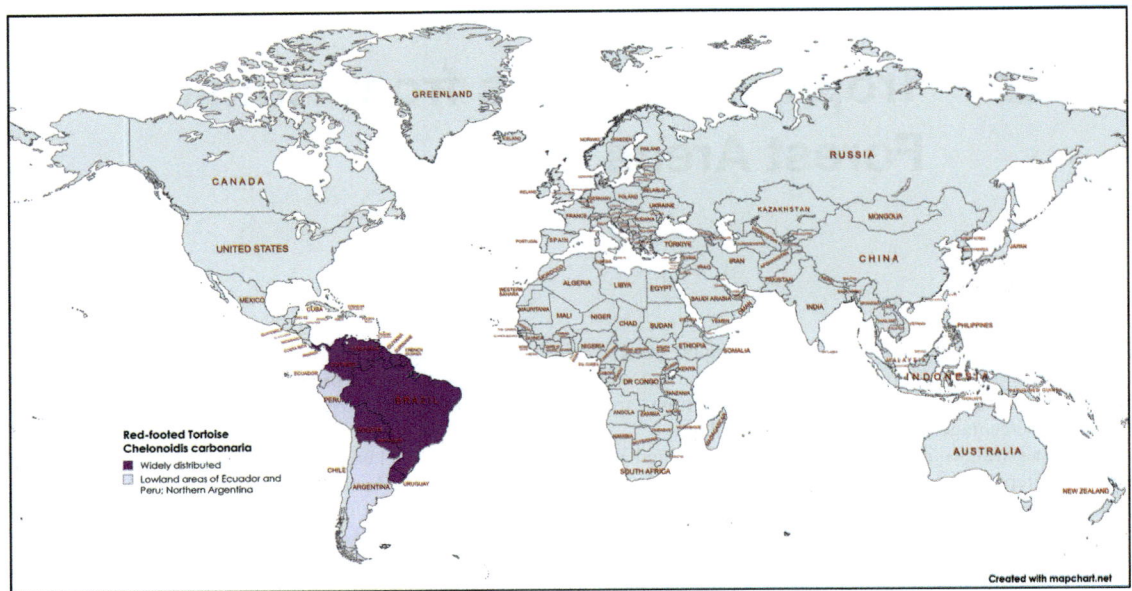

Fig. 15.1. Map of Red-footed tortoise locations. (https://www.mapchart.net/world.html)

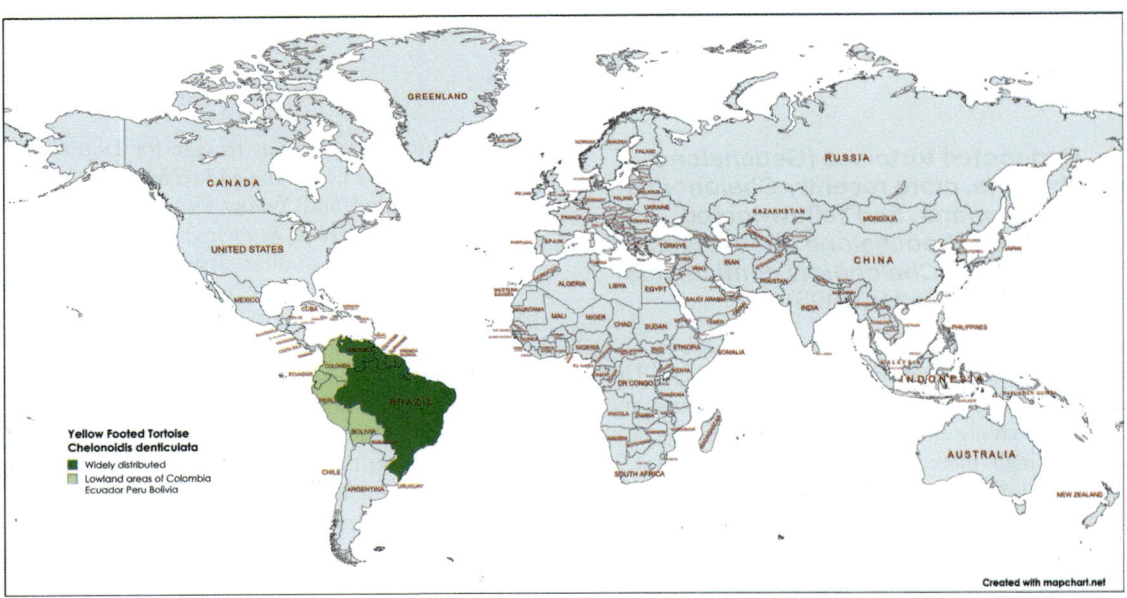

Fig. 15.2. Map of Yellow-footed tortoise locations. (https://www.mapchart.net/world.html)

which is essential if they are to stay healthy and well, particularly for the Yellow-footed species.

These tortoises must not be allowed to dry out. They need free access to water at all times. Due to the higher protein content of their diet as described below, they produce more nitrogen-containing wastes. They need water to be able to pass out these wastes in their urine as both uric acid and urea (Rendle, 2019). They are less well adapted to life in an arid environment, as they generally

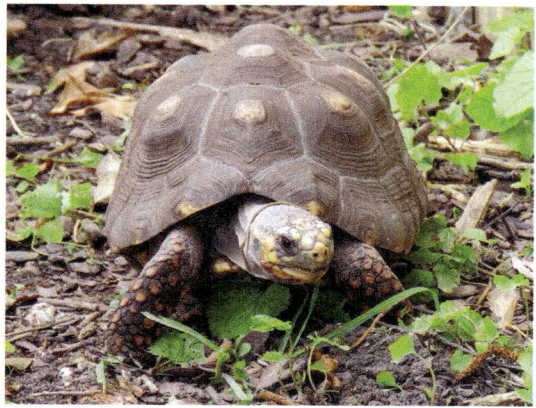

Fig. 15.3. Red-footed tortoise *Geochelone carbonaria* (more recently *Chelonoidis carbonaria*).

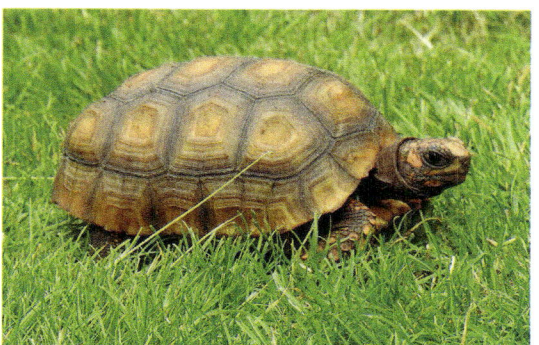

Fig. 15.4. Yellow-footed tortoise *Geochelone denticulata* (more recently *Chelonoidis denticulatus*) (James Sullivan).

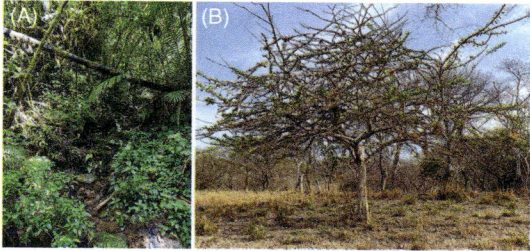

Fig. 15.5. (A) Rainforest habitat and (B) more open savannah scrub of South and Central America. The latter areas will be adjacent to more forested areas if used by Red-footed tortoises.

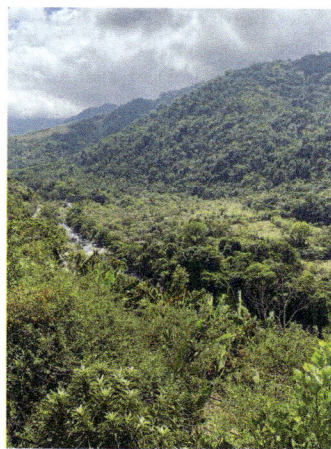

Fig. 15.6. Small open areas close to the cloud forest with good cover. The sky with heavy clouds indicates the frequent rainfall that occurs seasonally.

have access to water through rainfall and standing water in the natural environment.

Both Red-footed and Yellow-footed tortoises enjoy group living as they are more sociable than many other tortoises, which tend to be solitary in nature. These tortoises can live in small groups of 4–5 in captivity, given enough space and habitat choice within their accommodation. The balance should always be of more females than males. Red- and Yellow-footed tortoises have similar needs but the general principle of keeping species separately in captivity applies.

Where do Red-footed and Yellow-footed tortoises come from?

Red-footed and Yellow-footed tortoises come from Central and South America. They come from the northern regions of South America south to Paraguay and Brazil. They can be found in Argentina, Bolivia, Brazil, Colombia, French Guiana, Guyana, Panama, Paraguay, Trinidad, Suriname and Venezuela. They are also found in some of the Caribbean Islands, such as Trinidad (Figs 15.1 and 15.2). Although they may seem common in their countries of origin, we do not have data on the numbers remaining in the wild. Both species are listed as vulnerable by the IUCN as potentially threatened by over-exploitation (IUCN). They are protected from illegal trade by CITES listing (CITES, Appendix II).

The Red-footed tortoises live in slightly drier conditions of scrub and less dense woodland, which may be one of the reasons they are more commonly seen in captivity. Yellow-footed tortoises have a smaller range within their home countries, in more dense, humid forest (Highfield, 1996). Images of the range of natural habitats of these species are shown in Figs 15.5 and 15.6.

The main threats come from habitat loss for farming and other human developments. They are a source of food in some rural locations of South American countries such as Bolivia, often where human populations are economically deprived. Both Red-footed and Yellow-footed tortoises are exported from countries such as Colombia, Panama and Bolivia. This is largely for the pet trade, with the main importing states being the United States, Germany and Switzerland, although they are also taken into other European countries.

It is important to source these species ethically as they are still the subject of illegal trading. Captive-bred animals are available but often at a higher cost. Funding the trade in these threatened species by purchasing wild-caught animals is to be avoided at all costs.

How can you tell the difference between Red-footed and Yellow-footed tortoises?

Both tortoises are extremely attractive with beautiful markings on their head and legs. As you might expect from their names, the markings are red in Red-footed tortoises and yellow in Yellow-footed tortoises. This is the main difference between them. Their dark domed shells are similar in shape, and both have an elongated body shape. The head and limb skin patterns and coloration are very attractive. In *C. carbonaria* there is a potential subspecies often referred to as the Cherry-head which has particularly bright red-coloured patterns on the head.

Red-footed tortoises are around 30 cm in length and the average weight is around 12 kg. Yellow-footed tortoises are significantly larger, with 40 cm length being common, and individual animals having measured up to 70 cm and weighed 20 kg (Highfield, 1996).

Both species breed readily in captivity and lay several clutches of eggs each year. Red-foots lay 3–5 eggs whereas Yellow-foots may lay up to 15 eggs (Highfield, 1996). The mating and courtship rituals of the male involve rapid side-to-side head movements, biting, pushing and butting the female to encourage her to stand still. In the Red-footed tortoise vocalizations including clucking or clicking sounds are reported (Highfield, 1996) and in both species there are grunting sounds, which are also heard in other species.

What is the natural environment for Red-footed and Yellow-footed tortoises?

These tropical tortoises live in an environment that is radically different from that found in most of the countries in which they are kept in captivity. Red-foots can inhabit more open scrub, meadows and drier savannah areas, but still require high humidity levels through use of microclimates created by vegetation and are also found in rainforest and cloud forest areas. Yellow-footed tortoises are found only in the higher humidity locations of rainforest and cloud forest.

Rainforests and cloud forests provide shady but warm and humid habitats. Temperatures range between 22°C and 30°C, while humidity levels are high, at round 80–90% for much of the year. The open savannah will have slightly warmer temperatures but with opportunities for shade and higher humidity, as described above.

The substrate of the forest floor consists of loose soil, leaves, bark, detritus and humus. There is a mix of underlying soil and organic matter from dead and decaying leaves and animals. Fallen fruits and mushrooms are available as food sources, along with invertebrates as well as leafy green plants with flowers (see Chapter 5 on diet).

These tortoises are omnivorous. The forest floor provides a wide range of foodstuffs, including a variety of mushrooms, flowers, leaves, insects and tropical rainforest fruits. Because their diet is higher in protein than that of other species, tropical tortoises produce a more toxic nitrogen-containing waste. This urea requires more water to excrete, so Red-footed and Yellow-footed tortoises can often be found near water sources such as ponds, puddles and streams, in which they bathe and from which they drink. This is particularly true in drier areas of rainforests and in cloud forests, as the development into an omnivore lifestyle from being herbivores requires the availability of water for excretion of nitrogenous wastes (Rendle, 2019).

What is a suitable diet for Red-footed and Yellow-footed tortoises in captivity?

These tortoises should largely be eating weeds and growing plants along with mushrooms. They eat flowers and fruits (BCG caresheets) but these should be a small proportion of the diet (10–20%). They should also eat a very small amount of animal protein (5–10%) to ensure that they have access to

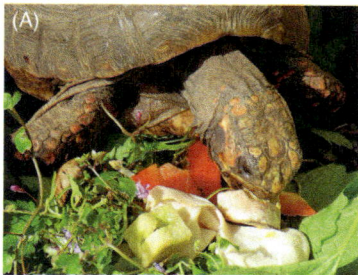 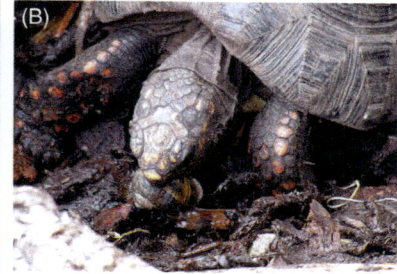

Fig. 15.7. (A) Red-foot eating a varied diet of plants, with mushrooms and fruit. Note that this female is selecting the mushroom as a desired food over the other available fruit and leafy greens. (B) Red-foot eating a snail.

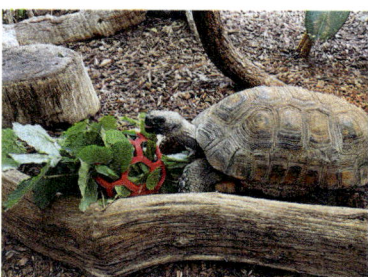

Fig. 15.8. Yellow-foot eating from an activity feeding toy, providing enrichment for this active species.

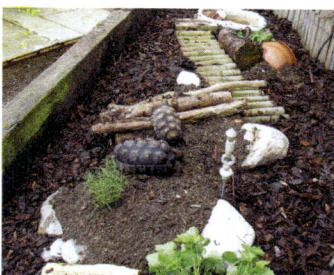

Fig. 15.9. Building an outdoor enclosure for Red-footed tortoises.

all essential amino acids in the diet (see Chapter 5 on diet), which should be given as a low-fat source. Examples are seen in Fig. 15.7.

Woodlice and other slow-moving insects and larvae can be eaten, along with snails and slugs. They will also take chicken and very small mouse pinkies. The latter have the additional benefit of containing bone and therefore calcium, as do snails with their calcium-based shells. Moskovits and Bjorndal (1990) found that these tortoises eat a huge range of plant leaves, grasses, flowers and stems along with fungi and animal protein from dried bodies of animals, snails, insects and faeces.

The availability and selection of food items chosen by these species suggests that their digestive systems are adapted to cope with a variety of food types (Bjorndal, 1989). They can digest the cell walls of plants (cellulose) using microbial fermentation in the lower bowel (Bjorndal, 1989).

It may be that presentation of food in an environmentally enriching way, to provide mental stimulation, is more important in these omnivores than we have previously realized (Lumbis and White, 2022) (see Chapter 8 on behaviour). Certainly my observations of Red-footed tortoises over the years suggest the need for an enriched environment.

It is advisable to supplement the diet with calcium two to three times each week, as for all species in captivity, to ensure that the diet contains sufficient calcium (see Chapter 5 on diets).

Red-footed tortoises will, in my experience, also particularly favour red food items, such as raspberries or strawberries.

What types of accommodation do these tortoises need in captivity?

Red-footed and Yellow-footed tortoises need access to warmth and light all year around. They do not hibernate. When the temperature outside is above 20°C these tortoises can be put into large outdoor enclosures during the day but must always be kept at similar temperatures overnight. Ideally the daytime temperatures for Red-foots would be 21–27°C to ensure that they remain within the preferred optimal temperature zone (POTZ) and for Yellow-foots 25–27°C (Varga, 2019).

When outdoor temperatures fall below 21°C these tortoises will need to be kept in large insulated outdoor buildings, e.g. insulated sheds or greenhouses, both day and night. The accommodation must be large enough to allow them plenty of space to move about. Indoors, Red-footed and Yellow-footed tortoises need free access to drinking water at all times and like to soak in deeper trays of warm water, approximately 5–8 cm deep. Once again, the best accommodation has linked outdoor and indoor spaces. This allows the tortoises to move indoors when the weather cools and to go outside to access more space when the temperature warms up.

The substrate needs to be humid and can be composed of combinations of soil, compost, coco-coir, bark and leaves. The substrate will need water adding to it regularly, to maintain humidity levels. Misting and use of a humidifier can be helpful, but a light sprinkling of water for these purposes will not be sufficient to maintain a damp substrate without pouring water onto the surface at least once per week. Recommended humidity levels for the two species are based on BSAVA data (Varga, 2019) as 50–60% for Red-footed tortoises and 70–80% for Yellow-foots.

Red-footed and Yellow-footed tortoises like to find shelters and safe places to rest. These tortoises do not bask as much as other species, as they are always warm in their natural habitat and light levels are often low. This means that they simply stay warm because the environment is always warm, without the need to bask as frequently as temperate species where there is greater variation in temperature on a daily and seasonal basis. Figure 15.9 shows an outdoor enclosure being prepared for two Red-footed tortoises.

These tortoises will thrive in captivity provided that their environmental needs are met. It is easy to get things wrong, however, and suitable temperature, diet and humidity are as vital as for any other species.

Hingeback tortoises – *Kinixys* species

There are three main species of Hingeback seen in captivity, on which the information below for captive maintenance is based:

- *Kinixys belliana* – Bell's Hingeback (Fig. 15.10)
- *Kinixys erosa* – the serrated or forest Hingeback (Fig. 15.11)
- *Kinixys homeana* – Home's Hingeback (Fig. 15.12)

Other species have been identified but are not commonly kept in captivity. There are also subspecies of *K. belliana* identified: *K. b. belliana* (as above), *K. b. nogueyi* (in western sub-Saharan Africa) and *K. b. zombensis* (in Tanzania and South Africa). Other *Kinixys* species (Vetter, 2002) include:

- *Kinixys lobatsiana* (Botswana and South Africa)
- *Kinixys natalensis* (Mozambique, South Africa, Estwatini)
- *Kinixys spkekii* (Botswana, South Africa, Estwatini, Zambia, Democratic Republic of the Congo, Angola).

There is clearly a great deal of further work to be done on the taxonomy and classification of this species.

Where do Hingeback tortoises come from?

Kinixys belliana lives in drier scrub, grassland and savannah areas (Fig. 15.13). *Kinixys erosa* and *Kinixys homeana* are forest tortoises living in the tropical regions of Africa as shown in the maps in Figs 15.14 and 15.15. Generally, in captivity, reasonably high humidity levels are advised, particularly for *Kinixys erosa* and *Kinixys homeana*.

The maps of their general distribution in Figs 15.13–15.15 show that there is much overlap with the different species living sympatrically within similar environments. The different species do occupy different niches and a variety of environmental conditions. The IUCN listings suggest that distribution is no longer as wide as suggested here by Vetter (2002), due to over-exploitation of these species. While they are dealt with collectively here it is important, as always, to know which species you have, to ensure that you tailor the captive environment to meet their needs as closely as possible (Highfield, 1996). Figure 15.16 shows forested areas in Zambia as an example of the natural habitat.

Trade in these tortoises is restricted by CITES as they are listed on Appendix II but some of the African home states carry out ranch breeding of the species. Some trade in these ranch-bred animals is permitted. The IUCN listing for *K. homeana* is 'critically endangered'. The data for *K. erosa* and *K. belliana* are insufficient to give a listing, providing an altogether very worrying situation. Luiselli and Diagne (2014) reported the high pressure being put on populations of *K. erosa*. They reported subsistence hunting by local people, who are desperately poor, as a major problem causing the decline of *K. erosa* along with deforestation due to land use for industry and agriculture.

It is again important to source these species ethically, as they are still the subject of illegal trading. Funding the trade in these threatened species by purchasing wild-caught animals is to be avoided at all costs.

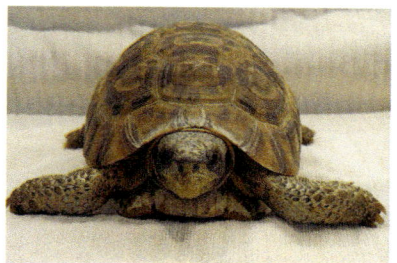
Fig. 15.10. *Kinixys belliana.*

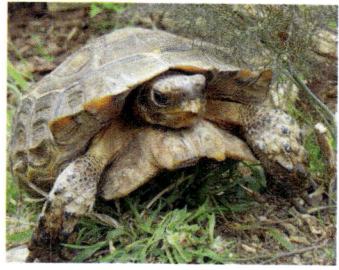
Fig. 15.11. *Kinixys erosa.*

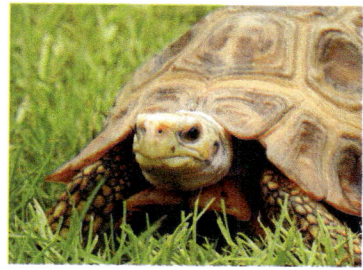
Fig. 15.12. *Kinixys homeana* (James Sullivan).

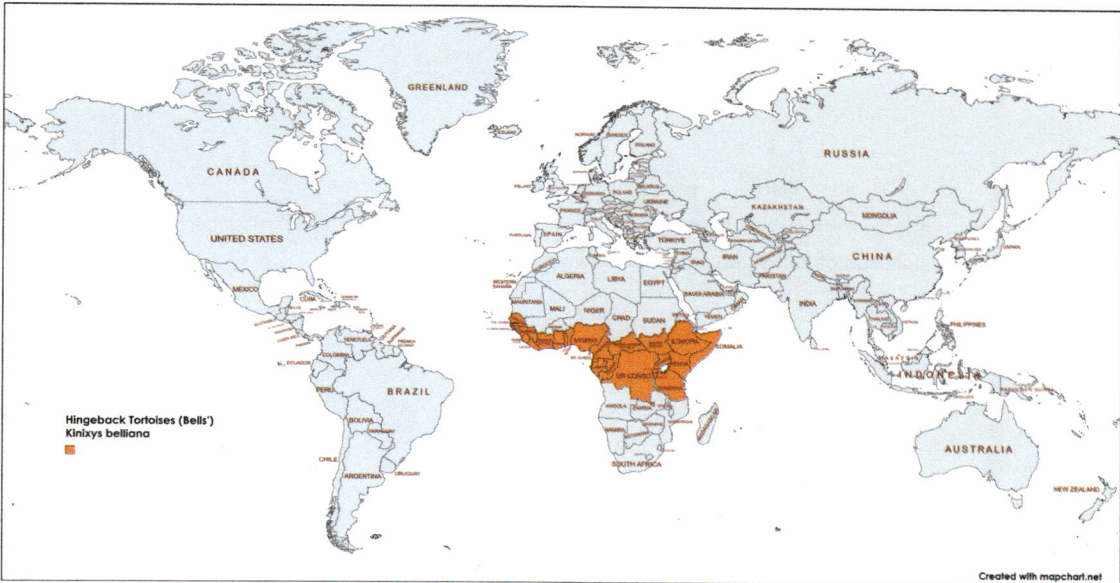
Fig. 15.13. Map of distribution for *Kinixys belliana.* (https://www.mapchart.net/world.html)

What makes the Hingeback tortoise distinctive?

These tortoises have one defining feature – which is where their name comes from. Both males and females have a hinge horizontally across the carapace. This becomes more mobile at egg-laying, allowing some movement of the shell for females to pass their eggs. Hingebacks are the only species where this is seen (Highfield, 1996). Other tortoises have a similar hinge, but in the plastron, between the femoral and abdominal plates. Because of this, Hingeback tortoises are a distinctive shape with a steep slope at the rear of the carapace after the hinge (Fig. 15.17).

Hingeback tortoises are elongate in shape. Because they are adapted to living in forest areas, as with Red-footed and Yellow-footed tortoises, they too have large eyes to enable better vision at low light intensities. Their eyes are therefore potentially more vulnerable to damage. Eye problems can easily result if humidity levels are too low, or if the temperature is not well maintained.

The *Kinixys* species all have the distinctive elongate body shape and shape of shell that results from the hinged carapace. Shell patterns are attractive and patterned to different degrees, as shown in Figs 15.10–15.12. *K. erosa* and *K. homeana* are darker species, while *K. belliana* is lighter with more distinctive patterns. The carapace is flat in *Kinixys*, as in Fig. 15.17. Figure 15.18 shows the differences between male and female *K. belliana*.

Hingebacks are around 15–25 cm in length, depending upon species, with *K. belliana* being larger than *K. erosa* and *K. homeana.*

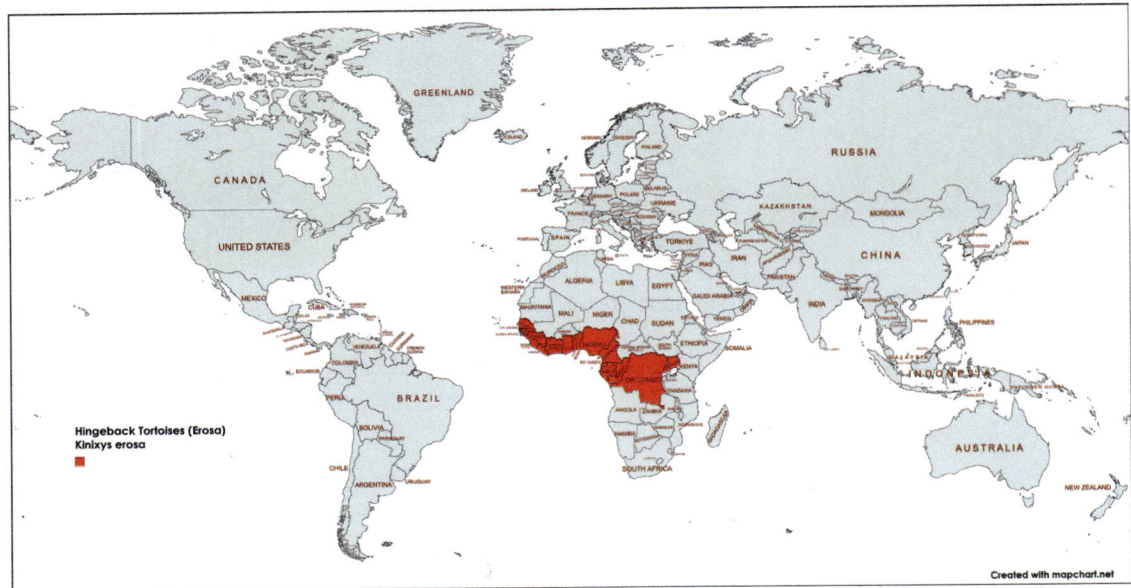

Fig. 15.14. Map of distribution of *Kinixys erosa*. (https://www.mapchart.net/world.html)

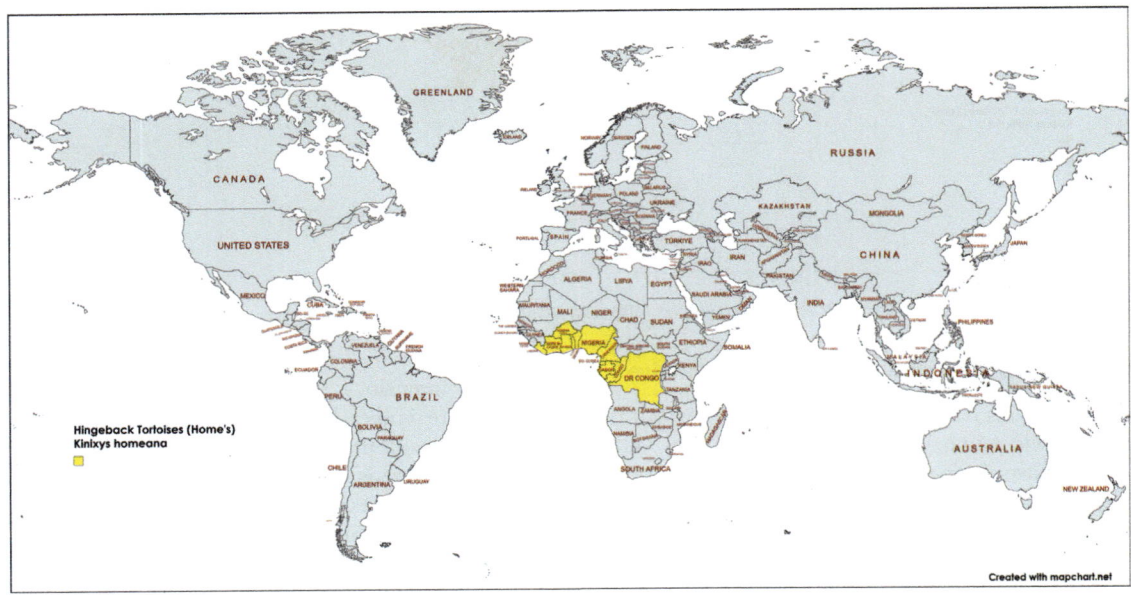

Fig. 15.15. Map of distribution of *Kinixys homeana*. (https://www.mapchart.net/world.html)

What is a suitable diet for Hingeback tortoises kept in captivity?

As Hingeback tortoises are omnivorous, they also need freely available water at all times, as described above for Red-footed and Yellow-footed tortoises. This is so that they can excrete, effectively, their more toxic nitrogen-containing waste, produced as a result of the higher protein content.

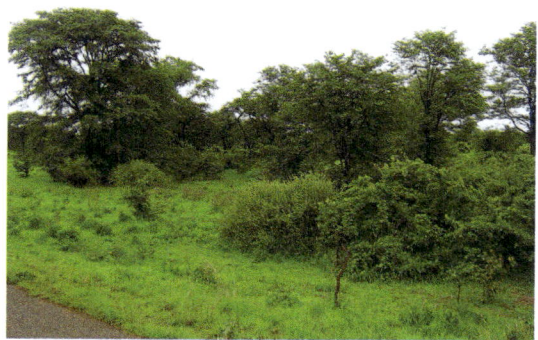

Fig. 15.16. Forest habitat.

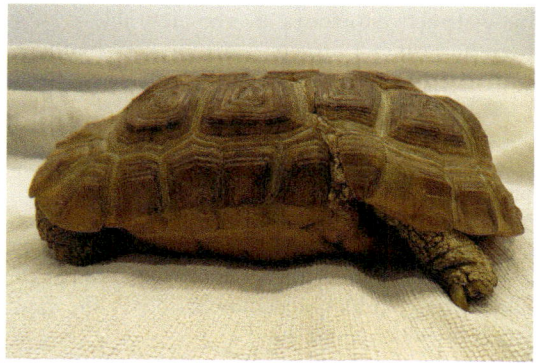

Fig. 15.17. Bell's Hingeback with very clearly shown hinge, with almost vertical rear carapace.

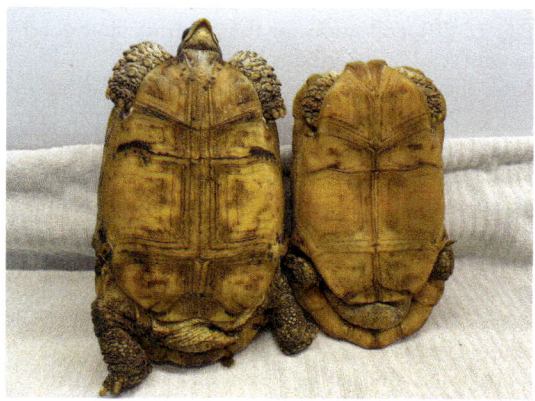

Fig. 15.18. *Kinixys belliana* female (left) and male (right) compared.

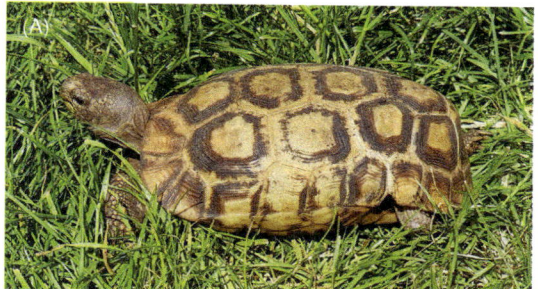

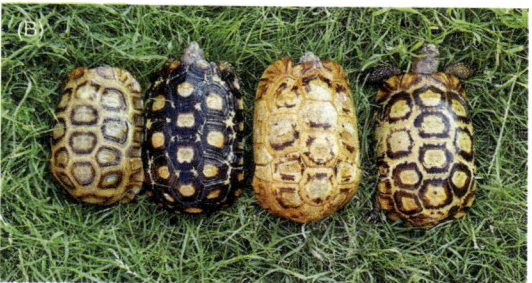

Fig. 15.19. Range of shell patterns in *Kinixys spekii* (James Sullivan).

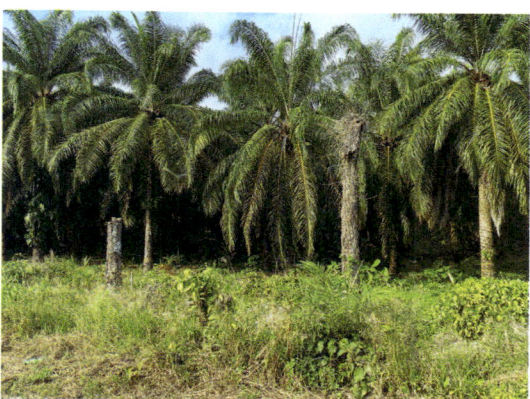

Fig. 15.20. Palm oil plantation in Central America.

It is likely that these species developed from herbivorous ancestors as a result of the need for sufficient calcium in the diet, obtained by eating animal bones and carcasses, and to compensate for limited vegetation in the dry season (Rendle, 2019).

These tortoises should largely be eating weeds and grown flowering plants from our gardens, along with mushrooms. Plenty of leafy green material is needed as the main constituent of the diet.

They also eat flowers and fruits (BCG Caresheets) but these should be a small proportion of the diet

(10–20%). They should also eat a very small amount of animal protein (5–10%) to ensure that they have access to all essential amino acids in the diet (see Chapter 5 on diet), which should be given as a low-fat source.

Woodlice and other slow-moving insects and larvae can be eaten along with snails and slugs. As described above, animal protein in the form of chicken or small pinkies can also be given (Rendle, 2019).

Again, these species may benefit from presentation of food in an environmentally enriching way, to provide mental stimulation, as mentioned above (Lumbis and White, 2022).

What types of accommodation do Hingeback tortoises need in captivity?

Kinixys species should be maintained separately, as stated above. *K. erosa* and *K. homeana* need more shade and even more opportunities to hide and retreat than *K. belliana*, although this is a requirement of all *Kinixys* species. *Kinixys spekii* is rare in captivity and has beautiful shell patterns, as shown in Fig. 15.19.

Hingeback tortoises are very shy tortoises, from my observations and those of others (Highfield, 1996). They like to find refuge and shelter, so suitable retreats and use of vegetation to provide cover are essential in their enclosures. They tend to be most active at dawn and dusk and spend large parts of the day hiding.

Hingebacks need access to warmth and light all year round. They do not hibernate. While smaller than the Red-footed and Yellow-footed tortoises, their accommodation needs to be sufficiently large for them to move around freely and walk during active periods in the mornings and evenings. This is when they are most likely to feed.

Use of misters, sprays and humidifiers may be helpful to increase humidity. Their need for high humidity levels can make them challenging species requiring a great deal of commitment. Free access to water for soaking is essential as this is an activity many of them undertake (Highfield, 1996) on a daily basis.

Ideally the daytime temperatures for *Kinixys* would be 24–28°C to ensure that they remain within the POTZ and humidity levels of 50–80% (Varga, 2019).

Male and female tortoises are distinguished from each other by a larger size in the female and a longer tail in the male, as shown in Fig. 15.18. Courtship and mating rituals involve the male attracting and engaging the female to encourage her to stand still through head movements, circling and shell ramming. Male *Kinixys* may be aggressive towards each other, which may prohibit them living together. Maintenance in breeding pairs, or singly with opportunities for mating, may be the most effective ways of maintaining these species in captivity. Clutches of four to eight eggs are usual and three to four clutches may be laid during the summer (Highfield, 1996).

These tortoises are not recommended for those new to keeping tortoises. They are specialist species with particular needs, which are often outside the capacity of more generalist keepers.

Conclusion

These attractive tortoises are very desirable as pets by enthusiasts but are not generally kept by those with a superficial knowledge of tortoise needs. Being tropical species means that they are awake and active all year round, which makes them more appealing to hobbyists and those with a passion for tortoises. The additional environmental requirements of year-round warm indoor accommodation and high levels of humidity make them more challenging for keepers. Once again provision of linked indoor and outdoor accommodation is the best option in colder climates.

If you decide to keep these species, acquisition of captive-bred individuals is essential to avoid contributing to the loss of wild populations (Luiselli and Diagne, 2014). The species are under a great deal of pressure from human activities, including farming practices such as palm oil production (Fig. 15.20), collection for the pet trade and development leading to habitat loss.

As the image of the palm oil plantation in Fig. 15.20 shows, these monocultures where only a single species of plant can grow are deserts in terms of biodiversity, with very little opportunity for any other species. When this type of planting is combined with use of pesticides and fertilizers, the outcomes for native wildlife are very poor, as we see the world over. This means that tortoise species face a bleak future without change to these farming practices.

Providing alternative forms of income for local people, so that they are not pressured into collecting animals for the pet trade, is another essential approach to preserving these vital ecosystems.

References and Further Reading

Bjorndal, K.A. (1989) Flexibility of digestive responses in two generalist herbivores, the tortoises *Geochelone carbonaria* and *Geochelone denticulata*. *Oecologia* 78, 317–321.

British Chelonia Group (BCG) Caresheets. The BCG 'for tortoise, terrapin and turtle care and conservation' (based in Walsham-le-Willows, Suffolk) publishes individual Caresheets on many Mediterranean and non-Mediterranean species, including: Spur-thighed, Marginated, Hermann's, Horsfield's, African Hingeback, African Spurred, Red-eared terrapin, Leopard, Indian Star, Pancake, Egyptian, Radiated, South American species, Soft-shelled species, USA Box turtles and Asian tortoises. Available at www.britishchelonia-group.org.uk/caresheets

CITES: Convention on International Trade in Endangered Species of Wild Flora and Fauna, Geneva. Website: www.cites.org

Highfield, A. (1996) *Practical Encyclopaedia of Keeping and Breeding Tortoises and Freshwater Turtles*. Carapace Press, London.

IUCN: International Union for Conservation of Nature, Gland, Switzerland. Maintains IUCN Red List of Threatened Species. Website: https://iucn.org

Luiselli, L. and Diagne, T. (2014) *Kinixys erosa (Schweigger 1812) – Forest Hinge-back Tortoise, Serrated Hinge-back Tortoise, Serrated Hinged Tortoise*. Chelonian Research Foundation Monograph No. 5 (part of Conservation Biology of Freshwater Turtles and Tortoises: A Compilation Project of the IUCN/SSC Tortoise and Freshwater Turtle Specialist Group.)

Lumbis, R. and White, C. (2022) Ch 5 Nutritional welfare. In: Rendle, M. and Hinde-Megarity, J. (eds) *BSAVA Manual of Practical Veterinary Welfare*. BSAVA, Quedgeley, UK, pp. 124–146.

Moskovits, D.K. and Bjorndal, K.A. (1990) Diet and food preferences of the tortoises *Geochelone carbonaria* and *G. denticulata* in northwestern Brazil. *Herpetologica* 46(2), 207–218.

Rendle, M. (2019) Ch 4 Nutrition. In: Girling, S.J. and Raiti, P. (eds) *BSAVA Manual of Reptiles*, 3rd edn. BSAVA, Quedgeley, UK, pp. 49–70.

Varga, M. (2019) Ch 3 Captive maintenance. In: Girling, S.J. and Raiti, P. (eds) *BSAVA Manual of Reptiles*, 3rd edn. BSAVA, Quedgeley, UK, pp. 36–48.

Vetter, H. (2002) *Turtles of the World Vol. 1, Africa, Europe and Western Asia*. Chimaira, Frankfurt

Vetter, H. (2005) *Turtles of the World Vol. 3, Central & South America*. Chimaira, Frankfurt.

16 Horsfield's (Afghan or Steppe) Tortoises

Abstract
This chapter looks at the features of the Horsfield's tortoise and its environmental needs. This is a small species that has become very popular in recent years as a pet tortoise, in part due to its size. This means that smaller enclosures can be used, which more people have space to provide. In addition, this species has not been listed at the highest level of protection by CITES (Appendix II), which has allowed more free trade. As a result, there has been much commercial farming of this species and export from native countries to Europe and the UK.

This small tortoise is lively and active under suitable conditions and is therefore appealing as a pet. Its needs, based on the environmental conditions in the home range, are only recently being understood. It lives at the extreme edge of parts of the globe that can sustain tortoises, which is why it is small. The chapter discusses the necessary provision in captivity to reflect the natural habitat, and the issues that can arise if these are not provided (health issues are covered more fully in Chapter 7 on common illnesses and diseases). This tortoise species is being badly maintained by many uninformed owners, some of whom have received very poor husbandry advice. As Horsfield's are being commercially bred on a large scale, inexperienced owners are taking on juvenile tortoises. In many cases, the animals are being badly maintained on a poor diet, which is leading to significant health issues (due to abnormal growth) and many welfare concerns.

The Horsfield's tortoise is a major concern from a welfare perspective for the many individual animals involved, but also more widely in terms of natural populations, which are being over-exploited. These issues are discussed at the conclusion of this chapter.

What are Horsfield's tortoises? – *Testudo horsfieldi* (more recently *Agrionemys horsfieldi*) (Vetter, 2002)

Horsfield's tortoises have become very popular pets. The images in Fig. 16.1 of an adult female and male indicate the size and gender difference. Adult Horsfield's tortoises are smaller than Mediterranean tortoises, as shown in Fig. 16.2.

Their small size adds to their appeal and many people think that they are more likely to fit easily into the average home. Despite their small size, Horsfield's tortoises still need plenty of space and an enriched environment. They can make very engaging pets if kept in the right conditions. They do hibernate/brumate and the same principles apply as for Mediterranean tortoises in terms of suitable hibernation provision and duration.

Adult female tortoises are around 180 mm in length and weigh 1200 g. Adult males are smaller at a length of 145 mm and weighing 650 g. The Horsfield's is round in shape with a less domed carapace than the Mediterranean species. They have a group of enlarged scales on the inner thighs in addition to the tail spur.

The shell is pale yellow in colour with darker markings. As with other species, the shell colour becomes very pale when these tortoises are overfed. This is due to insufficient time for the dark pigmentation in the shell to be taken up by the rapidly growing scutes. This creates a very pale coloration typical of overfed individuals suffering from shell pyramiding, soft shells or shell collapse (Fig. 16.3).

There is only one species of Horsfield's tortoise, *Agrionemys horsfieldi* (Vetter, 2002), from the northern Asian countries, as shown in Fig. 16.4, although two other very similar species are identified within the home range: *Agrionemys baluchiorum* identified in Iran and south-west Pakistan; and *Agrionemys kazchstanica* from southern central Asia (Vetter, 2002). Note that the range only includes the southernmost areas of Russia adjacent to the Central Asian countries.

Recently there has been much commercial farming of this species and export from native countries to Europe and the UK. One of the main factors allowing trade in this species from the countries of origin has been the breakup of the Union of Soviet Socialist Republics (USSR). This ceased to be a sovereign state at the end of 1991, and the strict

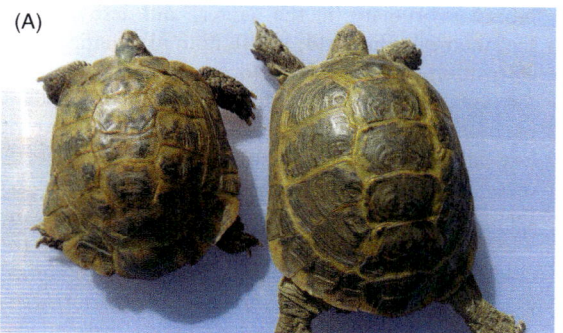 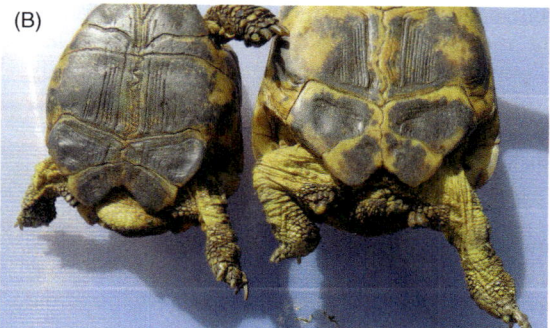

Fig. 16.1. (A) Male and female Horsfield's adults for size comparison and (B) undersides for tail comparison, showing the horny tip (similar to Hermann's tortoises) and thigh spurs (similar to Spur-thighed tortoises).

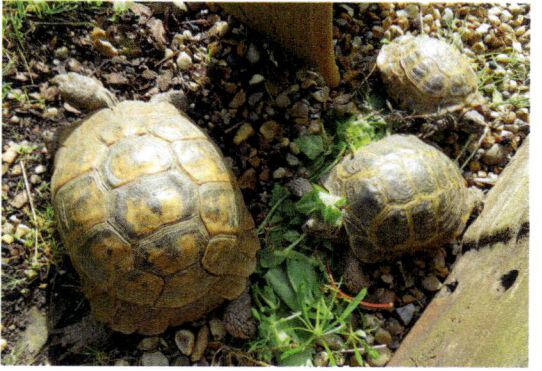 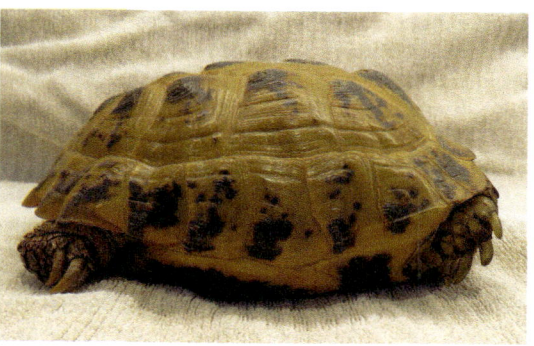

Fig. 16.2. Comparison of Mediterranean tortoise (female Spur-thighed *T. graeca ibera*, left) and Horsfield's female (centre) and male (right), showing size differences. Note these tortoises live separately as they are of different species, and are only together for the photo.

Fig. 16.3. Pale juvenile that has been fed a poor diet with insufficient calcium and/or overfed.

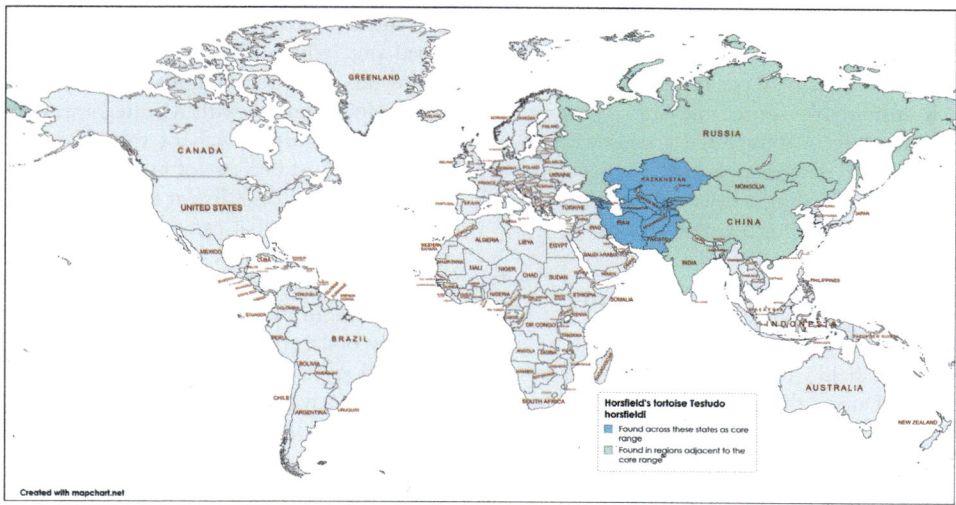

Fig. 16.4. Map of locations of Horsfield's tortoise. (https://www.mapchart.net/world.html)

controls exerted on human populations through the regime in the USSR were removed. This has allowed trade to take place that was previously prohibited in the 15 countries within the USSR, such as Kazakhstan, Uzbekistan, Azerbaijan, Turkmenistan and Georgia.

The negative consequence of this trade for *T. horsfieldi* has been huge. Data from the CITES database and Defra, the Government department in the UK responsible for animal movements, showed that around 17,000 *T. horsfieldi* were imported into the UK between 2020 and 2022. These wild-caught animals came from their home range, mainly from Uzbekistan, with smaller numbers from adjacent countries. This is just one northern European country in only 2 years. Undoubtedly this situation is being repeated across many countries where tortoise keeping takes place. Unsurprisingly, therefore, the IUCN lists this species as vulnerable due to the considerable over-collection and exploitation currently taking place in the 2020s (IUCN).

Currently the trade in Horsfield's tortoises is not as restricted as that for the Mediterranean species, but pressures on their natural populations have increased significantly in the past 30 years for the reasons given above. In the UK, certification through Article 10 certificates does not apply to this species. There are similar restrictions in Europe, but this species is listed under Appendix II on CITES and Annex B in Europe, which does not give such high levels of protection as the Mediterranean species have received.

It is always going to be more sustainable to buy a captive-bred tortoise than a wild-caught animal. It is important, as well as ethical, therefore, to research the provenance of any tortoise carefully prior to purchase. Only then can you be sure that you have the best chance of your new pet being both healthy and from a sustainable source. Buying a juvenile tortoise that has been captive-bred comes with its own difficulties, as described below. Very careful attention to diet and feeding is essential to ensure the best health and welfare of growing tortoises.

What is the natural environment of Horsfield's Tortoises?

In the wild, Horsfield's tortoises tolerate extremes of temperature. During the winter, temperatures fall below 10°C consistently, while freezing overnight temperatures are not uncommon. In the summer, temperatures can reach over 40°C. In the same year wild Horsfield's tortoises are likely to both hibernate/brumate (in the winter) and aestivate (in the summer) (Highfield, 1996). Both hibernation and aestivation are periods of dormancy. These allow tortoises to survive when there is not enough available food, or when the temperature becomes either too low (hibernation) or too high (aestivation) for normal metabolic processes to take place. Utilization of these mechanisms extends the range of habitats in which these tortoises can survive, allowing them to colonize areas that would otherwise be uninhabitable. In this species, the habitat extends into northern regions of central Asia only by utilizing these adaptations. In the UK, temperatures are never likely to reach those that require aestivation, at 38°C and above. However, this could be seen in mainland Europe or North America, where these tortoises have become popular tortoise pets in recent years.

Horsfield's tortoises live on the open steppes and surrounding grassland and scrub areas of Central Asia. The landscape is rocky, hilly and mountainous. These areas are home to a wide variety of grass types and wildflowers (Fig. 16.5).

Horsfield's tortoises are great climbers and diggers. Being small, they are relatively agile compared with other species common in captivity. They walk great distances to find sufficient food. This species can also dig very long tunnels and burrows in order to survive the very hot and very cold extremes of temperature of the natural environment. Without being able to do so, the species could not survive in much of its natural range. Being below ground reduces the extremes of temperature to which the tortoises would otherwise be exposed.

Many natural predators (which at one time would have included leopards, lynx and wolves) have been wiped out, which allowed this species to flourish before the more recent impacts of human activity and exploitation. As with Mediterranean and other species of tortoise, much of the habitat has been degraded or lost because of human activities.

Horsfield's tortoises live at the extreme edge of the parts of the globe that can sustain tortoises. There is a minimum requirement for these ectotherms in relation to sunshine and suitable temperatures throughout the year. In the wild they may be active for only 3 months of the year (Lagarde *et al.*, 2003), an aspect of their biology only recently discovered. When keeping this species in captivity this is an important consideration in terms of activity and the ways in which we hibernate/brumate this species. These aspects of Horsfield's biology have not yet been incorporated into guidance on keeping this species.

What is a suitable diet for Horsfield's Tortoises?

The diet for Horsfield's tortoises should be similar to that of Mediterranean tortoises, with very high fibre and calcium levels provided. The suggested Ca:P ratio for this species is 3.5:1 (Rendle, 2019). Fruit or any high-protein foods such as peas, beans, sweetcorn and animal products should all be a complete no-no for this species. Similarly, tomatoes are too acidic, and cucumber, which has little nutritional value, should not be fed. Lettuce such as Romaine and lamb's lettuce are a last resort, as described in Chapter 5 (diets).

To thrive and stay well Horsfield's tortoises need green leaves, together with the tough stems and the flowers of a wide variety of plants. These will include a selection of weeds and some cultivated garden plants (as described in Chapter 13 on Mediterranean tortoises) (Lagarde et al., 2003; Wegehaupt, 2009, 2021; King, 2020). Without the high fibre this diet provides, the tortoises can quickly show symptoms of diarrhoea as their gut microbes are put out of balance.

My Horsfield's tortoises seem to be particularly fond of plantain, deadnettle, sowthistle and bristly oxtongue, all of which are high in fibre (Fig. 16.6) (see Chapter 5 on diet).

Research into the time spent foraging and feeding in this species, where food is often scarce in an arid dry environment, showed that they spent only 15 minutes a day foraging (Lagarde et al., 2003), which indicates that the Horsfield's can gain the energy and nutrients needed with very little effort. This means that they can remain inactive for much of the time, an essential adaptation to extremes of temperature as discussed above. The research showed that Horsfield's tortoises do not feed on grass to any extent, but feed on plant species that are toxic to mammals, such as poppies (*Papaver* spp.) and buttercups (*Ranunculus* spp.). This allows them to feed in areas that are also grazed by mammals, as they are not choosing the same plants as food items (Lagarde et al., 2003).

What is a typical day for a Horsfield's tortoise in captivity?

As these tortoises are small, they can warm up quickly by basking in the sunshine. This results in them becoming very active, moving quickly to find food, and exploring their environment. Being small, however, means that as well as warming up quickly, they cool down fast. These smaller tortoises, where the cycles of warming and cooling are faster and the cycles take place more frequently, are more susceptible to negative effects of exposure to temperatures outside the preferred range of 20–30°C during the daytime.

It is important, therefore, that they are provided with the support necessary for maintenance of their preferred body temperature zone (POTZ) as needed throughout the day. They can tolerate low overnight temperatures, but in the wild this would signal them to start to hibernate/brumate. Control is needed in captivity to ensure that any hibernation is well planned and prepared for (see Chapter 12 on hibernation). Hibernation should be carried out as described for Mediterranean tortoises, for up to 8 weeks. In the wild, repeated hibernations could take place during the cold months of the year, but this is not advised in captivity.

Horsfield's tortoises will burrow into their substrate as part of their thermoregulation processes and will make use of microclimates within their environment. They need opportunities to walk and bask to gain radiation from the sun both for warmth and for the generation of vitamin D3, needed for calcium uptake. They also use hides and retreats to cool down and to provide refuge and a sense of security (Highfield, 1992; 2003). Scrapes are made often under bushes for night-time. It is important for all these reasons that the substrate is loose and dry enough to burrow and tunnel without the tortoise having to expend too much energy. Figure 16.7 shows an example of an outdoor enclosure.

What types of accommodation do Horsfield's tortoises need in captivity?

In captivity this species has similar needs to those of Mediterranean tortoises (Highfield and Highfield, 2008; 2009). The main requirement of Horsfield's tortoises is a sandy, dry substrate together with low humidity levels. Unfortunately, they can easily succumb to respiratory infections if forced to live in cold damp environments. As much time as possible should be spent outdoors where they have access to natural sunlight and good ventilation. When kept in cooler climates, they, like Mediterranean tortoises, need access to an indoor space. Although they can tolerate colder weather, they do not do well in cold and wet conditions.

Horsfield's tortoises are extremely good climbers and have a justified reputation for being the Houdinis of the tortoise world, as they are great escape artists (Fig. 16.8). Because of this their enclosures must be

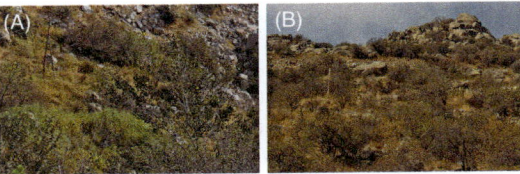

Fig. 16.5. Central Asian natural habitat of rocky hillsides with more open grass areas.

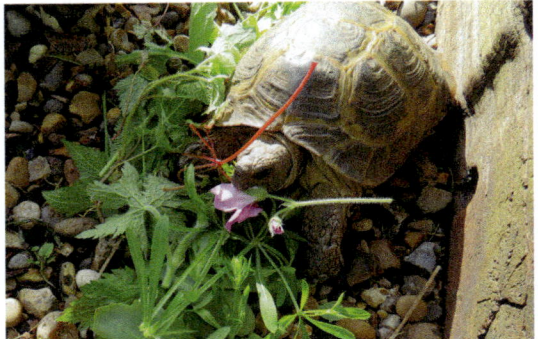

Fig. 16.6. Female Horsfield's tucking into a hardy geranium (cranesbill) flower within a meal of sowthistle, plantain, Herb Robert, goosegrass, sedum, deadnettle and bristly oxtongue.

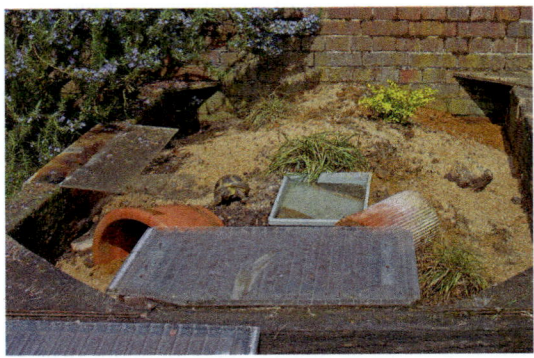

Fig. 16.7. Horsfield's in outdoor accommodation showing: sandy loose substrate; places to bask under polycarbonate and Perspex®; planting for cover and creation of microclimates; a sunken bath for free access to water; slopes and obstacles for climbing; very solid enclosure walls; and covers over the corners of the walls.

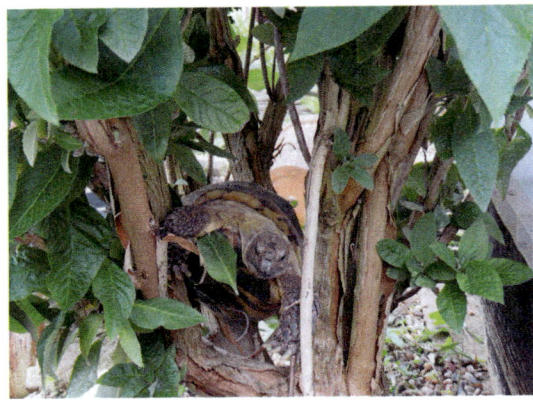

Fig. 16.8. Horsfield's climbing up a buddleia tree in an escape bid.

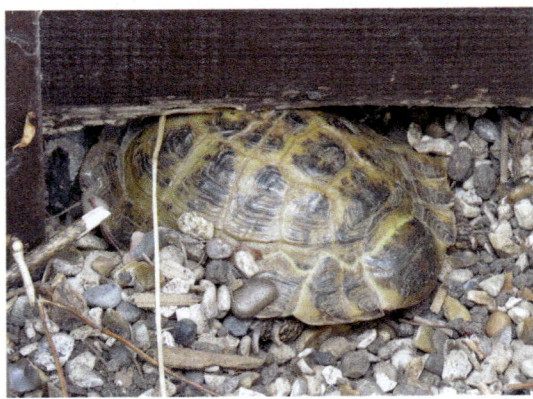

Fig. 16.9. Horsfield's burrowing in an enclosure.

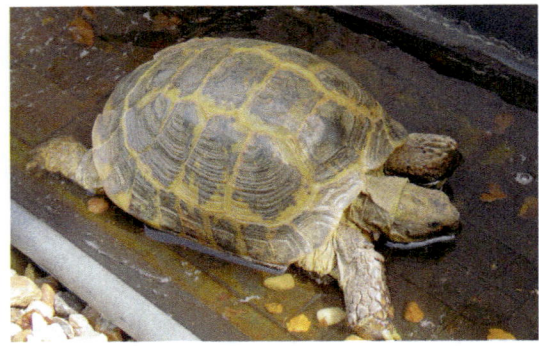

Fig. 16.10. Horsfield's in a bath.

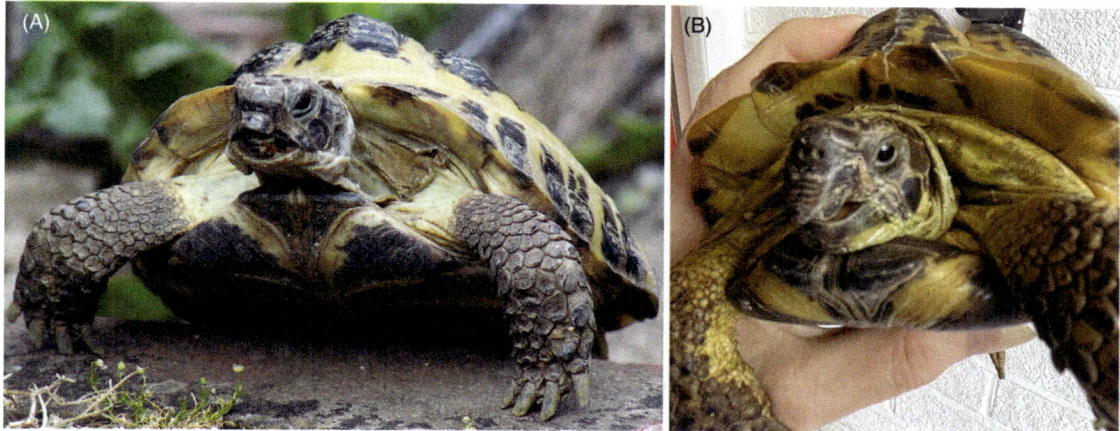

Fig. 16.11. (A) Overgrown beak and collapsed shell. (B) Severe beak overgrowth.

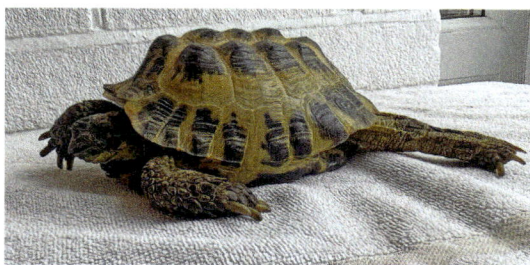

Fig. 16.12. Severe pyramiding.

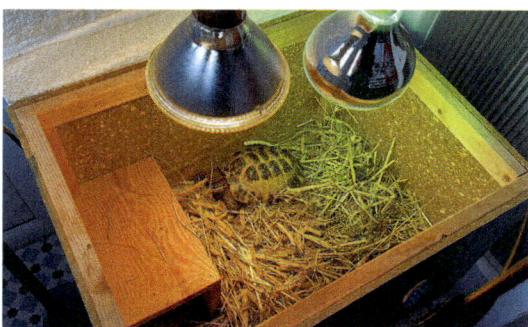

Fig. 16.13. Totally inadequate indoor enclosure. It is too small, has substrate that is a fire hazard and is not suitable for tortoises.

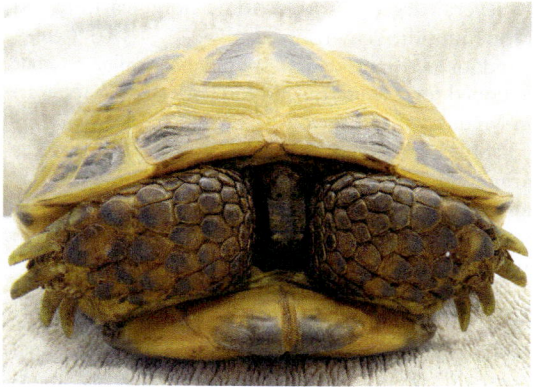

Fig. 16.14. Horsfield's tortoise, withdrawn into the shell, showing the enlarged, hard, protective scales on the front legs.

onto the wall and out. From a very early stage, Horsfield's juveniles are also great climbers.

Horsfield's tortoises are adept at wedging themselves into the corners of their enclosures, then using these corners to scramble upwards. Once they have achieved this feat, they will carry out the same action repetitively until they have successfully clambered out. Covering the corners of any square or rectangular enclosure with wooden or Perspex® triangles is therefore recommended (Fig. 16.7).

As mentioned, Horsfield's are also great at digging and tunnelling (Fig. 16.9). When creating an enclosure, the solid boundaries should be dug into the substrate (to a depth of at least 20 cm) to prevent them escaping the safety of their enclosure (see Chapter 3 on the captive environment).

very secure, with solid sides of a good height at least twice their length. The internal edges of their enclosures must be kept clear of rocks, shrubs and other plants. I have watched my Horsfield's male clamber into a shrub planted too near the edge of his enclosure and then use this to hoist himself up

Horsfield's tortoises should be provided with accessible drinking water at all times. Even though adapted for life in arid environments, the additional stress of captivity requires us to ensure that they do have access to water at all times (Fig. 16.10).

Enclosures should be created for enrichment with a variety of environmental options provided. A suitable enclosure will look similar to that of a Mediterranean tortoise, with a freely draining sandy substrate and plenty of opportunities to bask on surfaces such as stone, paving or concrete. Grass can be included in small areas but should not make up the main area of substrate. In colder climates grass holds too much moisture and creates a damp environment. Rocky, hilly areas for climbing are appreciated as part of environmental enrichment in the enclosure.

Covering some areas with polycarbonate or Perspex® can help increase localized temperatures by several degrees, so providing both warmth and a low humidity environment.

Indoor accommodation should be similar to that described for Mediterranean tortoises (see Chapter 13 on Mediterranean tortoises).

Problems of health and welfare in this species largely relate to poor diet. As mentioned, veterinarians are regularly seeing juveniles in particular who have pyramiding due to being overfed, not given sufficient calcium and given a diet lacking in fibre. Some of these animals are in terrible state. Figure 16.11 shows severe beak and shell deformities. In the rescue situation we regularly see deformed Horsfield's that can barely walk, with severe pyramiding or collapse of the shell as shown in Fig. 16.12. Some are extremely ill to the point of death, all due to poor husbandry (see Chapter 7 on common illnesses and diseases). The need for good husbandry, designed to suit the species, and an appropriate diet is emphasized by many veterinary authors in this field (McArthur, 1996, 2012; McArthur *et al.*, 2004; Chitty and Raftery, 2013).

Wholly inadequate enclosures are also a problem. Figure 16.13 shows a tiny indoor space that is far too small. The overhead lights may provide heat and light, but the tortoise has no chance of thermoregulating as there is no escape from them. The straw substrate is totally unsuitable for a burrowing species and gives no opportunity for access to microclimates to increase humidity. It is also a significant potential fire hazard.

Breeding this species is achievable. Mating is most likely in the spring after hibernation, once temperatures rise. The males can be very aggressive towards each other when females are available. The courtship and mating rituals involve head nodding and biting at the female's head and legs, sometimes to the point of injury and damage to the legs and head (Highfield, 1992; 1996; 2024).

Two or three clutches of two to five eggs may be laid. My female has usually laid two to three eggs when nesting. Provision of nesting sites for females is essential, as for the other species covered in this book. Hatching takes around 75 days and success rates are generally good.

Conclusion

This species of tortoise presents challenges in captivity. It is not as easy to keep as presented online and by retailers (Highfield, 2003; 2024). Adult tortoises are easier to keep than juveniles, especially for novice keepers. It is easier to get it right for adult tortoises, which are less susceptible to the effects of poor husbandry and diet, than for young tortoises. Unfortunately, the majority of Horsfield's tortoises being sold in the pet trade are captive-bred juveniles. While this is beneficial in terms of wild populations not being exploited (although sadly this is also still happening), it is a welfare disaster for many of the individuals involved.

As described, Horsfield's tortoises are only active for around 3–4 months each year. This is difficult for us to achieve in captivity. It is also not what many keepers want, as they enjoy interactions with their tortoises. We have no idea what the long-term effects of captivity will be on this species, which is relatively new to the pet trade for the reasons outlined above. Being active for 9–10 months of the year in captivity is very different from their natural lifestyle. They are active climbers and diggers but can also be quite shy tortoises, often using their hides and retreats. They are able to withdraw and protect themselves with large scales on the front legs (similar to those seen in the Egyptian tortoise, *Testudo kleinmanni*). Figure 16.14 shows a normal adult withdrawn into the shell.

Although often seen as a very good beginner's tortoise, they are in fact challenging in terms of being kept in suitable temperatures and humidity levels, away from combined cold and damp conditions (Highfield, 2024). Because they are adapted to live on very low nutrient levels, it is difficult to provide a diet in captivity that is high enough in fibre, low enough in protein and with high calcium levels. As small tortoises it is also really easy to overfeed them. Starting with an adult of this species would be preferable for new keepers than taking on a very young juvenile or a hatchling.

Sourcing this species from ethical sources is particularly difficult, as the numbers being traded are so high (see Chapter 20 on tortoise keeping in the past, present and future). If taking in an unwanted animal, do so through a responsible rehoming organization with whom you have a relationship. Taking on a juvenile is much more problematic and the advice would be to only buy directly from the breeder, so that you can see their set-up and be sure that the tortoise has not been wild-caught, ranch-farmed, or commercially bred.

References and Further Reading

Chitty, J. and Raftery, A. (2013) *Essentials of Tortoise Medicine and Surgery*. Wiley Blackwell, Chichester, UK.

CITES: Convention on International Trade in Endangered Species of Wild Flora and Fauna, Geneva. Website: www.cites.org

Highfield, A.C. (1992) The Horsfield's tortoise: *Testudo horsfieldi* (GRAY) 1844 – A brief review of its biology, ecology and captive breeding. (First published in *ASRA Journal*. Available now on Tortoise Trust website for historical publications at www.tortoisetrust.org/articles/horsfield2.html. Note that the up-to-date Tortoise Trust website is now www.tortoisetrust.com)

Highfield, A. (1996) *Practical Encyclopaedia of Keeping and Breeding Tortoises and Freshwater Turtles*. Carapace Press, London.

Highfield, A.C. (2003) Captive bred or illegal import? UK tortoise buyers need to beware. Available at www.tortoisetrust.com/illegal-imports

Highfield, A.C. (2024) The Horsfield's tortoise: *Testudo horsfieldii* (GRAY) 1844 – History in the pet trade, ecology and biology, captive breeding, misunderstood and some challenges in captivity. Available at www.tortoisetrust.com/articles/captive-care-of-the-russian-tortoise-testudo-horsfieldii

Highfield, A. and Highfield, N. (2008) *Taking Care of Pet Tortoises*. The Tortoise Trust Jill Martin Fund. Available from: www.tortoisetrust.org

IUCN Red List or Red List Index (RLI) https://www.iucn.org (accessed in 2024).

Highfield, A. and Highfield, N. (2009) *Keeping a Pet Tortoise*. Interpet, Dorking, UK.

King, L. (2020) *Edible Plants for Tortoises in the UK*, 4th edn. Available from www.books@tlady.clara.co.uk

Lagarde, F., Bonnet, X., Corbin, J., Henen, B., Nagy, K., Mardonov, B. and Naulleau, G., (2003) Foraging behaviour and diet of an ectothermic herbivore: *Testudo horsfieldi*. *Ecography* 26, 236–242.

McArthur, S. (1996) *Veterinary Management of Tortoises and Turtles*. Blackwell, Oxford, UK.

McArthur, S. (2012) *Chelonian Medicine: Improving Standards for Captive Chelonia in the UK*. Proceedings of Tortoise Welfare UK Conference, 17 November 2012.

McArthur, S., Wilkinson, R. and Meyer, J. (2004) *Medicine and Surgery of Tortoises and Turtles*. Blackwell, Oxford, UK

Rendle, M. (2019) Ch 4 Nutrition. In: Girling, S.J. and Raiti, P. (eds) *BSAVA Manual of Reptiles*, 3rd edn. BSAVA, Quedgeley, UK, pp. 49–69.

UK Government legislation via Animal and Plant Health Agency (APHA) and Department for Environment Food and Rural Affairs (Defra) (undated) Commercial use of endangered species: check if you need a CITES certificate. Available at www.gov.uk/guidance/endangered-species-certificate-for-commercial-use

Vetter, H. (2002) *Turtles of the World, Vol. 1, Africa, Europe and Western Asia*. Chimaira, Frankfurt

Wegehaupt, W. (2009) *Mediterranean Tortoises, Where and how they live in the wild*. Kressbronn, Germany

Wegehaupt, W. (2021) *Feeder Plants for Mediterranean Tortoises*. Kressbronn, Germany

17 Egyptian Tortoises

Abstract

This chapter describes the natural habitat and requirements in captivity of the beautiful Egyptian tortoise *Testudo kleinmanni*. As a small species, these tortoises are very susceptible to the effects of poor husbandry and inadequate environmental conditions. They do not hibernate/brumate. They have been traditionally described as a desert tortoise, but in fact live on the coast of North Africa in Egypt, Libya and Israel. These coastal regions have a different microclimate to the true desert inland areas.

Their coastal habitat is much more humid and has more vegetation than might be expected in a very arid region. It can be difficult for keepers to find up-to-date information regarding their requirements when kept in captivity. Discussion is included of the effects of increased humidity for part of the year, and how this might relate to breeding behaviour. Traditionally they have been reported as difficult to breed in captivity, but with seasonal changes breeding success can be greatly improved.

As a critically endangered species, red-listed by the IUCN since 2003 and listed on Appendix I Annex A (EU) by CITES since 1994, captive *T. kleinmanni* are an important conservation resource. If the breeding of captive animals proves to be successful it may be possible to ensure the continued existence of this lovely tortoise. It is difficult to see opportunities for the species to be returned to the natural environment soon, however, as pressures on their habitat remain. There are few conservation projects in natural locations. The market-driven desire to collect these tortoises for the pet trade remains problematic.

What are Egyptian tortoises?

Kleinmann's tortoise is the smallest tortoise found in the Northern Hemisphere. Female tortoises are larger than the males, as is typical in tortoises. Females measure up to 14 cm straight carapace length (SCL) and weigh up to 200–400 g (Biedenweg and Schramm, 2019). Males are narrower and have a longer tail. Again, this is typical of many tortoise species. Males are usually around 9 cm straight carapace length when fully grown and weigh up to 200 g. I have a very large female weighing 490 g but this is unusual.

The shells are highly domed (Fig. 17.1). They range in colour from ivory to pale gold or yellow with thin areas of dark brown patterning (Vetter, 2002). This colouring is an example of Gloger's rule (Gloger, 1833), which states that pale colouring helps regulate the impact of sunlight. Thus, a paler-coloured tortoise such as *T. kleinmanni* can stay in the desert heat for longer. Pale coloration is also an effective camouflage in the desert sand. The bottom of the shell is light yellow, often with two dark triangles on each abdominal scute.

My first encounter with this species was when someone locally gave me an adult male, which had clearly been wild-caught at some stage. Tut arrived here in October 1996 and has grown 20 mm in length, increased 120 g in weight, and mated with two adult females since his arrival. At that time not much was known about the natural habitat of these tortoises, or how to keep them in captivity. My set-up has changed significantly over these 18 years, as more information has become available. This is reflected in the sections below on accommodation in captivity.

Kleinmann's tortoise is a herbivorous species and depends on a variety of plants to provide a balanced diet. The diet changes seasonally, in a similar way to that of Mediterranean tortoises (see Chapter 13 on Mediterranean tortoises).

As these tortoises are adapted to live in the semi-desert coastal regions of North Africa, they are very well suited to survive in relatively harsh conditions, with limited food resources. Their small size allows them to find shade and shelter under relatively small plants and shrubs during very hot conditions. They do not hibernate, as the temperature never falls below the trigger temperature of 10°C. Being small also keeps their food demands within the limits of available resources. They will use burrows created by rodents when seeking shelter from very high temperatures and strong sunlight in the summer (Fig. 17.2). They have a good memory of their territories and repeatedly use the same shelters and retreats (Biedenweg and Schramm, 2019).

Where do Egyptian tortoises *Testudo kleinmanni* live?

In the wild, these lovely small tortoises are found along a coastal strip from Tripoli in Libya to the Negev Desert of the Sinai Peninsula in Israel, as shown in the map in Fig. 17.3. The strip extends from the Mediterranean coast to between 90 km according to Scheider and Schneider (2008) and 120 km inland from the Tortoise Trust (Highfield and Martin, 1994). The home range is therefore very small, which means that the entire habitat can be easily destroyed.

Kleinmann's tortoises inhabit scrub areas with mainly low-level vegetation to the east and west of the Nile delta. To the west, the region receives the highest precipitation in Egypt. This is 70–200 mm annually, with rainfall occurring during the winter months. With higher rainfall comes a richer flora, which is essential as a food source for these herbivorous tortoises. While the natural climate is hot and dry, at certain times of the year a sea mist rolls in early in the day, which increases humidity significantly, allowing more vegetation to grow. To the east, into the North Sinai region there is less rainfall, but again there are regions around salt marshes and where the dunes have stabilized with more vegetation (Highfield and Martin, 1994). The areas around the large coastal Lake Bardawil have previously been a location for Egyptian tortoises, but they are no longer present there (Schneider and Schneider, 2008).

The Egyptian tortoise is one of the smallest species of tortoise, and has been easy to locate and collect for the pet trade since the 1970s. Consequently, they have been brought almost to the point of extinction in their home countries of Egypt, Libya and Israel (EESP, 2006).

They are listed by CITES as Appendix I and in the EU as Annex A, which is the most restricted category, and trade in them is protected at the highest level. The species is on the IUCN Red List as critically endangered. Unfortunately, as they are so small, they are very easy to smuggle illegally. As trade continues in illegally collected animals, few remain in the wild in some regions (EESP, 2006; Zwartepoorte, 2007, 2015). They remain popular and the market for them remains strong. They can fetch high prices in markets in Egypt and more widely across North Africa. This makes them a tempting source of income for locals.

As far back as 1994, The Tortoise Trust reported that there were no animals found in a field survey in Egypt that year (Highfield and Martin, 1994). They identified as the causes of this loss as 'extensive (mostly irreversible) habitat destruction and widespread ecological changes caused by agricultural expansion, cultivation, over grazing and urban encroachment; and continued intensive collection for the pet trade by locals and professionals'.

In 2004, I was given an adult female tortoise by someone who had been watching a TV show about veterinary treatment at a hospital run by a large charity in the UK. There had been a recent item which showed an Egyptian tortoise being treated. When it was identified as a very highly regulated and protected species, the owner decided that they no longer wanted to keep the tortoise, which had apparently been found 'walking along a local high street'. The owner had visited Egypt for a holiday prior to giving the tortoise to me, from which you may draw your own conclusions. An adult female is shown in Fig. 17.4.

Combined with collection for the pet trade, habitat loss has decimated the endemic populations. The regions where tortoises live have been subject to high levels of human impact through farming and overgrazing. This has had a dramatic negative impact on the natural environment. There is much less vegetation in these regions, reducing the available habitat.

What is their natural environment like?

Climate

The climate as described by Biedenweg and Schramm (2019) is hot and dry in the summer, with cooler nights. In the winter, temperatures will be warm in the daytime and can be very cold at night. Daily summer temperatures range from 22°C to 32°C while in winter the range is 9–18°C. Daily fluctuations of 10–15°C can be experienced at certain times of the year. These large daily fluctuations provide the opportunity for very heavy dew to form overnight. This is essential for plant life to survive and is a source of water for the tortoises, who drink from plant leaves and rock surfaces.

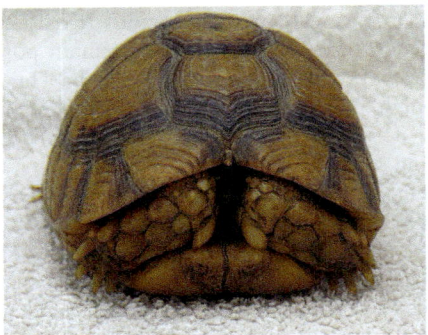

Fig. 17.1. *T. kleinmanni*, showing domed shell and enlarged, hard, protective scales on front legs.

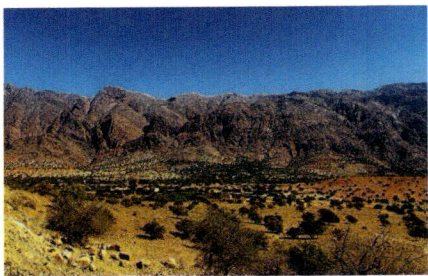

Fig. 17.2. Natural scrub-like areas up to 120 km inland used by this species (Corrine Wayends). Note the intensity of light in this area, where there is a very high UV index.

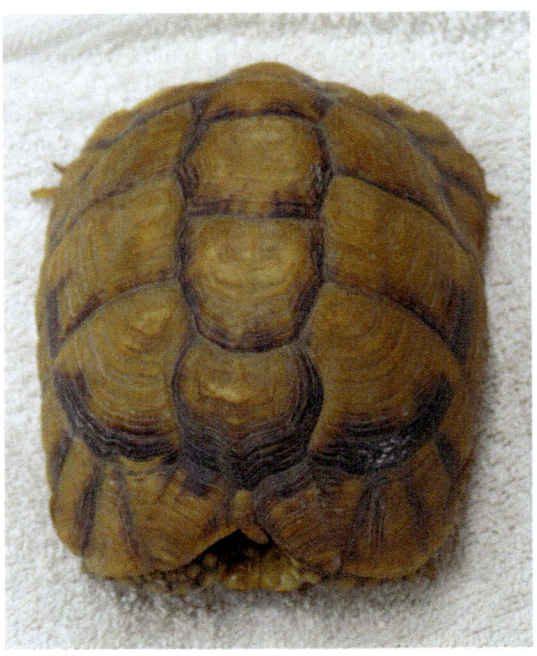

Fig. 17.4. Adult female *T. kleinmanni*. Note the slightly displaced nuchal scute above the head.

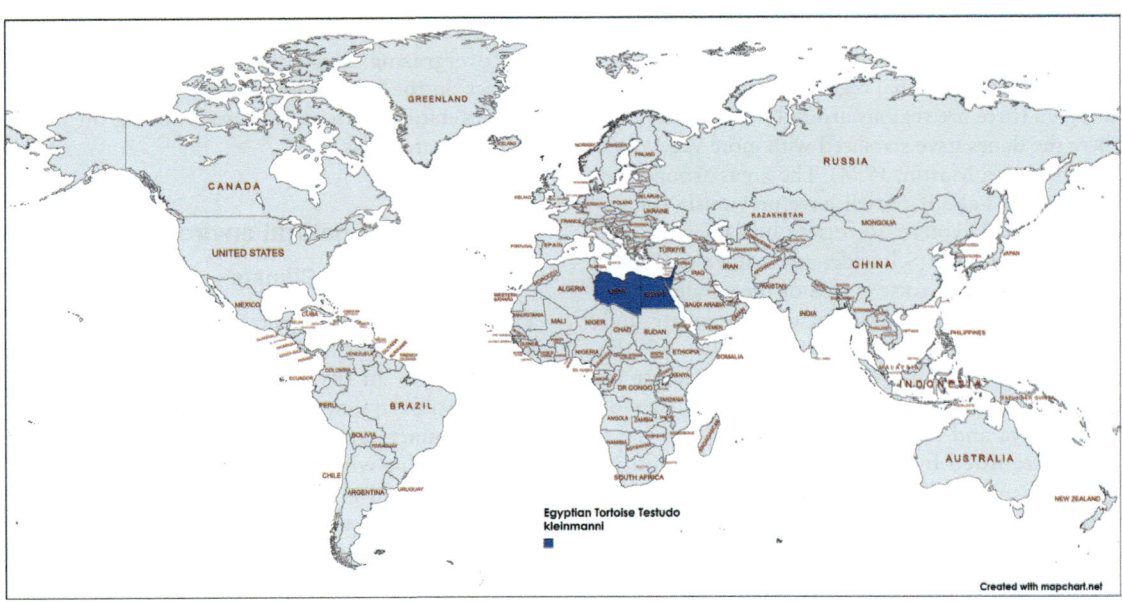

Fig. 17.3. Map of locations where *Testudo kleinmanni* is found. (https://www.mapchart.net/world.html)

Table 17.1. Plants identified as examples of food and for shelter (Schneider and Schneider, 2008; Biedenweg and Schramm, 2019).

Plant species	Food	Shelter/Retreats
Astragalus caprinus (vetch)	✓	✓
Artemisia monosperma (sagebrush)		✓
Atriplex leucoclada (oraches/amaranths)		✓
Coridothymus capitatus (wild thyme)		✓
Erodium ciconium (stork's bill/geranium)	✓	
Malva sylvestris (common mallow)	✓	✓
Mesembryanthemum nodiflorum (ice plant/stone plant)	✓	
Plantago albicans (plantains)	✓	
Retama raetam (white broom)		✓

Because of the sea mists that roll in, humidity remains relatively high throughout the year, reaching 60–68%. This is despite no rainfall in the summer months of June to August.

Daylength varies between 10 and 14 hours through the seasons. In the autumn, winter and spring, clouds and rainfall reduce the daily sunshine to 6–10 hours, whereas in the summer sunshine may last for 12 hours every day (Biedenweg and Schramm, 2019).

During very hot periods Egyptian tortoises aestivate. Aestivation is a period of dormancy seen in species where the temperatures rise to high levels during the summer (see also Horsfield's tortoises, Chapter 16). Egyptian tortoises can aestivate from June to September, as this is when temperatures rise and food becomes scarce.

Vegetation

The plants found in the home range are often halophytes, which are tolerant of salt. This is essential, as much of the humidity in the area comes from the sea. Salt marshes also increase salinity in the surrounding soil. Flowering plants such as *Halocnemum strobilaceum*, *Anthemis microsperma*, *Pancratium arabicum*, *Astragalus camelorum* and *Artemisia monosperma* are commonly found in the coastal areas of the Mediterranean and Red Seas, along with the evergreen shrub *Juniperus phoenica*. *Sonchus macrocarpus* (one of the sowthistle family) provides excellent tortoise food in a number of locations. Grasses such as *Bromus aegyptiacus* are found, together with succulents such as *Zygophyllum album*, all of which are potential food sources (Highfield and Martin, 1994).

Plants found here have been analysed as having low protein levels (17.3% average), high fibre (33–49%) and a very high Ca:P ratio (14:1). This makes them a perfect diet for herbivorous tortoises (see Chapter 5 on diets). As described previously, protein levels of 20% or less, fibre of 30% and a Ca:P ratio of 2:1 should be aimed for in providing a healthy diet for captive tortoises.

Terrain

Artemisia, or sagebrush, creates much of what could be described as a form of steppe habitat, but with less grasslands than might be expected in a traditional steppe, and more open areas of soil and sand broken up by shrubs and other plants. The area is largely flat or undulated and open with patches of scrub vegetation.

The region is also rocky in places, with hard compacted sand and gravel, as well as softer dune sand. This gives a varied substrate. Opportunities are provided for these small tortoises to find retreats, shade and higher levels of humidity within the areas covered with scrub-type vegetation. However, walking on the shifting sands of the inland dunes is impossible. This restricts tortoises to coastal areas where the substrate is hard enough to form a solid surface, aided by the roots of vegetation in the area.

In the wild, males have territories of 16.4 ha and females around half that size at 7.2 ha (Biedenweg and Schramm, 2019). These are much bigger ranges that those required by Mediterranean tortoises, probably because food is less available. Tortoises will need to walk much greater distances to find suitable food plants, especially in the late spring before aestivation. This high level of activity is an important consideration when creating captive enclosures for these busy tortoises.

How should Egyptian tortoises be kept in captivity?

In most countries where *T. kleinmanni* is kept in captivity, the climate is colder, wetter, and with less sunshine than their natural habitat. This often necessitates the use of an indoor enclosure, or terrarium, for much of the year (see Chapter 3 on the

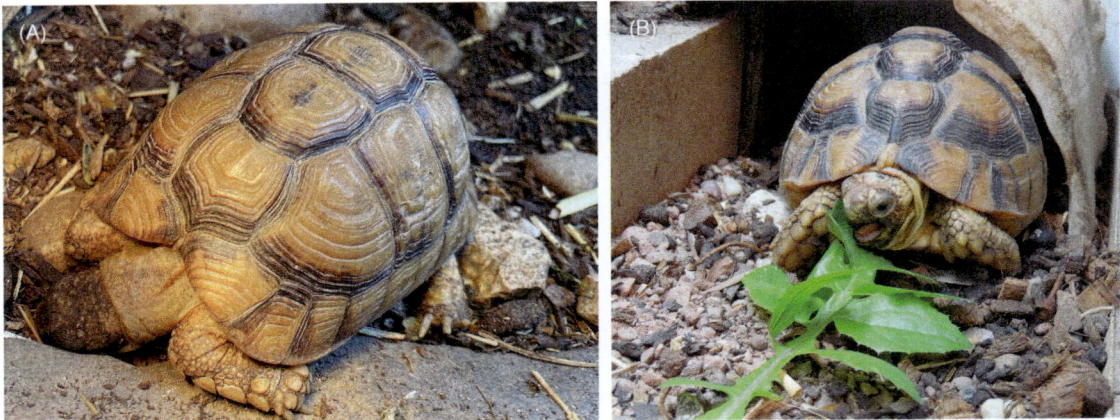

Fig. 17.5. Egyptian tortoise (A) resting and basking, and (B) eating with a healthy appetite.

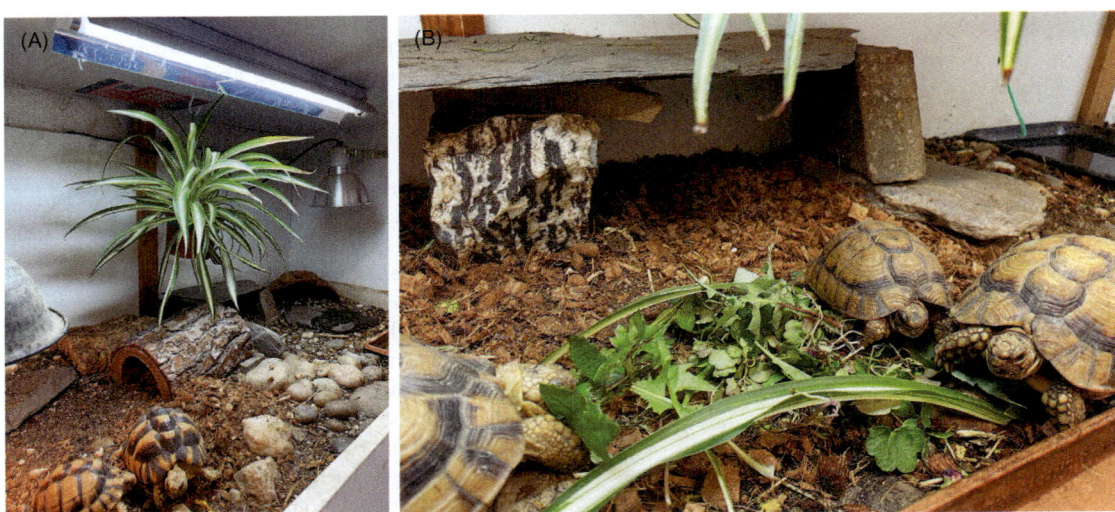

Fig. 17.6. Egyptian tortoises in sections of an indoor terrarium showing overhead UVB light source, basking light, water trays and infrared heater.

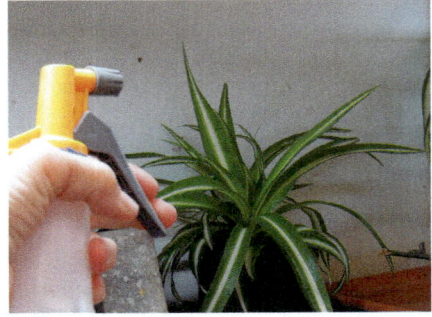

Fig. 17.7. Humidity can be increased using simple sprays or foggers/misters that can be electronically controlled.

captive environment). The available temperatures will otherwise not be warm enough when compared with those experienced by tortoises in the wild. If this is the case the range of normal behaviours will be restricted, with consequent harmful effects, which will also be damaging to health. Given their need for space to walk good distances daily, and their natural territory sizes, a large indoor area is needed. Good levels of artificial light (see Chapter 4 on artificial light and heat) are needed for this species, as it is adapted for high levels of light intensity and brightness, together with background heat. Background LED lighting (previously fluorescent tubes) providing suitable daylength and a natural light colour will be needed, together with basking spots for warmth and UVA and UVB wavelengths (Biedenweg and Schramm, 2019). Figure 17.5 shows Egyptian tortoises resting and eating.

The cost of setting up and maintaining such large indoor enclosures is considerable. Electricity and energy costs are not cheap in any month. This is a species for the enthusiast and real hobbyist, preferably with an interest in breeding this endangered species. Suitable sizes for a terrarium for Egyptian tortoises are 0.5 m² for two juveniles up to 6 cm SCL, or 1 m² for two adults 6–12 cm SCL (Biedenweg and Schramm, 2019). The terrarium cannot be too large – use as much space as you can to allow the maximum available walking area and as much variation providing environmental enrichment as possible, as shown in Fig. 17.6 of indoor enclosures.

The temperature range should be varied throughout the year to mimic the natural cycle in the wild. In the winter the temperatures will be cooler, with shorter days and some rainfall. In summer temperatures will be higher, with longer days and no rainfall. All of this we can try to mimic. The use of timers to control daylength is essential. These can be altered month by month. In addition, dimmers can be used to create a more natural sunrise and sunset. Alternatively, the timers can be sequenced so that lights come on separately over a period of time until the full set of lights is on. Temperature control through thermostats is also essential.

Egyptian tortoises are put into Ferguson Zone 3 (see Chapter 4 on artificial light and heat) based on their habits (Baines et al., 2016) – being active in the morning and evening only during the summer (unless they are aestivating, in which case they will be dormant in burrows). In autumn, winter and spring they will be more active and will expose themselves to the sun throughout the day. The natural environmental parameters by season indicate what we should be trying to achieve as shown in Table 17.2.

Temperature and UV gradients should allow the tortoises access to sufficient UVB and UVA, together with a suitable gradient for thermoregulation. Based on the data above, the tortoises need to be able to reach around 30°C when active and can cope with night-time temperatures down to around 15°C in the winter. Overhead infrared heaters can be used to good effect with thermostats to alter the temperatures seasonally. Examples of suitable products include those from Reptile Systems®.

Overhead lights provide background lighting and basking opportunities. Lighting using T5 lamps to create conditions as described based on the Ferguson Zone 3 is required. The Reptile Systems T5, for example, provides 12% UVB and a UVI of 4.1 and should be positioned 30 cm from the tortoises. The Arcadia® ProT5 UVB 12% desert lighting kit is another product providing similar parameters (Fig. 17.6).

Once again variation within the enclosure allows the tortoise to find the conditions necessary for it to achieve physiological homeostasis, which is the key to good health and success.

Humidity levels can be altered to mimic rain showers using a mister or fogger, or using a hose set as a spray if there is enough space (Fig. 17.7). The substrate can also have water added to it to prevent it drying out. I regularly water the substrate to ensure that it does not become too dry or dusty.

What type of substrate and furniture are needed?

For Egyptian tortoises an arid sandy habitat is needed if we are going to follow the principle of

Table 17.2. Natural environmental parameters, by season (from Biedenweg and Schramm, 2019).

Season/Parameters	Winter Dec–Feb	Spring Mar–May	Summer June–Aug	Autumn Sep–Nov
Hours of daylight	10–11	11.5–12	13–14	10.5–13
Hours of sunshine	6–7.5	7.5–9.5	10–12	7–9
Temperatures daytime (°C)	18–20	23–30	30–38	24–35
Temperatures night-time (°C)	10–15	15–22	22–26	17–24
Relative Humidity daytime (%)	55–65	50–65	50–65	55–60
Relative Humidity night-time (%)	70–80	65–80	70–80	65–75
Rainfall showers events	1–3 weekly	0–1 monthly	0	0–2 weekly

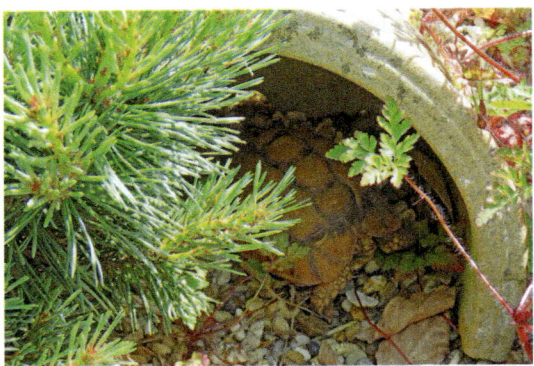

Fig. 17.8. Retreats, hides and shelters outdoors.

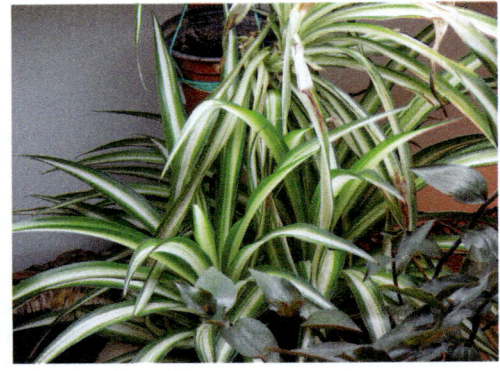

Fig. 17.9. Enclosure plants indoors: spider plant and tradescantia.

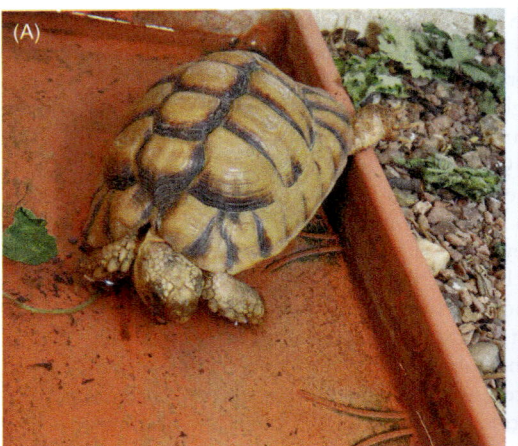
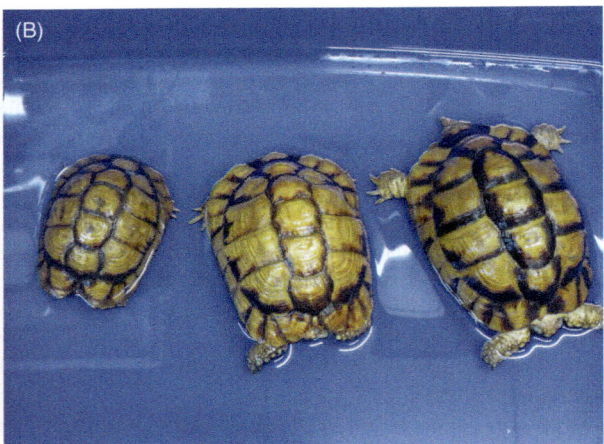

Fig. 17.10. (A) Water trays can be terracotta, or plastic, but should be sunk into the substrate for ease of access. (B) Placing the animals in a warm bath regularly allows the keeper to see any waste products.

trying to mimic the natural environment (a running theme throughout this book). Although the substrate should be sand-based in the captive enclosure, it does need to have sufficient loam added to provide a solid surface for walking. Loam is a fertile soil made of a mix of clay, sand and organic matter (humus). The proportions of loam to sand within the enclosure should be around 50–60% loam and 40–50% sand (Highfield, 1996). Some authors (Biedenweg and Schramm, 2019) suggest a mix of sand and loam powder (pulverized loam), which is available in Europe but not so readily accessible in the UK and some other countries. The sand recommended has often been washed playground sand, but I have always used building sand mixed with loamy soil and compost without any problems.

Keeping these tortoises on an entirely sandy surface limits opportunities for the creation of microhabitats. The addition of loam produces a more natural substrate and allows the sand to bind, creating a solid surface. The sand should be added to the enclosure first, moistened with water and then the loam or loam powder added and mixed thoroughly. The depth of substrate should be a minimum of 8 cm (Biedenweg and Schramm, 2019), with deeper areas fashioned into mounds. These may be used as nesting sites by females and provide some variation in the topography.

There should be open areas for walking and basking, together with retreats and hiding places for shelter and shade (Fig. 17.8). The use of plants within the enclosure is beneficial. This allows microclimates to be created, including areas of increased humidity.

There should be rocks, roots and branches for hiding under, together with broken plant pots and solid shelters and shade. In addition, plants can be put directly into the substrate for shade and increased humidity in some areas to create microclimates (Fig. 17.9). Plants that are used as browse and food can be put into plant pots sunk into the substrate, to allow some access for eating without destruction of the whole plant. Areas can be cordoned off to allow the plants to recover and regrow after grazing, and then to give access again on a rotational basis.

Access to water can be achieved through the provision of shallow water bowls, such as terracotta trays sunk into the substrate (Fig. 17.10). These should be of similar depth and size to the small puddles that may form after rain in the natural environment. Tortoises will drink from wet vegetation if plants within the enclosure are watered and they will take moisture from any surface on which water collects, including each other's shells (Biedenweg and Schramm, 2019).

What is the diet of Egyptian tortoises?

These herbivorous tortoises need a high-calcium, high-fibre, low-protein diet. This is best provided by offering a variety of plants, particularly those found in their natural habitat if these are available. Any plants grown in the enclosure will need to be replenished and usually supplemented with leaves and flowers. Care must be taken to ensure that the plants are not poisonous to tortoises.

As Egyptian tortoises are herbivorous the diet should be entirely based on plant leaves, stems and flowers. This can include wild herbs such as thyme, marjoram and chamomile. Suitable wild plants and weeds found in Europe and the UK include plantain, mallow, dandelion, sow-thistle, hawkbit, cat's ear and hawk's beard. These are all high fibre, with a high Ca:P ratio, and so are suitable for Egyptian tortoises.

The food naturally available will vary in moisture content during the seasons. Fresh food should be available, together with dry food in all seasons except summer, when dry food alone can be given. Water should always be available. Even though this is a deviation from natural conditions, if the tortoises are not aestivating in the hot months (if the local temperatures are high enough) they will need water. Because the captive environment can mimic, but never replicate, the natural conditions, water should always be available to avoid additional stress, which might lead to dehydration.

In winter, additions to the diet to supplement indoor plants could include dried flowers and soaked Pre-Alpin® cobs or Arcadia® Freshly Pressed Tortoise Food (see Chapter 5 on diets) which add variety, fibre and calcium to the diet.

Is it easy to breed Egyptian tortoises?

Until recently this species has been considered difficult to breed in captivity, although some examples of captive breeding were seen in the 1980–1990s in Egypt, Europe, the USA and the UK (Highfield and Martin, 1995). As the species is relatively rare in captivity, records of breeding are limited. As with all species, the adult tortoises must be in good health and condition if they are to reproduce, as well as being kept in optimal environmental conditions and in groups that live together harmoniously.

The European Studbook Foundation (ESF) spearheads a project to maintain captive populations and to encourage breeding between genetically healthy, viable populations, using zoo and private collections (Zwartepoorte, 2007, 2008, 2015). The programme began in 1997, having been established in the Netherlands. Henk Zwartepoorte coordinated this work until his death in 2016. I have four *T. kleinmanni* that are part of this programme. Two juvenile males arrived here in 2013 from Germany and a male and a female

Table 17.3. Suitable food plants which do well in a well-lit terrarium (The Tortoise Table; King, 2020; Wegehaupt, 2021).

Common name	Species
Creeping inchplant, spiderwort	*Callisia* (Commelinaceae family)
Bromeliads, e.g. Pink Quill	*Tillandsia cyanea*
Stonecrops	*Crassula* spp.
Aloes, e.g. Zebra plant	*Aloe* spp.
Cacti, e.g. Christmas, Easter	*Schlumbergera* spp.
Devil's tongue	*Sansevieria* spp. (Asparagaceae family)
Grasses, e.g. Blue grass	*Festuca* spp.
Spider plant, Acrospira	*Chlorophytum* (Asparagaceae family)
Spiderwort	*Tradescantia*

from the Netherlands. All remain healthy and well and show active mating behaviour at different times of the year.

In 2001 the European Endangered Species Programme (EEP), coordinated through the European Association of Zoos and Aquaria (EAZA), began a breeding programme. This has been headed up by Rotterdam Zoo since 2002 (EAZA, 2024).

The intention of these conservation programmes is to breed animals in captivity in order to avoid further collection from the wild. Unfortunately, the numbers involved are currently very small and so are unlikely to have a significant impact on populations as a whole. Nonetheless the contribution is significant. There were 407 ESF Studbook individuals reported in 2015 kept by 45 private keepers (Zwartepoorte, 2015). Much of the breeding work is done in European zoos. By dispersing the animals, and including private collections in the projects, there is mitigation against losses of large numbers of animals kept in one location. For example, deaths caused by a contagious disease affecting that individual group could otherwise result in the loss of the whole group.

The Egyptian tortoise mates in a similar way to other *Testudo* species. The male will sniff, chase and ram the female in an attempt to get her to stand still. Mating takes some time, during which the male will vocalize a high-pitched 'brrr, brrr' sound which is not heard in other *Testudo* species. Once he is mounted on the female, the penis introduces sperm as with other tortoise species. The female can hold this sperm for 2 years and use it to fertilize eggs at a later date.

Suitable nesting areas must be provided for females, who usually lay up to three eggs. Incubation periods of 70–143 days have been reported (Biedenweg and Schramm, 2019) with a common duration being around 100 days. Hatchlings weigh around 5 g, which is remarkable – a fully formed, independent baby tortoise at such a small size and weight! Further general details on breeding are given in Chapter 11.

What is the future for Egyptian tortoises?

As a critically endangered species, IUCN red-listed and CITES listed as Appendix I Annex A, any animals in captivity are important, as the wild populations are all but gone in many areas. The pressures described here on habitats are accelerating through climate change and more intense human activity in very populated areas. Additional pressures on land use currently include tourism and the associated infrastructure, alongside military uses, particularly in Israel. In Egypt the species is all but extinct (Zwartepoorte, 2015), numbers are very few in Israel and the only populations of any size are in Libya (Biedenweg and Schramm, 2019).

The market for this species continues to exist, making collection a strong driver for locals with limited incomes and resources. Selling one tortoise can provide a huge boost to the family income in these locations. Sadly, Egyptian tortoises are still available on the internet, with prices of US$1000–4000 quoted per animal, often with no reference to trade restrictions, or the need for certificates or licences. Any return to the wild would therefore need to be in secure locations. Large numbers of Egyptian tortoises continue to be confiscated from the illegal trade. For example, in 2017, 3000 tortoises, including *T. kleinmanni*, were stopped by the Libyan Wildlife Trust on route to the markets in Egypt. In the same year 1900 Egyptian tortoises were seized in a separate incident near Benghazi, Libya, also on the way to Egyptian markets (Biedenweg and Schramm, 2019).

Currently there are reserves and rescue projects (Zwartepoorte, 2015) such as the recovery project in the Zaranik Conservation area in North Sinai desert, established and supported by the local Sweirki Bedouin tribe and coordinated by Nature Conservation Egypt (Biedenweg and Schramm, 2019). The El Omayed Biosphere Reserve west of Alexandria is another example where a combination of tortoises is protected *in situ*, in their natural habitat, alongside captive individuals in fenced areas (*ex situ*). Linking these *in situ* and *ex situ* breeding programmes forms the basis for the conservation and recovery of the Egyptian tortoise in Egypt (Zwartepoorte, 2015).

Since 2000, the breeding programmes of both the EAZA and the ESF have been coordinated (Zwartepoorte, 2015). This type of cooperation and communication is essential for future successes.

Reintroduction into protected areas of limited size is essential in preventing reintroduced animals being collected for the pet trade again. Involvement of the local human population, to engage them in the conservation and field work, has been key to increasing the level of interest in the species and to provide alternative income for local people as trackers and observers. Without this element no research, conservation or reintroduction will be successful in the long term.

Conclusion

Egyptian tortoises are a very attractive species to keep as pets. Their husbandry requirements have been described, including their dietary needs. It can, however, be difficult to meet those needs throughout the year and doing our best for this species can be a lot of work. Making a commitment to provide the captive environment in which they can live well, breed and survive to a good age is essential prior to obtaining these one of these tortoises. In most countries where this species is kept as a pet, there will be many months each year when the outside environment is not warm enough for them, which means that indoor enclosures need to be as large as possible and well designed.

T. kleinmanni is not a tortoise for beginners or inexperienced keepers. Their needs are similar to those of Mediterranean tortoises (see Chapter 13 on Mediterranean tortoises) but their small size, huge conservation significance and their fragility in the face of disease make them a challenge. They do not hibernate, as previously stated, and this also presents a challenge for keepers in colder climates.

While in some ways a very suitable tortoise for the pet industry (for example, their small size allows greater scope to provide adequately sized captive enclosures), the ethics of keeping such an endangered species should give us all pause for thought.

Like other very threatened species, the source of any individual kept as a pet should be very carefully researched. All local legislation restricting trade, along with international regulations, must be adhered to. These tortoises should not be available for sale in the pet trade as they are so endangered. We should ask ourselves why we want to keep such species and consider carefully the benefits of trying to improve the potential success of the species, by engaging with the ESF for example, and breeding for the benefit of the species.

References and Further Reading

Baines, F., Chattel, J., Dale, J., Garrick, D., Gill, I., Goetz, M., Skelton, T. and Swatman, M. (2016) How much UVB does my reptile need? The UV Tool, a guide to the selection of UV lighting for reptiles and amphibians in captivity. *Journal of Zoo and Aquarium Research* 4(1), 42–63.

Biedenweg, F. and Schramm, R. (2019) *The Egyptian Tortoise Testudo kleinmanni Lortet 1883. A Fascinating Little Beauty*. Tartaruga-Verlag Ricarda Schramm, Grebenhain, Germany.

CITES: Convention on International Trade in Endangered Species of Wild Flora and Fauna, Geneva. Website: www.cites.org

EAZA and EEP: EAZA = European Association of Zoos and Aquaria. EEP = EAZA Ex-situ Programmes (population management programmes). Reptile EEPs include *Testudo kleinmanni, Emys orbicularis, Chelonoidis nigra* species complex, *Uroplatus henkeli, Mauremys annamensis, M. mutica, M. nigricans* and *M. sinensis, Astrochleys yniphora* and *Chelodina mccordi*. EAZA website: www.eaza.net

EESP: European Endangered Species Programme. TESTUDO KLEINMANNI Egyptian tortoise Husbandry and breeding guidelines Version 2, 2006. Species coordinator: Henk Zwartepoorte, Rotterdam Zoo 23.5.2007

ESF: European Studbook Foundation. Private non-profit organization in Europe, headquarters Sneek, Netherlands, with country coordinators elsewhere. Conservation of reptiles and amphibians through captive breeding, especially endangered species. Website: https://studbooks.eu

Gloger, C.W.L (1833) *The Evolution of Birds Through the Impact of Climate* [in German]. Breslau: August Schulz. pp. 11–24. ISBN 978-3-8364-2744-9. OCLC 166097356

Highfield, A. (1996) *Practical Encyclopaedia of Keeping and Breeding Tortoises and Freshwater Turtles*. Carapace Press, London.

Highfield, A.C. and Martin, J. (1994) *Status of the Egyptian Tortoise Testudo kleinmanni in Egypt*. Tortoise Trust Web.

Highfield, A.C. and Martin, J. (1995) *Captive breeding of the Egyptian tortoise Testudo kleinmanni*. Tortoise Trust. Available at https://www.tortoisetrust.org/articles/kleinmanni.html

IUCN: International Union for Conservation of Nature, Gland, Switzerland. Maintains IUCN Red List of Threatened Species. Website: https://iucn.org

IUCN Red List or Red List Index (RLI) https://www.iucn.org (accessed in 2024)

King, L. (2020) *Edible Plants for Tortoises in the UK*, 4th edn). Available from books@tlady.clara.co.uk

Reptile Systems EU: sub-brand of Aquarium Systems (www.aquariumsystems.eu) offering wide variety of reptile-keeping equipment, care guides and expertise (www.reptilesystems.eu)

Schneider, C. and Schneider, W. (2008) The Egyptian Tortoise, *Testudo kleinmanni* Lortet, 1883 in Libya. *Salamandra* 44(30),141–152.

The Tortoise Table App: available from www.thetortoisetable.org.uk

UK Government legislation via Animal and Plant Health Agency (APHA) and Department for Environment Food and Rural Affairs (Defra) (undated) *Commercial use of endangered species: check if you need a CITES certificate*. Available at www.gov.uk/guidance/endangered-species-certificate-for-commercial-use

Vetter, H. (2002) *Turtles of the World, Vol. 1, Africa, Europe and Western Asia*. Chimaira, Frankfurt

Wegehaupt, W. (2021) *Feeder Plants for Mediterranean Tortoises*. Kressbronn, Germany

Zwartepoorte, H. (2007) *Studbook and Breeding Programme: Egyptian or Kleinmann's tortoise Testudo kleinmanni*. Annual report 2006, European Studbook Foundation (ESF). Available at https://studbooks.eu/site/assets/files/annualreports

Zwartepoorte, H. (2008) Egyptian tortoise – linking captive population management with wild population protection. Turtle Survival Alliance, August, 22–23. 59.

Zwartepoorte, H. (2015) Captive breeding the Critically Endangered Egyptian tortoise Testudo kleinmanni Lortet, 1883, for an in situ recovery project in Egypt. International Zoo Yearbook 49(1), 42–48.

18 What It Takes to Be a Tortoise Keeper

Abstract

This chapter highlights the areas of 'expertise' that are beneficial for tortoise keepers to have, in order to do the best possible job when caring for tortoises.

Whether the keeper is able to take a DIY approach, or utilizes the skills of professionals, will have an impact on costs. Setting up enclosures, whether indoors or outdoors, can be expensive. The more economically and financially sound any given tortoise keeper is, the more resources can be obtained and provided.

In this chapter the range of subject areas and practical skills needed to set up the most effective captive environments (often in less-than-ideal conditions) are described and discussed. Where tortoises are kept in captivity in their natural locations, the requirements for the creation of artificial environments will be reduced. For example, keeping Gopher tortoises (*Gopherus polyphemus*) in Florida will be less of a challenge than keeping them in the northern United States or northern Europe. This is true for all the tropical species.

The skill set needed for a tortoise keeper to meet the needs of captive tortoises is underpinned by the need to understand the biology of tortoises as reptiles. A good knowledge of the specific requirements of the individual species of tortoise being kept is also essential.

Knowledge set

An effective tortoise keeper should be up to date with the latest husbandry and welfare practices. Keeping up to date requires access to evidence-based research. There are many online forums and websites for tortoise keepers where good practice, ideas and experience can be shared. You need to check that the tortoises referred to belong to the species you actually keep. For example, people who use US websites often find information relevant to Gopher or Red-footed tortoises, but not Mediterranean species as they are less commonly kept.

Using the common names for tortoises can also be confusing, depending on where you live. So, to be sure of which species, you need to know the scientific name for your tortoise. As an example, a fairly recent and widely used term these days is the 'Greek tortoise'. In Europe and the UK this often refers to tortoises from Greece, unsurprisingly. The species often associated with Greece is the Marginated tortoise, *Testudo marginata*, although the other Mediterranean species, Hermann's (*Testudo hermanni*) and Spur-thighed tortoises (*Testudo graeca* spp.) also live there. The term 'Greek tortoise' is also used to describe the Spur-thighed tortoise *Testudo graeca* in both the USA and Europe. This is just one example of where a common name may lead you to treat your tortoise as a *Testudo marginata*, when it is actually *Testudo graeca*.

Not all of the information available online, through social media and in print is evidence-based, however. Sources may reflect outdated, entrenched ideas and now debunked practices that were previously accepted as the norm. Previously, for example, it was common in the UK to drill holes in the shells of tortoises, to tether them with string or rope so that they did not wander off and get lost. This was in the days before keepers understood the need to create tortoise gardens and terrariums that mimic as far as possible the natural habitat (see Chapter 3 on the captive environment). Keeping tortoises in such a way is now considered inhumane (the drilling of the hole usually damages both shell and bone, which is painful as well as damaging, as shown in Fig. 18.1).

This practice also restricted the tortoise's life to a very small area; damage was often caused if the string wrapped around the tortoise's leg, causing wounds and, in the worst cases, the loss of a limb; and the tortoise was unable to live any kind of

© CAB International 2025. *Tortoise Husbandry and Welfare*. (J. Williams)
DOI: 10.1079/9781800623736.0018

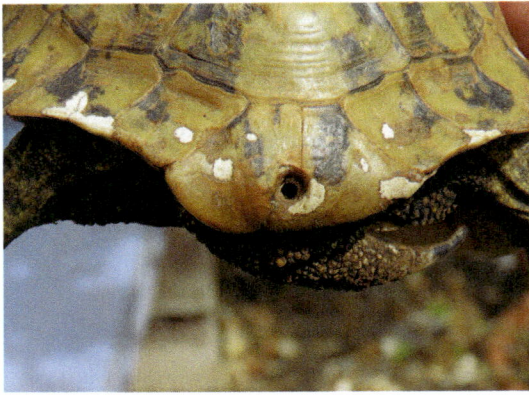

Fig. 18.1. Tortoise shells with holes drilled through both shell and bone, the latter seen as the white ring around the edge of the hole.

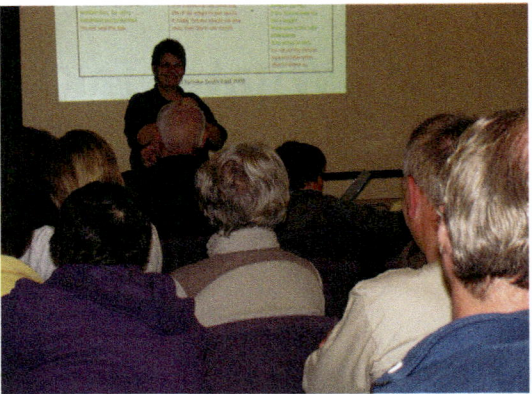

Fig. 18.3. Tortoise South East one-day workshop, for around 20 delegates, on hibernation/brumation, held in Essex, UK.

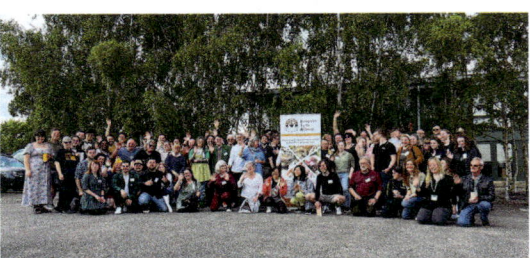

Fig. 18.2. European Turtle Alliance Conference 2024, which included presentations on conservation, husbandry and welfare from the UK, the USA, Europe and Bangladesh, to around 120 delegates from all over the UK. The conference took place over 2 days and included presentations from the zoo community, private breeders, research and conservation projects, and those involved in rescue and rehabilitation.

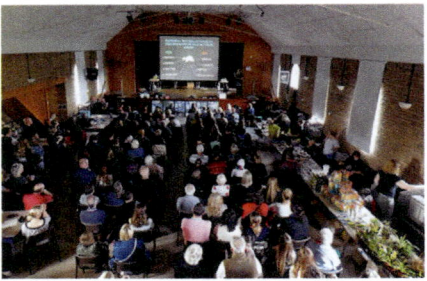

Fig. 18.4. The Norfolk Tortoise Club (UK) meeting attended by around 100 people is a great example of a very active, well-supported local group.

reasonable life as set out in the Five Domains. The Five Freedoms (Mellor, 2016a, b; Yeates, 2022) and Five Domains, as they are now described, list the 'freedom and opportunity to express normal behaviour'. Clearly this freedom was not available to tortoises that were kept tethered.

Another myth about the diet and feeding of Mediterranean tortoises was the notion that they ate dog or cat food. The idea that these foods were good for tortoises was a commonly held view in the early years of them being kept as pets in the UK and Europe, which started in the 1950s. The tortoises loved these foods, and of course chose them (as high protein and high fat) above any greens or healthy weeds they were offered. This had massive health and welfare issues, leading to some tortoises refusing to eat anything other than cat or dog food. This very rich diet caused problems such as fatty livers, kidney failure due to high protein levels in the blood, bladder stones and the very painful condition of gout (see Chapter 7 on common illnesses and diseases). Many of these tortoises died an early and painful death as a result. As discussed throughout this book, herbivores such as Mediterranean species need a high-fibre, high-calcium, low-protein diet if they are to stay healthy and well. Dog and cat food should not feature on the menu at all. Unfortunately, this outdated information is still available.

I once looked after a very elderly female Spur-thighed tortoise, *Testudo graeca whitei*, living in the UK, who had been given a 'Sunday roast' every week for the past 45 years she had lived with her owners. This meal included roast beef, cooked

Table 18.1. Useful organizations.

Organization	Website
Animal and Plant Health Agency (APHA) (UK)	www.gov.uk/government/organisations/animal-and-plant-health-agency
British and Irish Association of Zoos and Aquariums (BIAZA) (UK)	https://biaza.org.uk
European Association of Zoos and Aquariums (EAZA)	www.eaza.net
British Chelonia Group (BCG) (UK), for tortoise, terrapin and turtle care and conservation	www.britishcheloniagroup.org.uk
Convention on International Trade in Endangered Species of Wild Flora and Fauna (CITES)	www.cites.org
Emys Centre (Switzerland) – turtle protection and recovery centre (Association Protection et Récupération des Tortues, PRT) in Chavornay, Switzerland	www.tortue.ch
European Studbook Foundation (ESF)	https://studbooks.eu
European Turtle Alliance (ETA)	www.eta.org.uk
Garden State Tortoise (USA)	www.gardenstatetortoise.com
International Union for Conservation of Nature (IUCN)	https://iucn.org
Norfolk Tortoise Club (UK) – tortoise rescue, welfare, rehoming	www.tortoiseclub.org.uk
SOPTOM Turtle and Environmental Protection Station (France) – Station for the Observation and Protection of Tortoises and their Environment	www.tortuesoptom.org
The Nature Conservancy US	www.nature.org
The Nature Conservancy Canada	www.natureconservancy.ca
The Turtle Conservancy (USA)	www.turtleconservancy.org
Tortoise Welfare UK – tortoise rescue, welfare, rehoming, education, support and advice	www.tortoisewelfare.co.uk
Tortoise Trust (UK)	www.tortoisetrust.org.uk
Tortoise South East (UK)	www.tortoisesoutheast.co.uk
Turtle Island (Austria)	www.turtle-island.org
Turtle Survival Alliance (TSA) (USA)	www.turtlesurvival.org

Table 18.2. Useful sources of evidence-based published information.

Source	Publications and websites
British Herpetological Society (BHS)	*Journal of Herpetology*
British Small Animal Veterinary Association (BSAVA) Publications – e.g. *BSAVA Manual of Reptiles*	Various publications, e.g. *BSAVA Manual of Reptiles* www.bsava.com
CABI publications	www.cabi.org/what-we-do/cabi-publications
International Society for Anthrozoology	Journal *Anthrozoos* https://isaz.net/
Elsevier/Science Direct	*Journal of Veterinary Behavior* www.sciencedirect.com/journal/journal-of-veterinary-behavior
British Chelonia Group (BCG)	*Testudo* – Journal of the British Chelonia Group www/britishcheloniagroup.org.uk/testudo
The Tortoise Table edible plant identification App (UK)	www.thetortoisetable.org.uk
The Turtle Conservancy	*The Tortoise* www.turtleconservancy.org

vegetables such as peas, beans, carrots and cabbage, roast potatoes, Yorkshire pudding and of course gravy. All these food items are totally unsuitable in the diet of a herbivorous Mediterranean tortoise. When I mentioned this to her owners, and that in the wild these animals would be as likely to come across such foods as they would be to come across a nice glass of Châteauneuf-du-Pape to go with it, I was told that Penny loved her Sunday roast and that she seemed fine on it.

Table 18.3. The tortoise keeper's skills set.

Skills and expertise	Types of job or activity
Taxonomist	You need to be able to identify the species of tortoise(s) that you are caring for. This is essential if you are to effectively mimic the animal's natural environment and living conditions when setting up enclosures, as well as providing a suitable diet and enrichment opportunities. All of these will vary from species to species.
Ecologist	You need to be aware of the natural relationships between the physical environment and the things that live there. Understanding the relationships and interactions between organisms and their environment is essential when creating tortoise habitats.
Botanist/Naturalist	As many tortoise species are herbivores, you need to be able to identify suitable food plants and know which plants are toxic to tortoises. You should have a knowledge of which plants are suitable for shade and shelter too. An understanding of the size, habitat and environmental conditions plants need can really help when creating naturalistic habitats and microclimates for tortoises.
Ethologist	Understanding the natural behaviour of the tortoises you care for is key to knowing that you are providing the right conditions for your tortoise, as it cannot explain its needs to you. Behaviour is the best indicator of good health. Providing opportunities for most naturally occurring behaviours is fundamental to meeting tortoise needs. A tortoise that is behaving abnormally is either ill or is being deprived of the correct environmental conditions. First you must have an understanding of what is 'normal' for your tortoise. Without this you will not be able to identify what is abnormal.
Physicist/lighting and heating technician	Providing suitable artificial light and heat sources is essential when keeping tortoises in countries that are too cold or too wet for them to exist in the wild. Knowledge of lighting requirements and the ability to set up lighting and heating systems safely is required. The following aspects need to be borne in mind: The type of lighting and heating sources needed will vary with species. The positioning of sources to provide suitable temperature gradients and to provide adequate areas of lighting is crucial when designing accommodation. Placing outdoor enclosures in the best natural light and temperatures is a fundamental starting point.
Landscape gardener	Outdoor enclosures must be safe and secure, and should provide enrichment opportunities and sufficient choice for tortoises to access their environmental needs. When designing outdoor enclosures, hard landscaping in terms of enclosure boundaries, and the structures within, have to be considered.
DIY enthusiast	Creating indoor and outdoor accommodation may require a number of basic practical skills such as carpentry, fixing equipment to the structures created. Forward thinking will be needed to ensure that all available resources are used to their best effect. Safely setting up equipment and knowing your own limitations is important – it may be necessary to call in professional advice and expertise, particularly when setting up electrical equipment. Keeping animals and humans safe is absolutely critical, as the potential for injury or a fire can be significant.
Conservationist	As keepers of often endangered species of tortoises, we have a moral duty to ensure that any tortoises we own have been responsibly sourced. It is easy to unwittingly make financial payments for animals without fully understanding or meeting the relevant legal requirements of ownership. Legislation, certificate and registration requirements, together with CITES listings and trade rules, are all subject to change, sometimes very quickly. Checking government websites and international listings of endangered species before making any purchase is highly recommended. We can help the conservation efforts for some species, for example by breeding individuals through schemes such as the European Studbook Foundation. We would not want to contribute to the demise of any species by collecting individuals obtained illegitimately or illegally. Collectively we all have a responsibility to avoid contributing to the extinction of species, to climate change or to habitat destruction through our actions.

Sharing ideas with other keepers can be hugely beneficial, but only if those ideas represent best practice. In many cases, tortoise keepers, not knowing any better, will advise the use of methods that they have adhered to for a long time, without fully understanding that these might actually be detrimental to the health and well-being of their tortoises. There is often an assumption that because

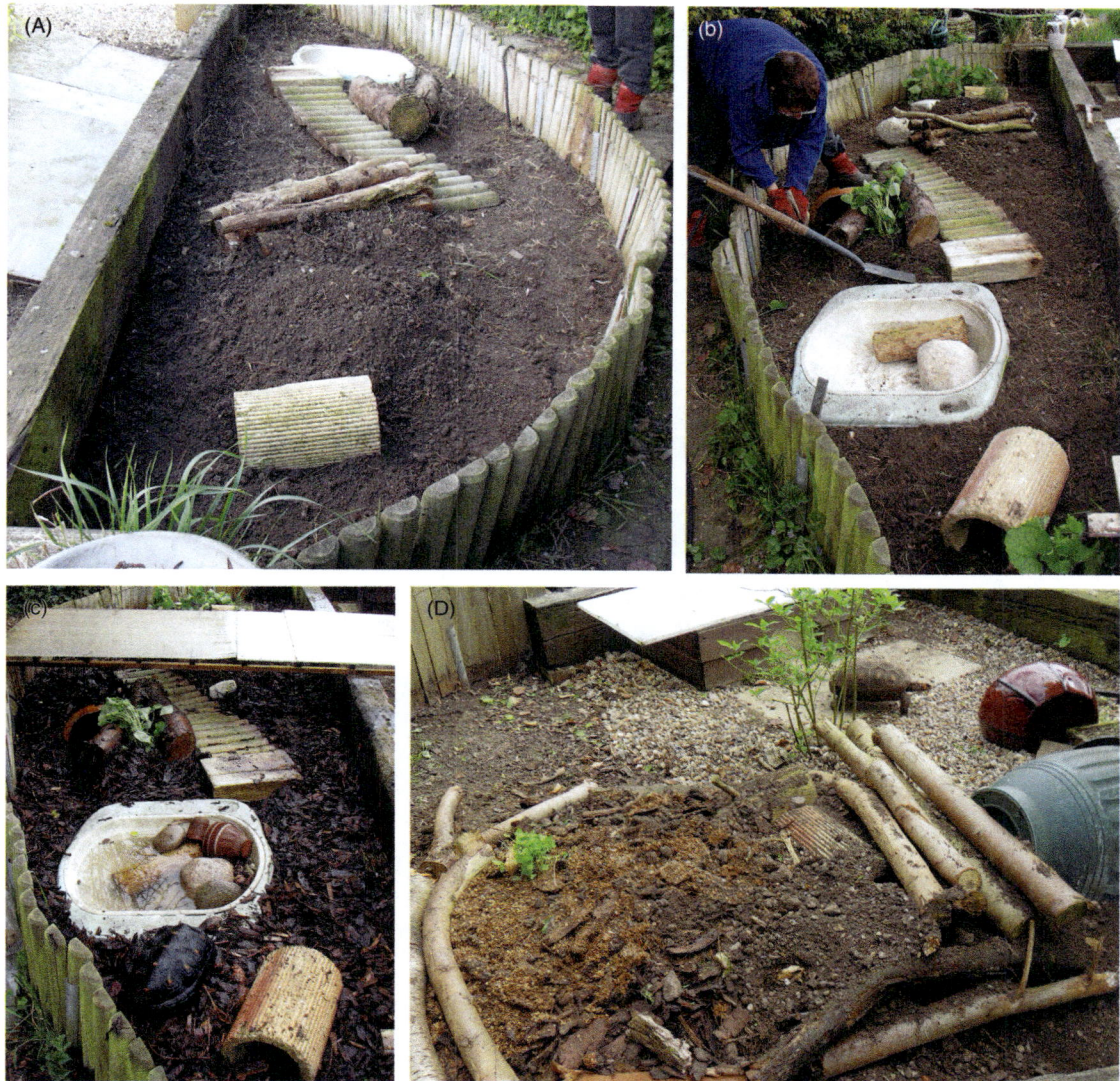

Fig. 18.5. Red-footed tortoise enclosure being created, with bath, a soft humid substrate that can be used for nesting, opportunities to increase temperature under polycarbonate, enriched surfaces and calcium carbonate rocks.

a particular practice has been carried out for many years 'and the tortoise isn't dead yet', this means that it is a practice that should be stuck with, even in the face of other more modern or more scientific evidence to the contrary.

For example, UK keepers who report that 'for over 40 years their tortoise has happily been hibernated/brumated in the garden shed for 5 months of the year' (or more), are unaware of the research into how these tortoises live in the wild. This research shows that hibernation should be for a considerably shorter time period if the tortoise is to remain healthy. In fact, hibernation should be similar in length to that in the wild, at around 8 weeks for most hibernating species (McArthur *et al.*, 2004; McArthur, 2012). Keepers who subject their tortoises to much longer hibernations may not realize that their tortoise has in fact been gradually slowing down, being less active and feeding less well, when out of hibernation. This leaves the tortoise more susceptible to disease and illness, resulting ultimately in an early death. Of course,

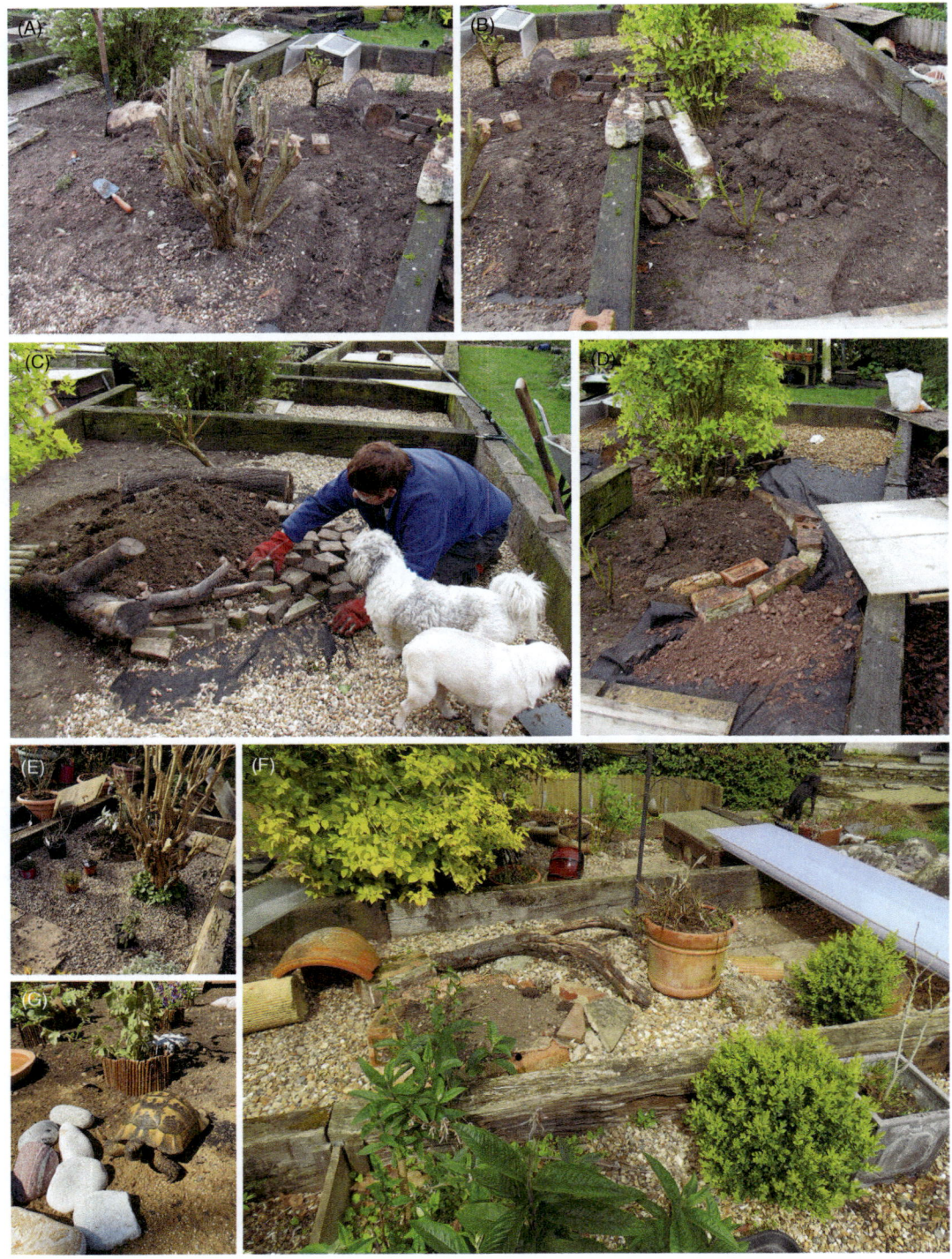

Fig. 18.6. Mediterranean tortoise enclosures being created with varied substrates, opportunities for digging and nesting, planting for forage and to create microclimates and increased humidity, basking areas, hides and retreats.

in such long-lived species an early death can be decades later.

It often takes a long time for poor husbandry to kill a tortoise. They can survive but not thrive under regimes with poor husbandry for many years. For many species of tortoise, life expectancy is 100 years or more. Tortoises who die in captivity prior to 80–100 years are usually tortoises who have experienced bad husbandry. If you have managed to keep a tortoise alive for 20 years this does not imply that it has had a long life.

Attending conferences and meetings (face-to-face or remote) can provide good avenues for chatting with other keepers and getting ideas, such as the ETA conference whose attendees are shown in Fig. 18.2. It is important to engage with reputable organizations, however, as these are the key to good experiences and to gaining positive, current, accurate and useful information on tortoise keeping, such as Tortoise South East whose workshop is shown Fig. 18.3 or the Norfolk Tortoise Club whose meeting is shown in Fig. 18.4.

Some useful organizations to consider engaging with, where sources of information are evidence-based, are listed in Tables 18.1 and 18.2.

Many of these information sources are referenced in the individual chapters of this book. These are all reputable organizations who report on evidence-based research, and many are peer-reviewed publications.

Keeping up with recent book publications can be expensive. Libraries can be very helpful in this regard. A list of useful books is provided at the end of each chapter in this publication. Reading scientific articles online can also be more cost-effective, where these are available free. YouTube, Instagram, Facebook and other social media platforms can also be useful sources of information, but they are not regulated in terms of the content. They can be beneficial, or can be harmful, in terms of the advice given.

The organizations suggested above are more likely to provide accurate information than some other sources. They are all involved in educating owners and keepers, involving local people where tortoises are indigenous, and have a focus on a scientific approach to husbandry, care and welfare.

Practical skills sets

Keeping tortoises gives those of us who love and admire these animals a great deal of pleasure. As a hobby and interest, tortoise keeping affords great rewards – doing a good job of keeping them healthy and well brings an enormous sense of satisfaction. Some keepers have just one tortoise, others keep larger numbers, or have collections of several species, at which point the interest can become all-consuming (and very expensive).

Keepers can spend large amounts of time, energy and money continuously striving to keep their tortoises in the best possible conditions. Indeed, this is what we should all be doing – given that these animals are completely dependent upon us to provide all their daily needs. Once taken into captivity, or having been born into captivity, these tortoises have lost many of their free choices. They cannot select their environment to meet their needs as they would in the wild. We have to provide the suitable environment (Highfield, 1996). They cannot find food unless we provide it and they can only eat what we provide. Time, energy, money and imagination are all essential when creating captive environments to suit the needs of individual animals, as shown in Fig. 18.5 where a pen for Red-footed tortoises is being created.

Effective tortoise keepers need to develop sufficient levels of skill in all of the following areas when creating indoor and outdoor accommodation for tortoises in captivity. If keepers do not feel confident that they have or can develop the skills necessary, professional help should be sought, particularly for those areas which have health or safety implications (Biedenweg and Schramm, 2019). Table 18.3 identifies the key areas of practical skills involved in setting up tortoise enclosures, which are being put to good use in Fig. 18.6 when building pens for Mediterranean tortoises. If in any doubt at all regarding your own competence, particularly around electrical products and installations, seek professional help.

Your safety and that of your tortoises are the highest priority when carrying out these building and maintenance projects.

Planning and preparation are everything

'If you fail to plan then you plan to fail,' as Benjamin Franklin allegedly rightly said. If you are reading this book as a prospective tortoise keeper – doing your research before getting a new companion – well done! It is much better to think through how much of your home the tortoise will need to occupy, how much of your garden will need to be given up in order to make a tortoise enclosure and to consider the costs involved in keeping tortoises **before you get one**.

Preparation and set-up are both essential before you start. Obtaining a tortoise as an impulse buy is a very bad idea. In many countries, reptile events, where animals are sold off-the-cuff to potential owners, have been restricted or banned. This is to prevent impulse buys, which often lead to the animal being rejected or abandoned (in many cases having been neglected) because the implications of keeping such a pet have not been thought through beforehand.

Deciding on what you can offer a tortoise, putting that in place and then obtaining the animal from a reputable source is much the best plan. These animals will outlive a human, given the right conditions, so preparation for the long term is also something we all need to consider as tortoise keepers. When we reach a stage when we can no longer care for our tortoises, we need to have thought about the next keeper who will be able to do the best for our tortoises.

This is often a very difficult decision, and one which many of us will struggle with at some stage of tortoise ownership. I have taken in tortoises from elderly owners, or those who have become too ill to care for their animals, many times in the past 30 years. It is much better for an owner to make the decision themselves to rehome, having thought this through and chosen someone suitable and informed, rather than leaving the decision to a relative who has no knowledge or links with tortoise people.

The process is emotionally distressing for many keepers, having had the tortoise in their lives (and with their family) for perhaps 50 years. To take this step requires a good deal of selflessness and a real desire to do the right thing by the tortoise. It also requires a high level of trust in the person being given the tortoise. Owners need to feel confident that their tortoise will continue to be cared for. Establishing a relationship with an owner is often key to this. This is where local groups and organizations can be so valuable, in establishing links and providing opportunities for networking at the community level.

Conclusion

Developing the knowledge and skills sets needed to do a good job as a tortoise keeper may look daunting from the information in this chapter. However, it is much better to be prepared for the demands of ownership than to stumble upon them through trial and error, often at the expense of the tortoise. This chapter sets out those requirements. Reptiles and tortoises, in particular, are fascinating animals. Without that feeling and commitment to do the best for them, we may not be driven to provide for their needs. The more we know about them, the more there is to know about the best practices we should put in place as keepers.

Reptile rescue centres often have huge demands placed on them. Suitable new homes may be limited or unavailable. Fortunately, the days of taking a tortoise home in a brown paper bag are long gone – but new challenges emerge as we see an increasing variety of tortoise species traded around the world. Taking ethical issues into account and addressing the challenges involved in meeting a tortoise's needs has become (and continues to become) more complex.

We have an increasing responsibility to these hugely important animals, in a world where climate change and loss of biodiversity are becoming more and more significant. The safe maintenance of tortoises in captivity is likely to become even more important as the natural world changes. Private collections are inevitably going to become more vital as contributors to breeding and conservation programmes coordinated by zoos and other organizations. One example is the European Studbook Foundation (ESF), which coordinates breeding programmes in Europe, enabling breeding stock to be spread out, thus mitigating against some of the challenges associated with the spread of disease through collections.

Whether you own one tortoise, or many, the responsibility on all of us as keepers is to:

- Source tortoises responsibly without negatively impacting the future of the species
- Know the species
- Know the individual animals
- Do our very best to create the most suitable enclosures we can in captivity
- Use husbandry techniques that give the tortoises maximum opportunity to live long, healthy lives.

References and Further Reading

Sources of information and helpful organizations are listed in this chapter in Tables 18.1 and 18.2.

Biedenweg, F. and Schramm, R. (2019) The Egyptian Tortoise *Testudo kleinmanni* Lortet 1883 A Fascinating

Little Beauty. Tartaruga-Verlag Ricarda Schramm, Grebenhain, Germany

Highfield, A. (1996) *Practical Encyclopaedia of Keeping and Breeding Tortoises and Freshwater Turtles*. Carapace Press, London.

McArthur, S. (2012) *Chelonian Medicine: Improving Standards for Captive Chelonia in the UK*. Proceedings of Tortoise Welfare UK Conference 17 November 2012

McArthur, S., Wilkinson, R. and Meyer, J. (2004) *Medicine and Surgery of Tortoises and Turtles*. Blackwell, Oxford, UK

Mellor, D.J. (2016a) Updating animal welfare thinking: Moving beyond the 'Five Freedoms' to 'A Life worth Living'. *Animals* 6, 21.

Mellor, D.J. (2016b) Moving beyond the 'Five Freedoms' by updating the 'Five Provisions' and introducing aligned 'Animal Welfare Aims'. *Animals* 6(10), 59.

Yeates, J. (2022) Ch 1 Animal ethics and welfare. In: Rendle, M. and Hinde-Megarity, J. (eds) *BSAVA Manual of Practical Veterinary Welfare*. BSAVA, Quedgeley, UK, pp. 1–17.

19 Health and Safety for the Tortoise Keeper and Tortoise

Abstract
This chapter looks at elements of the physical environment we create for tortoises in captivity that require special attention from a health and safety perspective. This includes anything electrical, which requires us to follow all safety guidelines and instructions on equipment, and to ensure the safety of our tortoises by restricting any access to any electrical fittings or cables. We should also be prepared to call in professional help for any electrical installations beyond our capabilities.

Within the physical environment, aspects of the enclosures created that may have associated health risks are discussed, including water features and access to water.

The chapter also looks at issues of biosecurity for both tortoises and humans, including the need for good hygiene when handling tortoises and when preparing food. The potential for disease transmission through pathogens is discussed along with the need for us as keepers to be aware of the possible zoonosis risks to our health.

All things electrical

Lighting should be positioned safely in relation to the tortoise. The basking lights should be overhead. They should be at a suitable height to provide the necessary temperature needed to maintain the preferred body temperature, but far enough away from the tortoise to prevent burns (see Chapter 4 on artificial light and heat). The surface underneath the lamps should be flat so that there is the least possible opportunity for any animal to fall onto its back and overheat (Fig. 19.1).

Heat sources such as ceramic and infrared heaters should also be overhead and used with a thermostat to control temperatures. Underfloor heating or sidewall pads should be avoided, as the tortoise can come into contact with these and be in danger of burns or electrocution if there is any wear and tear to the fittings. The surface underneath heaters should be flat so that there is the least possible opportunity for any animal to fall onto its back and overheat (Fig. 19.2).

Lamp and heater holders need to be ceramic or heat-resistant, as they get very hot and plastic fittings can melt or catch fire. Always follow the manufacturer's specifications for fittings. Cables also need to be of a suitable specification, as they can also get hot near the heat or light source.

Cables should be away from the tortoises and safely secured to avoid any trip hazards for the keeper. Plugs should be kept away from the animals and made easily accessible for the keeper. Fuses should offer the correct level of safety and be used together with an electric circuit breaker for human and tortoise safety (Fig. 19.3).

The manufacturer's instructions should be followed and, if in any doubt, professional help from a qualified electrician should be sought.

Ensure that smoke detectors are fitted in case of a fire. Check all fittings regularly and replace any that are worn or damaged.

Any electrical fencing used as a predator deterrent in outdoor enclosures should also be well maintained and meet the correct specifications.

Receiving an electric shock is a potential hazard for keeper and tortoises if correct procedures are not in place. It goes without saying that the animals must not be able to touch or dislodge electrical fittings. All cables and fixtures must be secured and away from the tortoises. Tortoises can receive a shock if they touch exposed cables or fittings, as can humans.

A residual current device (RCD), is a very effective safety measure to have in your home to prevent a potentially fatal shock from touching something live, such as a bare wire. These devices can also be helpful in protecting against electrical fires. An RCD is a very sensitive safety device that

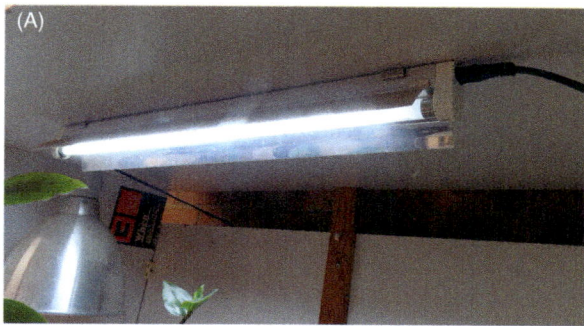
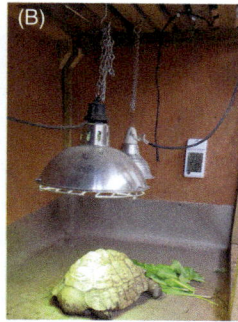

Fig. 19.1. (A) Overhead fluorescent/LED lighting with reflector for increased efficiency. (B) Overhead basking spotlight, with protective grill across, which can reduce amount of light (see Chapter 4 on artificial light and heat) but is safer in terms of reduced access to the hottest part of the light. The metal chain allows the height to be altered to suit the tortoise and type of light to ensure that it is not close enough to overheat or burn the tortoise. The metal is non-combustible (so a safe material) with flexibility of use, for suspending lights or heaters.

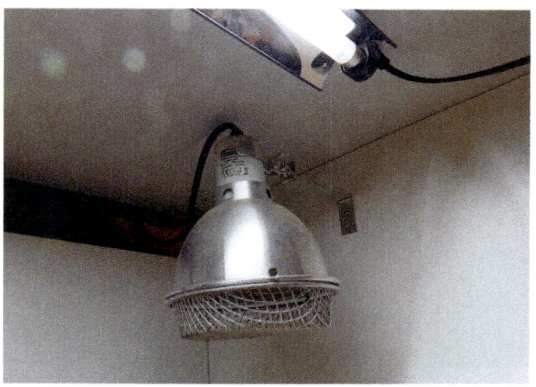

Fig. 19.2. Overhead heating attached to side-wall and clearance above, with protective grill for additional safety.

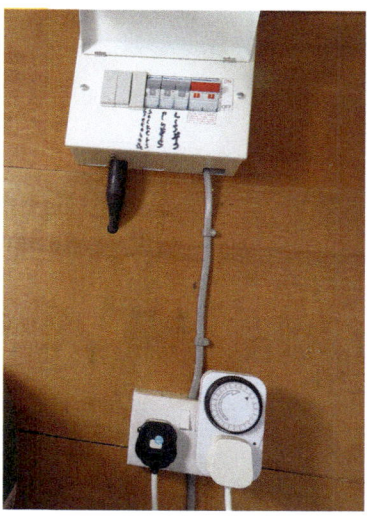

Fig. 19.3. Securing cables and fittings is essential. This fuse board has an RCD fitted for additional safety.

switches off electricity automatically if there is any fault, and to protect against the risks of electrocution.

Access to water

Water and electricity do not make safe companions unless well fitted and with a distance between them. Electrical fittings must always be well away from water sources. Tortoises need easy access in and out of shallow water trays (Highfield, 2008; Highfield and Highfield, 2009). The depth and size of the tray will depend on the tortoise. Trays should be sunk into the substrate and made of strong solid material that can be easily cleaned. Tortoises can fall onto their backs in their water, which can make the water a drowning hazard if it is too deep. Plastic or terracotta plant drip trays make very good shallow baths. The water temperature should be lukewarm – dip your elbow in to check or use a thermometer.

Creation of habitats and enclosures

Creating safe enclosures is key to tortoise health. Solid enclosure sides are needed to reduce the tortoise's attempts to escape. Scrabbling at the sides

Health and Safety

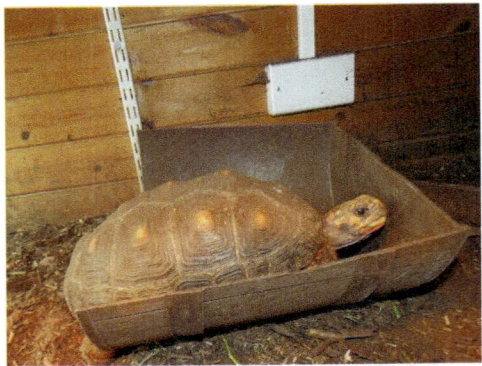

Fig. 19.4. All inclusions in the enclosures should be safely located and fitted, as should electrical fittings – not like this.

of the enclosure could lead to injury (particularly if the sides are made of wire) or the tortoise falling onto its back.

Internal furniture and enrichment provision should be secure to prevent this from happening. Figure 19.4 shows a Red-footed tortoise trapped in a hide, which should not happen.

The use of camera systems to allow observation from a distance can be a huge advantage in terms of observing natural behaviour without human interference.

Indoor enclosures

Indoor provision needs to be in a suitable building that is safe from predators and theft. It must be

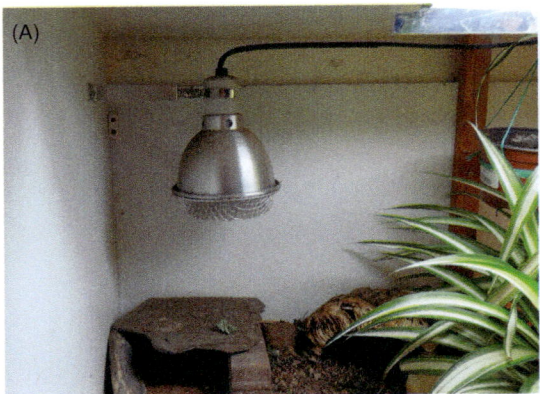
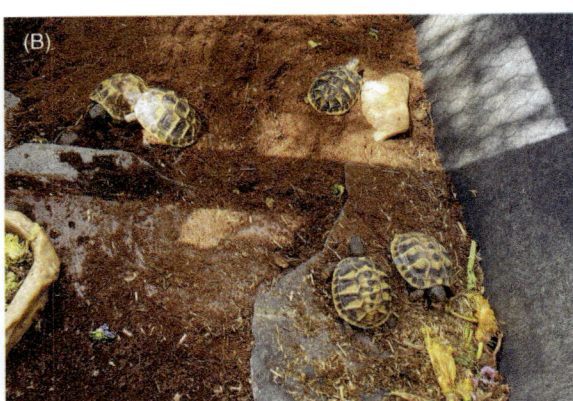

Fig. 19.5. (A) Indoor enclosure with solid sides high enough for the tortoise not to be able to climb out. This is the rear of the terrarium, made of wood coated with laminate for easy cleaning. The front will need to be low enough to allow easy access for cleaning and for ventilation. (B) Open sides and/or top are the best design to achieve this, as shown in an outdoor enclosure for juveniles made from a large heavy-duty fish container.

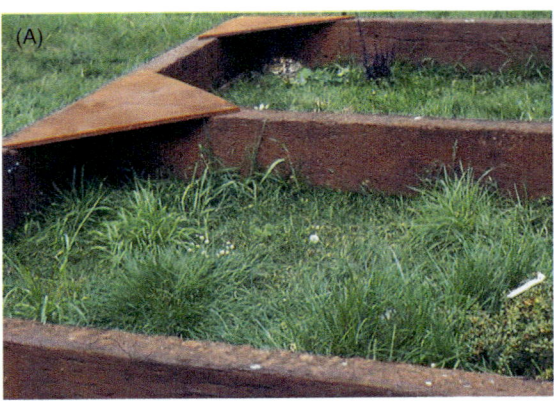
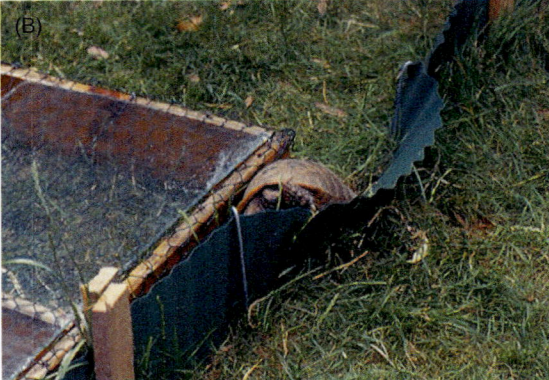

Fig. 19.6. Outdoor enclosures showing (A) secure corners and (B) escapee with inadequate fencing, which is too low and not solid.

252   Chapter 19

possible to achieve and maintain suitable temperatures for the species of tortoise being kept.

Indoor enclosures should be made of wood, or laminated wood, and must be built to fit the available space, giving the tortoise the maximum area in which to walk. Laminated surfaces have the advantage of being waterproof and easy to clean (Fig. 19.5A). Alternatively, the wood can be made waterproof with sealers or varnish, or it can be covered with a pond-liner.

Smoke detectors should always be installed and regularly tested in rooms and buildings where tortoises are kept. Fire is always a potential hazard where there are heaters and hot lamps in use.

The possibility of fire as a hazard exists when there is a chance of hot lights or heaters coming into contact with combustible materials. Materials that can easily catch fire include paper, wood, cardboard, clothing, some plastics, sawdust, hay, straw and woodchips. This is particularly so if these materials are dry. Some of the materials listed may be considered by keepers as suitable substrates for tortoises. For this reason alone (and there are other welfare reasons, as described in Chapter 3 on captive environments) they are not. Substrates must always be non-combustible, which is why soil and sand, sometimes combined with compost, coco-coir or bark (depending upon the species), should be chosen. Paper should never be used near heaters or lights, as the risk of fire is very high.

The risk of clothing catching fire should also be remembered: when carrying out maintenance, repairs or fitting of heat and light fixtures, everything should be turned off and cool, for the safety of the keeper.

Outdoor enclosures

Outdoor enclosures must be solidly constructed from tough materials (Fig. 19.5B). Tortoises are surprisingly strong and often much better at digging and climbing than we imagine, especially the large species such as Sulcatas. Walls of wood such as railway sleepers and scaffold boards, or concrete blocks and bricks can all be positioned to create safe, secure enclosures. Corners should have protection so that the tortoise cannot climb up the sides (Fig. 19.6A). Generally, the height of the sides should be twice the length of the tortoise, with escapees likely where the sides are too low or lacking strength, as seen in Fig. 19.6B. The sides should be sunk into the soil to prevent digging underneath.

Tortoises should be kept safe from predators such as rats, foxes, raccoons, mink, coyote and dogs, or large birds such as raptors or corvids. It is a good idea to increase security for juveniles, as their small size makes them more vulnerable to predation. A strong mesh cover can be placed over the enclosure.

Where electric fencing is used as a deterrent to predators, all legal requirements and safety guidance should be followed in terms of location and use. These systems can present a hazard to both humans and the tortoises if not installed correctly. When used properly they can be very effective in protecting tortoises and turtles (and their nests) against predators such as racoons and foxes (Geller, 2012).

Other forms of protection from predators include ultrasonic pest repellents. Red-blinking lights can be used, particularly at night, to mimic the appearance of an animal's eyes. This may deter any approaching predator. Motion detectors can be used to alert the keeper to the approach of predators or thieves, but only if they are monitored or linked to an alarm.

The use of camera systems allows the keeper to observe tortoises from a distance, which is useful for welfare and for behaviour observations. In addition, such cameras can be a deterrent to theft and a record of any such event. Similarly, the cameras can be used to record the presence of predators.

Protection against loss or theft, with the added benefit of being able to identify your tortoise if found, is provided through microchipping. Microchipping of tortoises once they have reached a certain size, for example 60 mm length in the UK, is required before they are bought or sold, if they are listed as CITES Appendix I or II Animals, and/or EU Annex A, depending upon species. The smallest type of microchip is used, as the tortoise is relatively small, and it is inserted in the back left leg (Fig. 19.7).

If a microchip is not available, but you would want to be able to identify your tortoise if lost or stolen, take very detailed photographs of the carapace, front and rear of the tortoise. You will also need a photograph of the plastron, which also has a unique pattern from which your tortoise could be identified, as shown in Fig. 19.8.

Biosecurity and health of the tortoise

(See also Chapter 7 on common illnesses and diseases.)
There are two areas of concern here:

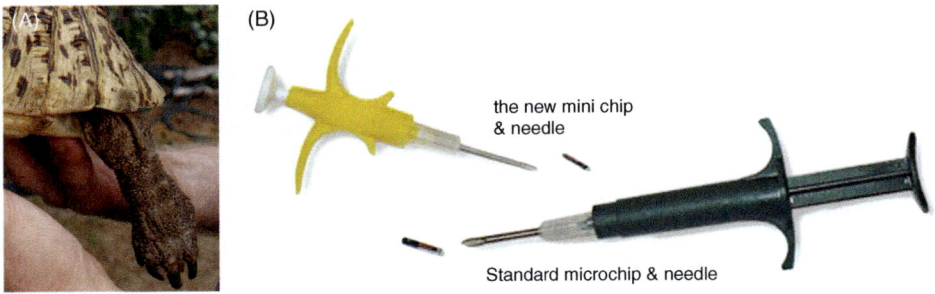

Fig. 19.7. (A) Position of microchip in leg. (B) Example of microchip insertion equipment (Eleanor Lien-Hua Tirtasana Chubb).

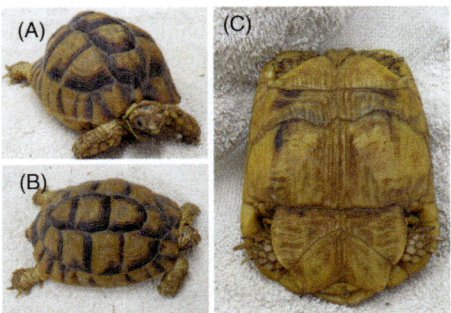

Fig. 19.8. Identification photographs of an Egyptian tortoise.

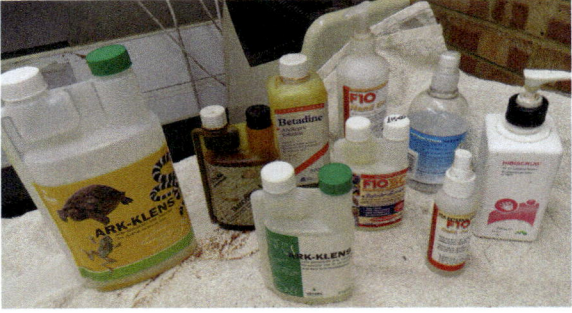

Fig. 19.9. Cleaning products: Hibiscrub®; Tamodine®; Betadine®; Arklens®; F10®.

1. Harmful organisms (pathogens) can cause disease in tortoises. These organisms exist in the environment and so good hygiene measures are essential to ensure that high levels of pathogens do not build up in enclosures, or in food or water. Keeping clean, well-maintained tortoises is the best way to ensure both their health and safety and that of the humans around them.

2. Keeping more than one tortoise means that, potentially, diseases can be passed from one to the other. The general principle is that tortoises of different species should not be kept together. This ensures that disease is unlikely to be transmitted from one to the other. Hand-washing when handling is essential, as you move from one enclosure to another. When introducing new tortoises, a 6-month minimum quarantine is essential, ideally 12 months, so that any disease can be manifest and identified (Highfield, 1996).

There are some very infectious diseases that are easily passed between tortoises. These include the bacterial *Mycoplasma* infections (*Mycoplasma agassizi*) linked to upper respiratory tract disease (URTD) or runny nose syndrome (RNS), and tortoise herpesvirus, which is a very serious, usually fatal disease (100% death rates are reported). Unlike the human herpesvirus, which is often only a mild infection, tortoise herpesvirus infects many organs, causing lesions, swelling, respiratory and liver damage. Infections of testudine intranuclear coccidiosis (TINC) have been reported in tortoises in recent years. One species of which we are aware, *Cryptosporidium*, can be transmitted to humans through water. Of course there may be others yet to be discovered.

Use of safe cleaning products such as Hibiscrub®, Tamodine, Arklens (Vetark®) and F10 to ensure that enclosures are clean is vital, without causing harm to the tortoises.

Zoonosis and health of the keeper

Some pathogens can be passed from tortoises to people – hence the need for good hygiene when handling tortoises. The use of gloves when handling

Table 19.1. Common pathogens that may cause disease in humans (note this list is not exhaustive but includes the more common pathogens).

Pathogen	Notes
Tuberculosis (*Mycobacterium tuberculosis*) or TB	TB is a serious illness, which may cause no symptoms in its early stages. The early signs of infection include persistent cough as the disease affects the lungs. If left untreated, other parts of the body can become infected and ultimately the disease can be fatal. Other symptoms include fever, weight loss and exhaustion. This bacterium is spread through close contact with an infected animal.
Intestinal pathogens such as *Campylobacter*, *Salmonella* and *E. coli*	Tortoises can shed *Campylobacter*, *Salmonella* and *Escherichia coli* bacteria in their faeces without any signs of disease themselves. A tortoise may appear to have normal faeces, with no sign of diarrhoea for example, but still be passing these types of pathogen. Good hygiene and husbandry in enclosures is very important to prevent faeces build-up in enclosures. Similarly, good hand hygiene after handling tortoises is essential, especially before eating or drinking. These organisms are present in food and in the environment. They can pass through the gut of tortoises without being destroyed, hence they can be passed out in faeces. Handling of waste products from your tortoises should always be carried out with good hygiene practices, wearing gloves for example.
Cryptosporidium	This bacterial species can be transmitted to humans through water. Boiling water can kill the organism. Hand-washing with soap and hot water can also remove the risk of contamination.
Leptospirosis	*Leptospira* bacteria are common in water and soil. Infection occurs from the urine of rats and mice, which, if present in water or soil, can be passed to humans through the skin of the nose, mouth or eyes, or through a wound in the skin. It is important to protect tortoises from the presence of rodents, as they can cause significant damage. Their presence in enclosures can allow this bacterium to be present within the enclosure.

is good practice. Alternatively, the use of suitable hand sanitizers, either alcohol-based or water-based, is essential. One of the simplest ways to destroy bacteria and other pathogens is washing hands with soap (e.g. Hibiscrub) and hot water.

Tortoises may carry pathogens without showing any signs of illness themselves. This makes it even more important that we look after our own health as we care for our tortoises (Rendle and Jones, 2022 p. 214).

Tortoise food should be kept away from human food as a general principle. Where the tortoise is eating plant material, and in particular naturally growing plants and weeds, the risk is less than if the tortoise requires meat, or other animal products, as part of the diet. Animal products themselves can also be a potential source of infection to humans. Where tortoises are being fed small mice, pinkies or other small rodents, scrupulous hygiene is required. Keeping such foods frozen until they are needed is a safe approach, but again these food items should be stored away from human food. Care must be taken when defrosting, and hands sanitized after handling such foods.

Some pathogens can be transmitted in water, so it is essential to always wash your hands using soap after handling or cleaning your tortoise enclosures and water sources.

Some examples of diseases that may be passed to humans include the pathogens in Table 19.1. If in any doubt seek medical advice and be sure to mention that you are a reptile keeper when describing symptoms to a health professional.

Conclusion

Human and tortoise health and safety should always be the first considerations and top priority when handling and interacting with our pets. We should avoid over-handling anyway (Rendle and Jones, 2022), bearing in mind the needs of the tortoise and that these are wild animals not in any way domesticated. But from a hygiene perspective, limiting physical interactions is beneficial for both animal and human.

Safety considerations are paramount, and minimizing risk should be the starting point for all our activities with tortoises. Whether we are building or maintaining enclosures, carrying out husbandry with the tortoises or planning breeding programmes, safety in terms of the physical environment and in terms of disease reduction should be key to our actions.

The highest possible levels of hygiene should be employed when removing tortoise waste products and uneaten food. Good hygiene, in particular hand-washing, is absolutely essential in ensuring that we do not contract pathogens from our pets. Only by using good hygiene techniques can we give ourselves the best possible chance of ensuring our own good health.

Similarly, we need to maintain hygiene when handling different species and between groups of tortoises. It is important to prevent the spread of disease within one location, and between collections if we take in new animals or some of our animals are involved in breeding programmes elsewhere.

Fortunately, the recorded incidence of disease being passed from tortoises to humans is low, but there is little research in this area. It is likely, therefore, that there have been transmissions that have not been noted. There are relatively few recorded pathogens that can pass disease from tortoises to us, which also reduces the risk. With sensible, simple hygiene techniques we can keep ourselves safe from any disease our tortoises may have. We can also keep our tortoises healthy by preventing transmission of disease between individuals.

References and Further Reading

CITES: Convention on International Trade in Endangered Species of Wild Flora and Fauna, Geneva. Website: www.cites.org

Geller, G.A. (2012) Reducing predation of freshwater turtle nests with a simple electric fence. *Herpetological Review* 43(3), 398–403.

Highfield, A. (1996) *Practical Encyclopaedia of Keeping and Breeding Tortoises and Freshwater Turtles*. Carapace Press, London.

Highfield, A. and Highfield, N. (2008) *Taking Care of Pet Tortoises*. The Tortoise Trust Jill Martin Fund. Available from: www.tortoisetrust.org

Highfield, A. and Highfield, N. (2009) *Keeping a Pet Tortoise*. Interpet, Dorking, UK.

Rendle, M. and Jones, B. (2022) Ch 9 One Health. In: Rendle, M. and Hinde-Megarity, J. (eds) *BSAVA Manual of Practical Veterinary Welfare*. BSAVA, Quedgeley, UK, pp. 209–229.

20 Tortoise Keeping – Past, Present, Future

Abstract

This chapter summarizes tortoise keeping in the past 50 years, looks at the current situation in brief and speculates on the potential ways in which tortoise keeping might develop into the future. As wild animals, not domesticated in any way, animals such as tortoises being kept as pets brings with it many ethical questions.

A trade in exotics where animals are commercially bred on a large scale for profit, or taken from the wild, is problematic in terms of conservation and species loss. The role of retailers is considered and whether they can be encouraged or regulated to do more in educating potential and novice keepers. Sales through online outlets can lead more easily to impulse buys, which are less likely to be beneficial in outcome for individual tortoises. Currently this is a huge global industry worth billions of dollars. Approximately 13,000 exotic species are currently traded, some of which are very challenging to care for. Some consideration is given to potential control of this trade, and whether this can be effectively achieved, as many species of tortoise are now listed by the IUCN as endangered or critically endangered.

This chapter considers the ethics of keeping tortoises as pets. Should we keep them at all? What are the potential gains and losses for individual animals and for the species? The issues considered apply to private keepers, as well as those in establishments with larger collections, such as zoos. The role of breeding programmes is also considered, along with the work of rescue and rehabilitation centres, who are left to cope when overproduction leads to unwanted pets. The reasons for relinquishment are also considered in the current economic climate.

The innovative ways in which some projects are using technology and other means to carry out research in the field to identify the status of some species is discussed. The impact of such research on their listing on CITES and the IUCN, so that they more accurately reflect their wild populations, is discussed. The other pressures on tortoise populations, due to a range of human activities, are mentioned briefly.

The need for ethical sourcing of tortoises as pets is included, along with consideration of the 'One Health' concept when considering the relationships between tortoises and humans, and their value and benefit to humans. What is the cost to the tortoises?

How did pet tortoise keeping start?

Pet keeping has been a part of human culture for at least 12,000 years (Yeates, 2022). In the 19th century collection of specimens without consideration of welfare was common in the UK (Ritvo, 1994). In developed countries, pet keeping on a large scale across much of the population did not really increase until after the Second World War. Stability following the war led to increased prosperity and disposable income. This meant that larger numbers of people could afford to own a pet.

Keeping exotics such as tortoises began on a much smaller scale, but tortoises have always been particularly popular in the UK. This followed the Victorian era (1837–1901) when there was a national obsession with collecting specimens (both dead and alive) of newly discovered species from all over the world. Charles Darwin's travels to the Galapagos Islands early in the period (1831–1835), together with publication of his journals in 1838, brought tortoises to the attention of many people. When he published his revolutionary theory *On the Origin of Species through Natural Selection* in 1859, his observations of Galapagos tortoises were included (Darwin, 1859).

The keeping of tortoises as pets increased rapidly in the UK through the 1960s and into the 1980s. All of the animals would have been wild-caught. It was not until 1984 that a ban on the importation of Mediterranean tortoises (which made up the vast majority of pet tortoises at that time) came into force across Europe. Wild populations had been decimated by local people, collecting for the pet trade. Mediterranean tortoises were almost at the point of extinction in some areas.

Trade in some species was severely restricted following the creation of the Convention on International Trade in Endangered Species (CITES) by the United Nations General Assembly. This was passed in 1973 and came into force in 1975.

CITES rules require documentation for the import, export and sale of listed species, and may also limit the numbers of animals of particular species. This control of trade made tortoises more valuable than they had previously been.

Those species that were not protected by the 1984 importation ban were the most heavily traded. This meant an escalation in the trade in species from Africa and Eurasia as alternative sources for pet keeping were sought. The Tortoise Trust reported in 1992 that 'between 1965 and 1971 a total of 119,319 Horsfield's tortoises were received at UK ports'. This species has not been included in the importation ban and does not require documentation for importation (Highfield, 1992).

By the late 1990s, huge numbers of tortoises were being imported commercially for the pet trade. At that time a large number of African Spurred tortoises (*Centrochelys sulcata*) were imported. In 1991 another ban on importation of tortoises was implemented across Europe, adding 18 species to the Mediterranean species already listed.

Table 20.1. Species listed on the European 1984 tortoise importation ban (Vetter, 2002; 2004; 2005; 2006).

Name	Species
1. Hermann's tortoise	(*Testudo hermanni* spp.)
2. Spur-thighed tortoise	(*Testudo graeca* spp.)
3. Marginated tortoise	(*Testudo marginata*)
4. Aldabra Giant tortoise	(*Aldabrachelys gigantea*)
5. Galápagos Giant tortoise	(*Chelonoidis nigra*)
6. Radiated tortoise	(*Astrochelys radiata*)
7. Bolson tortoise	(*Gopherus flavomarginatus*)
8. Burmese Star tortoise	(*Geochelone platynota*)
9. Angulated tortoise	(*Chersina angulata*)
10. Indian Star tortoise	(*Geochelone elegans*)
11. Madagascar Flat-tailed tortoise	(*Pyxis planicauda*)
12. Egyptian tortoise	(*Testudo kleinmanni*)
13. Leopard tortoise	(*Centrochelys pardalis*)
14. Bell's Hingeback tortoise	(*Kinixys belliana*)
15. Elongated tortoise	(*Indotestudo elongata*)
16. Forsten's tortoise	(*Indotestudo forstenii*)
17. Impressed tortoise	(*Manouria impressa*)
18. Ploughshare tortoise	(*Astrochelys yniphora*)
19. Red-footed tortoise	(*Chelonoidis carbonaria*)
20. Yellow-footed tortoise	(*Chelonoidis denticulata*)

In 2002 the UK Government Department for Food and Rural Affairs (DEFRA) commissioned a report from TRAFFIC. This report, *Selling Like Hot Cakes* (Pendry and Allan, 2002) revealed that the on-going legal and illegal trade in tortoises into Great Britain was much larger than had been realized.

The TRAFFIC report noted that up to 2000 animals (80% of imported tortoises) were wild-caught. Of course, these are the numbers of legal imports; the numbers of animals being illegally traded cannot be known.

From the year 2000 onwards, the numbers of captive-bred tortoises increased, due to the importation restrictions, but the demand for tortoises did not diminish. Legal and illegal importation continued, as it does today on an ever-increasing scale it would seem.

What did tortoise keeping look like up to the 2020s?

From the 1960s in the UK a huge number of households had a pet Mediterranean tortoise. These animals often did not live long, because so little was known about how to care for them. This trend followed in Europe, and in both locations many tortoises died in the cold wet climate. Many more died from excessively long hibernations/brumations, as in the early days tortoises were considered to be 'garden' pets. Even if it was cold and wet, they stayed outdoors with no support. Often left to hibernate in the garden they went into hibernation earlier, and came out later, than in their natural habitat (see Chapter 12 on hibernation).

There was little information available for tortoise keepers about their natural environment or their needs. The concept of pet welfare was in its infancy. Tortoises were freely available in pet shops across Europe until 1984 and it was not uncommon for crates of them to be seen stacked outside shops in London and other cities, or sold at markets.

Once sold, they would often be thrust into a thick brown paper bag to be taken home. Due to the stress of being carried and moved it was not unusual for them to urinate in the bag, which then fell apart. By the time the buyer had reached home, walking or on public transport, the tortoise had fallen out of the bag, to survive as best as it could on the streets of London or another city.

Many tortoises were kept free-ranging in a garden, which was often not secure. It was common for them to dig out or escape through gaps in fences.

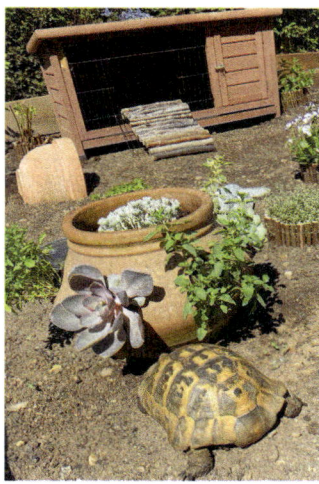

Fig. 20.1. 'Garden tortoise' in enriched garden.

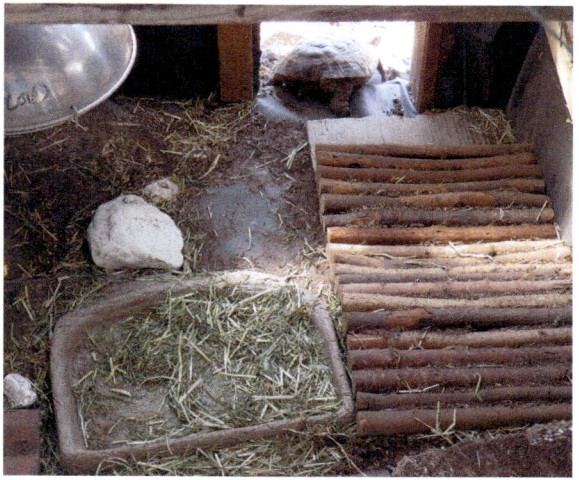

Fig. 20.3. Tortoise indoor enclosure with artificial heat and light, allowing this Horsfield's tortoise access to its outdoor enclosure – the ideal arrangement.

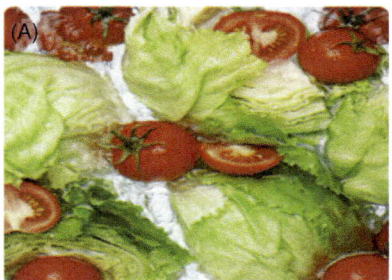
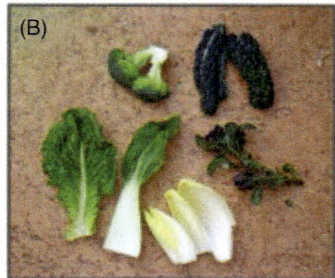
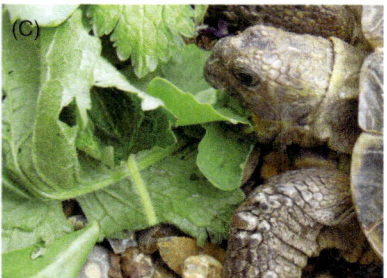

Fig. 20.2. (A) and (B) Poor diet choices for herbivorous tortoises were common and some tortoises are still fed in this way (Eleanor Lien-Hua Tirtasana Chubb). Lettuce and tomatoes were standard fare, with shop-bought salads and unhealthy brassicas (see Chapter 5 on diets). Even worse choices were dog and cat food; peas and beans; crab sticks and pizza. (C) A much more natural diet for a herbivore.

They may have been provided with a small wooden house in which to shelter from the worst of the weather, but this was largely useless in terms of meeting any other environmental needs. Figure 20.1 shows a modern enriched tortoise garden, with a wooden house for shade and shelter but also access to lights in indoor accommodation.

Gradually through the late 1980s and into the early 2000s, awareness grew of a tortoise's need for artificial heat and light. However, many owners were still completely unaware of this. Pet shops largely did not provide useful information at the point of sale (there is still no requirement in most countries to provide reliable information about the care and health of animals sold as pets).

Hibernation/brumation periods were generally very long, 5–6 months in some cases, depending on the winter temperatures in the northern part of Europe and in the UK. This is where the majority of tortoises were in captivity until recently.

Diet was often poor. Many tortoises were fed solely on shop-bought salads and greens, along with fruit such as strawberries and raspberries in the summer (Fig. 20.2A and B). The diet also included very high-protein foods such as peas, beans, or cat and dog food. Human foods were also fed – sometimes bread, pizza (as a result of the Ninja Turtles craze) or even cooked dinners containing meat, potatoes and gravy. Figure 20.2C shows a much more natural diet.

Table 20.2. Five Freedoms and Five Opportunities and Provisions for tortoises (text in green relates to giving the tortoise agency).

Five Freedoms	Provisions for physical health and well-being including choices which provide agency for the tortoise	Five Opportunities and Provisions for mental health and emotional well-being including agency for the tortoise
1. Freedom from hunger and thirst	Ready access to fresh water and a suitable diet to maintain full health	Opportunity for satisfaction through dietary choices from a varied diet from which to choose
2. Freedom from discomfort	An appropriate environment that allows sufficient choices to maintain health	Opportunity for some control within the environment to allow achievement of motivations related to access to habitat requirements
3. Freedom from pain, injury and disease	Prevention through environmental choice, rapid diagnosis and treatment	Opportunity for pleasure, development and health through enjoyable experiences and beneficial interactions
4. Freedom and opportunity to express normal behaviour	Sufficient space, facilities and presence/absence of own kind	Seasonal environmental provision to allow daily, seasonal and breeding behaviours
5. Freedom from fear and distress	Providing conditions, handling and treatment that avoid mental suffering	Opportunity for interest and confidence by providing conditions that allow mental satisfaction and enjoyment

The lack of owner understanding of tortoise needs with regard to preferred body temperature, the need for support with additional heat and light, and the potential effects of living within a group or entirely alone, was very high. Figure 20.3 shows a modern set-up with the tortoise having access to indoor and outdoor accommodation.

Yeates (2022) highlighted the control an owner, keeper, caregiver or guardian has over a pet when creating the home environment. The negative impact that humans can have on animal welfare was largely not considered in the late 20th century where tortoises were concerned. The direct harm we can cause through lack of resource control, behavioural restrictions and manipulation, the fear and anxiety we can create and the lack of agency of the animal were considerations not even on the agenda for the majority of pet owners. Sadly, this is still the case for some owners.

The minimum requirements necessary for maintaining the welfare of any animal are encompassed by the Five Freedoms. This was developed by the Farm Animal Welfare Council in the UK (1979).

Yeates (2022) adapted these into Five Opportunities with reference to tortoises. These are summarized in Table 20.2.

These Freedoms, Provisions and Opportunities are important considerations for anyone keeping a pet tortoise.

The Five Freedoms have been further developed into Five Domains by Deane and Valentine (2022), and Mellor (2016), defining four areas of physical well-being (nutrition, environment, health and behaviour) plus a fifth, mental state. Deane and Valentine (2022) set out what these physical and functional aspects to life look like and how the accompanying emotional experience and mental state are as important to animal welfare. Table 20.3 is adapted from this work.

The Five Domains concept moves forward the idea of maintaining physical well-being, and includes mental health and emotional state. Paying attention to the quality of a tortoise's life means that it is more likely to thrive rather than just survive. The tortoise should have a life that is worth living, even if that life is in captivity and not in the environment for which it was designed.

Yeates (2022) noted that tortoise supply chains, devised to meet market need, have very negative impacts on welfare. The trade in wild-caught tortoises has a high mortality rate and is not sustainable (Pendry and Allan, 2002). Captive-bred animals from large-scale commercial breeders (as shown by the number of eggs in Fig. 20.4 and the juveniles in Fig. 20.5), small businesses and hobbyists are often transported in unsuitable ways, especially with the advent of online sales. Breeders in Eastern Europe, for example, have websites boasting of hatching 30,000 eggs from a range of different species, every year. This sort of scale is not sustainable and reflects a very high mortality rate of hatchlings and juveniles.

Table 20.3. The Five Domains and their impacts on physical and mental states, as adapted for tortoises.

Physical Functional Domains		Affective Experiences Domain	
Physical State		**5. Mental State**	
1. Nutrition		**Nutrition**	
Restrictions	**Opportunities**	**Negative**	**Positive**
Water intake	Drink enough water	Thirst	Quenching thirst
Food intake, food quality, food variety	Eat enough variety of food in the right quantities	Hunger, malnutrition, overfeeding, malformation during development	Pleasures of foods with different tastes, textures, smells
			Normal growth and development
2. Environment		**Environment**	
Unavoidable conditions	**Available conditions**	**Negative**	**Positive**
Thermal extremes	Preferred Optimum Temperature Zone	Thermal chilling or overheating	Thermoregulation for homeostasis
Unsuitable substrates	Suitable substrates	Lack of suitable microhabitats and burrowing	Additional microhabitats and burrowing, retreats and egg-laying
Close confinement	Larger enclosures	Frustrations and repetitive pacing and walking	Opportunities to walk good distances in a varied enclosure
Inappropriate light intensity and quality	Required light intensity, duration and wavelengths	Abnormal growth and development	Normal growth and development
Environmental monotony	Environmental enrichment	Boredom and frustration	Sense of well-being and exploratory behaviours
Unpredictable events	Predictability	Anxiety, fear and stress, agitation	Sense of well-being and calmness
3. Health		**Health**	
Unwanted pressures	**Pressures alleviated**	**Negative**	**Positive**
Acute and chronic disease	Care and attention to prevent disease	Discomfort, pain, physiological stress	Well-being and good health
Acute, chronic, husbandry injuries	Care and attention to prevent injuries	Discomfort, pain, physiological stress	Well-being and good health
Poisons	Prevention of access	Fatal	Good health
Obesity/Anorexia	Suitable diet	Debilitation	Well-being and good health
4. Behaviour		**Behaviour**	
Agency impeded by	**Agency exercised by**	**Negative**	**Positive**
Unavoidable environmental stressors	Varied, engaging enriched environment	Frustration, anxiety, stress	Calmness, secure
Unavoidable threats or ability to escape	Refuges, retreats provided	Fear, stress, anxiety	Agency and control create calmness
Restricted choices	Opportunities for movement, foraging, exploration	Agitation, frustration	Agency and control create calmness
Barren environment	Opportunities for movement, foraging, exploration	Agitation, frustration	Agency and control create calmness
Limitations on sleep and rest	Sufficient sleep/rest	Exhaustion	Active and lively
Constraints on access to other individuals or too much access	Suitable mating and breeding opportunities	Frustration and agitation	Sexual and reproductive requirements met

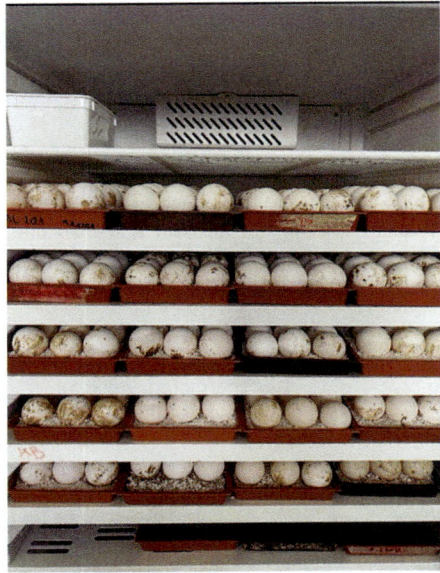

Fig. 20.4. Large-scale commercial breeding from hatching of many eggs in incubators such as this (Dillon Prest).

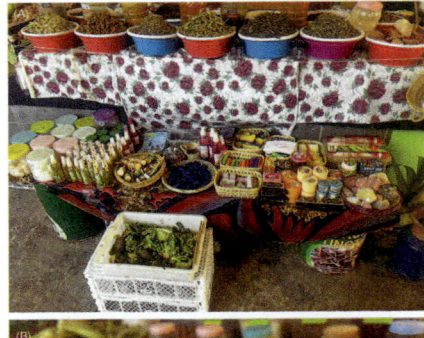

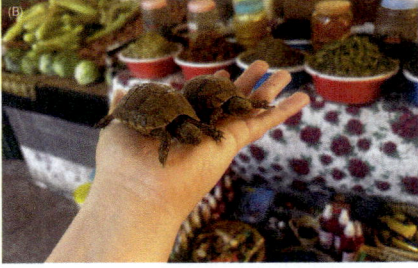

Fig. 20.6. Tortoises for sale illegally in markets in Morocco in 2024 (Corrine Wayends). Here the stall sells tea and herbs ... oh, and tortoises. Two juvenile Spur-thighed tortoises with a very uncertain and potentially short life.

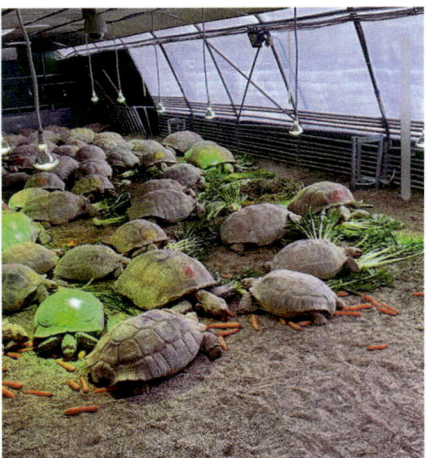

Fig. 20.5. Commercial breeding and raising of species that are difficult to care for or at risk of abandonment, such as Sulcatas (Dillon Prest).

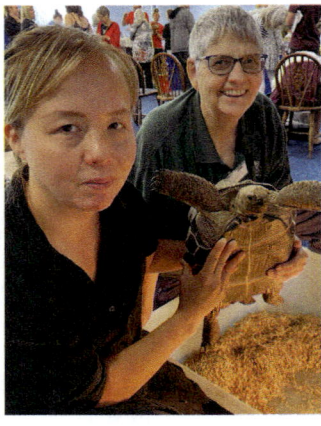

Fig. 20.7. Conferences or local events can be good sources of up-to-date information.

Poor conditions are often seen in retail outlets, with inaccurate information provided to potential buyers (Fig. 20.6 photos show juveniles being sold in a Moroccan market). Alongside this, substandard equipment and enclosures are often sold. Mixing of species and the keeping of large numbers of tortoises, as is common in breeding establishments, creates increased opportunity for disease to be spread (see Chapter 7 on common illnesses and diseases). If infected animals are then moved into other collections, the disease moves with them.

With the rise of the internet and social media from the 2000s to the 2020s, more hobby groups were formed. The standard of information given varied a great deal. Some gave good information; some gave very poor (or even dangerous) information. As there are no controls on information provided through the internet, it can be difficult for owners and prospective owners to identify evidence-based sources of information. There is still a great deal of out-of-date and inaccurate information out there. Much information is based on anecdote rather than information grounded in science. It can be difficult to keep up to date as our knowledge of tortoises increases, but we owe it to them to stay as informed as it is possible to be. Over all in my experience with many different tortoise keepers, the majority of people I speak to have a better understanding of their tortoise's needs than in the past, often by attending conferences or local events, such as the one shown in Fig 20.7.

What does tortoise keeping look like in the 2020s?

In recent years much more attention has been paid to the ethics of keeping reptiles such as tortoises as pets. More recent studies about tortoise cognition and ability to learn (see Chapters 8 and 9 on behaviour, and learning and emotions respectively) have increased awareness of the need to consider the Five Freedoms and Five Domains when considering welfare. The concept of agency for animals in captivity has only recently been applied to animals such as tortoises.

As Yeates (2022) suggested, tortoises need to be considered as either suitable or unsuitable pets. Toland *et al.* (2020) suggested that an improved alternative way of legislating to protect exotic pets being traded and kept would be for governments to 'positively list', that is, to allow only the keeping of animals that meet certain scientifically proven criteria. The considerations would be in respect of species, environmental and public health and safety protections. Jessop and Warwick (2014) and Warwick and Steedman (2021b) suggested a possible classification system where animals are assessed for their suitability as pets, based on how effectively their needs can be met in captivity. The proposed 'EMODE system' 'allows anyone to score animal species or types as easy, moderate, difficult or extreme in terms of how challenging they are to keep, according to managing their biological needs as well as human health and safety issues in the home'. While this is a rational approach, and may be seen as potentially beneficial when compared with simply banning the unsuitable species, such a system has yet to be introduced.

From a human perspective we want our pet to be a companion. What we want from that companion determines the suitability of the tortoise for this purpose. We might ask:

- Does the tortoise provide human companionship?
- Is it simply ornamental?
- Is there a risk to us from keeping wild animals, such as tortoises, in terms of zoonotic disease?

Looking at it from the tortoise's point of view:

- Does the tortoise find human companionship rewarding?
- Does the tortoise find being in close proximity to humans stressful?
- Is the tortoise able to enjoy the captive environment in the presence of humans?
- How is behaviour impacted by the presence of humans? (Warwick *et al.*, 2013)

The benefits gained from owning pets (as compared with working animals) are not always obvious. Serpell (2002) suggested that keeping pets may confer health benefits on their owners in terms of much-needed social support. The affection that many owners feel towards their tortoise may well counter the relatively high costs of pet ownership. Serpell identified the socially supportive potential of pets as hinging on 'their ability to behave in ways that make their owners believe that the animal cares for and loves them, holds them in high esteem, and depends on them for care and protection'.

Over many years I have spoken with owners who experience a very deep emotional attachment towards their tortoises. In some cases, the tortoise may have been a companion for 60+ years. This creates a bond that extends down through generations of the same family. The tortoise is 'always there', providing them with an anchor, stability in an uncertain world.

The majority of keepers I now come into contact with, in the UK and Europe, have both indoor and outdoor accommodation for their tortoise. There is a more widely held understanding that tortoises living in countries that are not their natural homes require support in the form of additional heat and light for at least part of the year. There is a general understanding that hibernation periods that are too long can lead to the death of the tortoise and should be avoided.

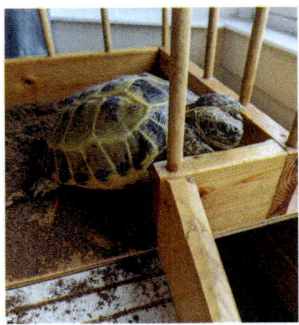 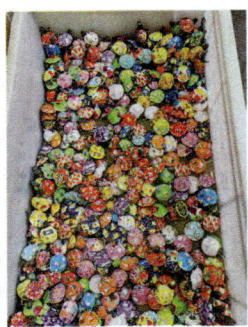 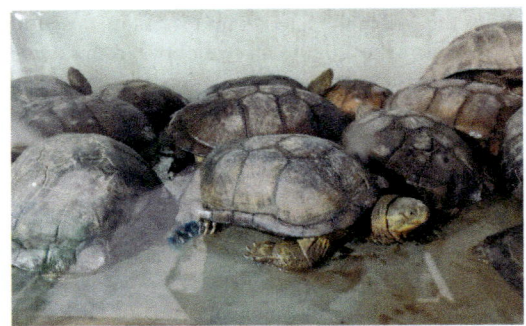

Fig. 20.8. Totally unsuitable indoor enclosure for Horsfield's tortoise, sold as a package with the tortoise, with balcony for human benefit – certainly not for the tortoise's benefit (Andy Lane).

Fig. 20.9. Painted turtles in huge numbers for the Chinese pet trade. How long does that take to paint, causing considerable stress for the turtle? (Dillon Prest).

Fig. 20.10. Tortoises and turtles for sale in markets in China on an industrial scale, mainly for food (Dillon Prest).

Captive collections and captive breeding have become increasingly important as we experience climate change and loss of biodiversity in the 21st century. Tortoise keepers already contribute to breeding programmes for endangered species, such as the European Studbook Foundation (ESF). It is clear that this sort of input to conservation will be increasingly important going forward (as described below).

Currently the numbers of captive-bred specimens are significant across Europe, where tortoise keeping is now a popular hobby. Commonly kept species from my experience and that of others within the tortoise-keeping community in the UK and Europe are:

- Horsfield's tortoises;
- Hermann's tortoises;
- Spur-thighed tortoises;
- Marginated tortoises;
- Leopard tortoises; and
- Sulcata tortoises.

In North America, tortoise keeping has risen in popularity with the species kept being more likely to be native to North and Central America. The most commonly kept tortoise species in the USA (as reported in a personal communication from Chris Leon of Garden State Tortoise) are:

- Red-eared sliders and yellow-bellied sliders;
- Box turtles (mostly wild-caught);
- Sulcata tortoises;
- Horsfield's tortoises (usually small males);
- Red-footed tortoises; and
- African side-necked turtles (*Pelusios* species).

In the Southwest USA, people commonly adopt and keep California desert tortoises (*Gopherus agassizii*). Radiated tortoises (*Astrochelys radiata*) are widely bred in the USA but are protected under the United States Endangered Species Act and cannot be bought or sold. Asian species are kept by fewer people and have a much higher value.

Currently there are hundreds of thousands of pet tortoises in the UK. The conditions under which they are kept is largely unknown. One species of particular concern is the Horsfield's tortoise (Highfield, 1992, 2003, 2024), which is being traded in huge numbers. Figure 20.8 shows an indoor enclosure sold with the tortoise.

Unbelievable numbers of wild-caught and captive farmed animals are shipped out of countries such as Uzbekistan annually, to meet the demands of being a cheap tortoise pet – basically a throwaway pet (Dillon Prest, personal communication). Farming, or ranching as it is called, involves capturing wild females, putting them into pens, waiting for them to lay and harvesting the eggs. This has negative welfare impact on the females and devastating consequences for local populations when carried out on a large scale. It seems to be the case that little has been learned from the situation created by over-collection of Mediterranean tortoises in the 1970s and 1980s. The CITES trade database for 2020–2022 showed 17,000 *Testudo horsfieldii* imports to UK, for example.

Any internet search will recommend Horsfield's as the best, hardiest, simplest pet tortoise, although they actually have very specific needs, as do all species, and that marketing pitch is simply not the case

(Highfield, 2024). This is reinforced by the numbers being given up for rehoming in the UK. The often very poor state in which these young animals are presented, due to poor diet, metabolic bone disease, shell pyramiding and so on, is shocking.

The numbers and conditions of pet tortoises kept in other parts of the world are unknown. In developing countries such as China and India, pet keeping is on the rise. Some of these animals are being treated as ornaments and objects while still alive, as shown by shocking images of painted turtles in Chinese markets (Fig. 20.9). The stress levels for these animals must be very high indeed (Warwick et al., 2013).

In China turtles are traded in unimaginable numbers for human food (Fig. 20.10). Species are not just those native to China or even Asia – many of these commercially bred and farmed animals are now from North and South America, as supplies of native species run out (Dillon Prest, personal communication).

As is the case in the UK, Europe and North America, little is known about the conditions in which tortoises are kept worldwide. Obviously, the owner, keeper, caregiver or guardian has complete responsibility for meeting their tortoise's needs. As with other companion animals kept as pets, the welfare implications for animals kept in people's homes is completely unknown.

'Pet trading and keeping globally involves at least 13,000 species,' as reported by Warwick and Steedman (2021a) 'and at least 350 million individual non-domesticated or "wild pet" animals annually.' Our appetite for pet keeping of these animals is very high, but this is not sustainable for the individual animals, the species or the planet as a whole going forward into the future.

What might tortoise keeping look like beyond the 2020s?

Climate change and loss of biodiversity in the 21st century are currently accelerating rather than being slowed in any significant way. The impact on natural habitats for tortoises will be significant. The greater the loss of habitat and the greater the pressure from increasing human populations living in these regions, the greater is the threat to species. Tortoises have been used for thousands of years by humans for a huge range of purposes (Young, 2003). As well as being pets, tortoises have provided (and in some case still provide) food, useful artefacts and tools, oils and other medicinal or cosmetic products. They are a valuable resource and commodity in countries where people have limited means of surviving. These pressures are likely to increase as the negative impacts of climate change and loss of biodiversity continue to accelerate.

The 'One Health' concept (Destoumieux-Garzon et al., 2018) is one to which we all need to pay attention, being based on three aspects of health and well-being. The concept is based on the notion that we need to take a holistic approach to these three inextricably linked parts:

- environmental health;
- human health; and
- animal health.

Human activities are now affecting every aspect of what is happening on the planet. The relationships between humans, animals and their environment are complex, and in many ways not well understood (Rendle and Jones, 2022). This is illustrated in Fig. 20.11, which is adapted from Destoumieux-Garzon et al. (2018), with an emphasis on the environment and the relationships between the three components.

The concept requires equal emphasis on the three components for us to effectively grasp the significant effects of our behaviours on animals and the environment. The inability to focus on all three parts is the cause of many of the problems being created by humans to the detriment of animals and the environment. We think that we are entitled to own any pets that we want, including wild animals such as tortoises, regardless of the consequences. We need to reconsider this and whether it is a sensible or rational approach to pet ownership.

Taking this concept a step further, 'One Welfare' extends the approach of (and partially overlaps) the One Health theme to promote the links between animal welfare and human welfare. The third part of this relationship is promoting environmentally friendly animal-keeping systems. The concept supports 'food security, sustainability, reducing human suffering and improving productivity within the farming sector through a better understanding of the value of high welfare standards' (García Pinillos, 2024). These are globally important objectives that we should all be concerned with.

Considering one aspect of the One Health and One Welfare agendas within the tortoise world illustrates some of the innovative approaches being taken and highlights the links between humans, animals and the environment. Conservation programmes and efforts to prevent species from becoming extinct in the wild are taking place all over the world. One

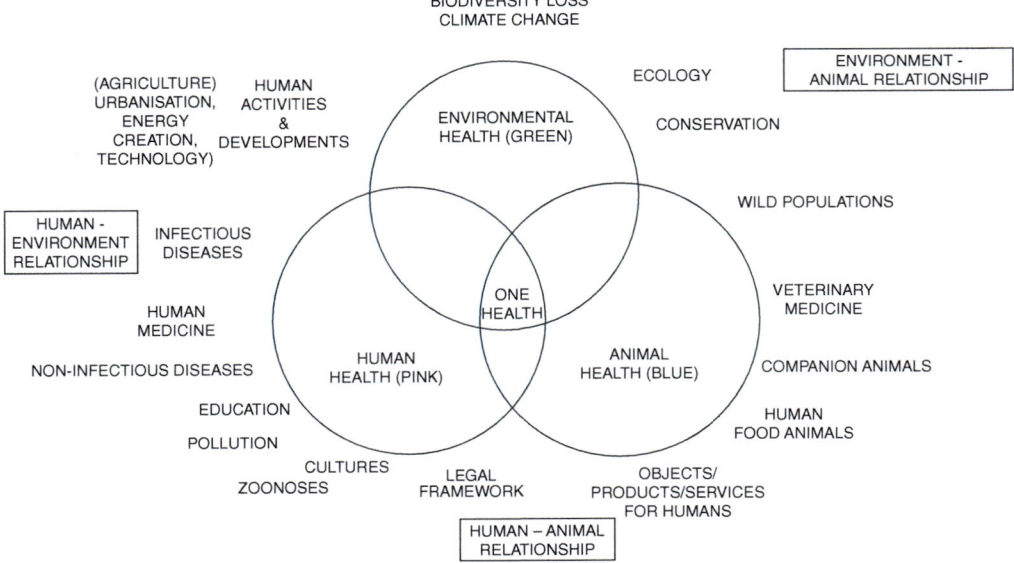

THE ONE HEALTH CONCEPT

Fig 20.11. The One Health concept, illustrating the complex relationships between human health, animal health and environmental health, and now developed into the One Health One Welfare concept (adapted from Destoumieux-Garzon et al., 2018).

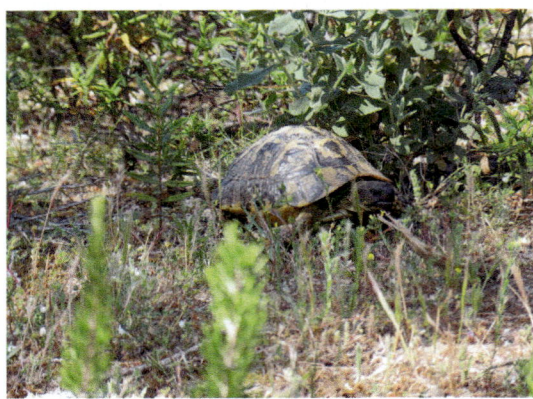

Fig. 20.12. Hermann's tortoise in the wild in the Mediterranean.

example is the work of Caesar Rahman and his colleagues in Bangladesh who are part of the Creative Conservation Alliance. The project aims to reintroduce the endangered Burmese Brown tortoise (*Manouria emys*) to an area of Bangladesh where the animal is all but extinct. The local population of largely subsistence hunters have wiped out the tortoise for food. This is an economically deprived area with an increasingly high human population. The project has centred on captive breeding and releasing

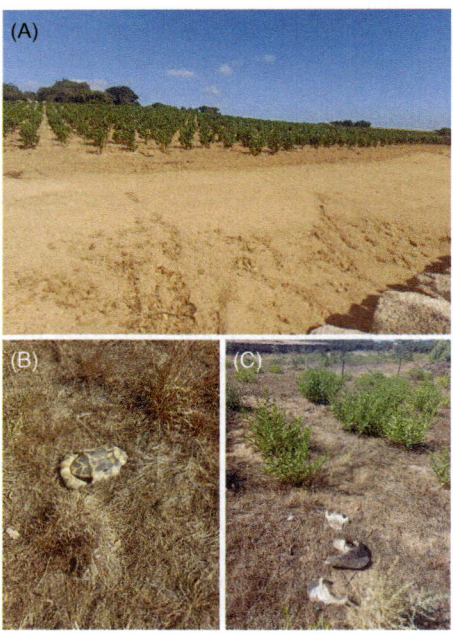

Fig. 20.13. Marginated tortoise habitat destruction and death of the previously stable population through agricultural development in Sardinia. The bones and shells are the remains of the tortoises that were not even moved from the site. (Dillon Prest).

the tortoises back into the local area. Clearly this could not happen without agreement of the local community, so that they maintain the tortoise and value them, rather than collecting and eating them.

In the Bangladesh project, radio transmitters were initially used to track and monitor the tortoises after reintroduction. These have a limited life, however, and can fall off. As a more sustainable way of continuing the monitoring, they have trained tortoise detection dogs to find the tortoises in the field. Similarly in Southern France, SOPTOM is researching the population of Hermann's tortoise, *Testudo hermanni*, following a devastating fire 3 years ago. The tortoises have been monitored for fatalities and injuries. The damaged tortoises have been treated at their centre, Village des tortues, before being released. This project has also used detection dogs for their research and reintroduction programme. Figure 20.12 shows a Hermann's tortoise in its natural habitat.

Conservation efforts have never been so important, given the current global problems of habitat loss, pollution levels, human overpopulation and the exploitation of wild animals for a variety of reasons. A very recent example in Sardinia illustrates that vigilance and monitoring continue to be vital in maintaining wild populations. The area in Fig. 20.13 shows the previously beautiful habitat utterly destroyed for agriculture. There had been a very healthy adult population of Marginated tortoises. These *Testudo marginata* were still living there when the destruction occurred, based on the bodies and remains seen here.

An innovative conservation project in the Mojave Desert of California is being carried out by conservationist Tim Shields (2023) to try to restore the population of the desert tortoise *Gopherus agassizii*. The tortoise population has crashed by 95% in the past 25 years, in part due to habitat loss and in part due to ravens. Human activity, including incursion into the edges of the desert for cattle feed-lots, has also led to an increase in raven numbers. The birds are intelligent and have worked out that the food and wastes available at the cattle feeding stations are an easy source for them. They are therefore present in much higher numbers where the tortoises live and breed.

Ravens can eat baby tortoises when they are young and their plastrons are still soft by rolling them onto their backs and pecking through the shell. Tim Shields has a number of ways to reduce raven populations and to protect this very important species. Within the desert, the Mojave tortoises dig burrows and long tunnels, which provide shelter for many other desert species. He has used lasers to disturb flocks of ravens, which do not like the green laser light. He has also used drones to remotely oil the raven eggs, thus preventing them hatching by blocking the pores in the shells. The really innovative use of technology comes in his third approach, which is to create artificial baby tortoise using 3D printing. These fake babies contain grape juice, which ravens dislike. When they peck at the tortoise a small explosive release of the juice scares them away. Tim Shields is also using small remote roving vehicles for monitoring tortoise populations and activities (Shields, 2023).

A documentary film made of the project ('*Eco-Hack! Saving desert tortoises from extinction*') has also greatly raised the profile on social media (Shields, 2023), illustrating another important element in successful fund raising and promotion of conservation projects.

Another, converse, problem is the introduction of invasive species into non-native countries. This is happening in northern Europe and the UK, and includes some chelonians. Their movement may impact on native species in different countries. One example in the UK is the Red-eared terrapin (*Trachemys scripta elegans*), which has been illegally released into rivers, ponds and lakes. Most of these animals have come from the pet trade and have been abandoned. These terrapins are voracious carnivores, happy to eat many species of indigenous wildlife, including newts, frogs, toads, small fish and a wide range of invertebrates. As yet, they have not been able to breed in the UK due to the cold weather during winter. This has limited their impact, as numbers have not been able to increase to any significant extent. However, the effects of global warming may lead to them being able to breed. This will change the population dynamics and the impact on native species will be significant.

For individual tortoise keepers, the impact of high energy costs is already being seen, with keepers unable to continue to pay for the additional heat and light their tortoise needs. The rescue centres and those involved in rehoming and rehabilitation are being overwhelmed with unwanted pets as this is written in the mid-2020s. The numbers become very high when this is combined with the existing factors leading to relinquishment, such as some species growing too large to be accommodated (Sulcatas), owners dying or becoming incapacitated as they themselves age, and animals becoming sick who require expensive veterinary treatment.

Keepers have greater available resources and access to information than past generations. The incredible

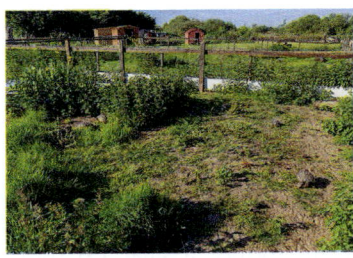
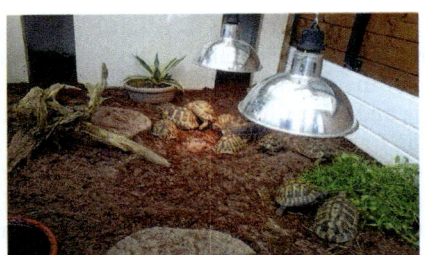
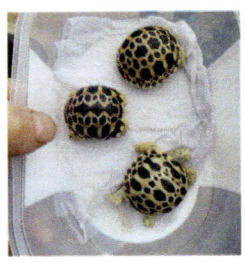

Fig. 20.14. Large Mediterranean tortoise enclosure in the UK shows how close to the natural environment we can get (Dillon Prest).

Fig. 20.15. Indoor enclosures making best use of available technologies and resources, with group of Mediterranean tortoises (Dillon Prest).

Fig. 20.16. Hatchlings of the critically endangered Burmese Star tortoises *Geochelone platynota* bred in the UK (Andy Lewis).

lengths that some keepers go to are inspirational, including creating buildings and enclosures that provide a high quality of care and a life worth living for tortoise in captivity. Figure 20.14 show a large outdoor enclosure giving environmental choices to tortoises.

The indoor enclosures being created use advanced technology to control temperature, daylength and humidity (Fig. 20.15). This can be altered on a seasonal basis to try to mimic the natural cycle of the natural environment. Developments continue in the creation of more effective artificial lighting to provide UVB and other wavelengths. Infrared heaters are becoming more efficient at providing heat at suitable wavelengths to mimic the sun, penetrating the skin and shell as the sun does.

New generations of tortoise keepers come along and there continue to be young people fascinated with these animals who will be the future of tortoise keeping. Past generations have learnt how to care more effectively for tortoises in captivity, and as new technology and more innovative approaches develop, understanding of their needs will continue to grow. The future remains uncertain for some tortoise species, but their importance as companions and pets continues undiminished.

Conclusion

Chelonians are greatly endangered across the globe. Of the 356 species identified, 148 are listed as threatened or endangered by the IUCN. They are classed as either vulnerable, endangered or critically endangered. They are described as 'The Great Survivors' (Gerlach, 2012) and have survived for over 200 million years. We must continue to strive to ensure that they survive this current era, the Anthropocene, the period of significant human impact on the planet.

The conservation of these valuable animals will involve captive breeding as well as attempts to restore habitats. Reducing their collection for the pet trade, or for the artefacts and products people so value, will be key to creating sustainable opportunities for continued populations. Conservation projects involving captive-bred tortoises are likely to increase in importance and level of contribution to the overall survival of species. Important breeding of endangered species is being undertaken by individuals, for example these Burmese Star hatchlings seen in Fig. 20.16.

As pet owners we have a responsibility to do our best for the animals we care for. This will become even more the case as we discover new ways to enhance their experiences in captivity and meet their needs. The more we know, the more there is to do in this regard.

We also have to consider whether we are in a position to offer the best opportunities for tortoises in captivity and whether we should take on tortoises as pets. They are fascinating animals and will continue to be in demand as pets, but we need to do more to manage the expectations of prospective owners. We need to educate owners and provide accurate information to help them do a good job of being a caregiver.

My life has been enriched from my experiences of keeping these incredible animals. I very much hope that this will be possible for future generations and that there is a real purpose for tortoises in captivity. Our responsibility for them goes way beyond pet ownership, and we should all be aware of the ethical responsibilities we have towards the individuals we care for and for the species as a whole.

References and Further Reading

CITES: Convention on International Trade in Endangered Species of Wild Flora and Fauna, Geneva. Website: www.cites.org

Creative Conservation Alliance: based in Bangladesh and dedicated to ecological and cultural preservation within Bangladesh's remaining wild places. www.conservationalliance.com

Darwin, C. (1859) *On the Origin of Species through Natural Selection*. John Murray/ Hachette UK, 24 November 1859.

Deane, K. and Valentine, A. (2022) Ch 2 Assessment and recording methods tool kit. In: Rendle, M. and Hinde-Megarity, J. (eds) *BSAVA Manual of Practical Veterinary Welfare*. BSAVA, Quedgeley, UK, pp. 18–71.

Destoumieux-Garzon, D., Mavingui, P., Boetch, G., Boissier, J., Darriet, F., Duboz, P., Fritsch, C., Le Roux, F., Morand, S., Paillard, C., Pontier, D., Sueur, C. and Yann, V. (2018) The One Health Concept: 10 Years Old and a Long Road Ahead. *Frontiers Veterinary Science* 5, 14.

ESF: European Studbook Foundation. Private non-profit organization in Europe, headquarters Sneek, Netherlands, with country coordinators elsewhere. Conservation of reptiles and amphibians through captive breeding, especially endangered species. Website: https://studbooks.eu

García Pinillos, R. (2024) One Welfare: The Concept (director@onewelfareworld.org) Conference Proceedings of the APBC (2024) One World, One Health, One Welfare.

Gerlach, J. (2012) *The Great Survivors*. Phelsuma, Cambridge, UK.

Highfield, A.C. (1992) The Horsfield's tortoise: *Testudo horsfieldi* (GRAY) 1844 – A brief review of its biology, ecology and captive breeding. (First published in *ASRA Journal*. Available now on Tortoise Trust website for historical publications at www.tortoisetrust.org/articles/horsfield2.html. Note that the up-to-date Tortoise Trust website is now www.tortoisetrust.com)

Highfield, A.C. (2003) Captive bred or illegal import? UK tortoise buyers need to beware. Available at www.tortoisetrust.com/illegal-imports

Highfield, A.C. (2024) The Horsfield's tortoise: *Testudo horsfieldii* (GRAY) 1844 – History in the pet trade, ecology and biology, captive breeding, misunderstood and some challenges in captivity. Available at www.tortoisetrust.com/articles/captive-care-of-the-russian-tortoise-testudo-horsfieldii

IUCN: International Union for Conservation of Nature, Gland, Switzerland. Maintains IUCN Red List of Threatened Species. Website: https://iucn.org

Jessop, M. and Warwick, C. (2014) Pets: to keep or not to keep – perhaps EMODE has the answer. Available at www.vettimes.co.uk

Mellor, D.J. (2016) Updating animal welfare thinking: moving beyond the 'Five Freedoms' towards a 'Life worth Living'. *Animals* 6, 21.

One Welfare World (no date) About One Welfare. Available at www.onewelfareworld.org

Pendry, S. and Allan, C. (2002) *Selling like Hot Cakes: An investigation into the trade in tortoises in Great Britain*. TRAFFIC International and Defra, UK

Rayment-Dyble, L. (2019) Ch 2 Reptile pet trade and welfare. In: Girling, S.J. and Raiti, P. (eds) *BSAVA Manual of Reptiles*, 3rd edn. BSAVA, Quedgeley, UK, pp. 26–36.

Rendle, M. and Jones, B. (2022) Ch 9 One Health. In: Rendle, M. and Hinde-Megarity, J. (eds) *BSAVA Manual of Practical Veterinary Welfare*. BSAVA, Quedgeley, UK, pp. 209–229.

Ritvo, H. (1994) Animals in nineteenth century Britain: complicated attitudes and competing categories. In: Manning, A. and Serpell, J. (eds) *Animals & Human Society: Changing Perceptions*. Routledge, London and New York, pp. 20–127.

Serpell, J.A. (2002) Anthropomorphism and Anthropomorphic Selection – Beyond the 'Cute response'. *Society and Animals (Journal of Human-Animal Studies)* 10(4).

Shields, T. (2023) *Eco-Hack! Saving Desert Tortoises from Extinction* (film). See: www.hardshelllabs.com/conservation-efforts; see also: *Practical Reptile Keeping*, November 2023; *BCG Newsletter* 277 (Jan./Feb. 2024)

SOPTOM Association: Station for the Observation and Protection of Tortoises and their Environment – rescue centre for damaged Hermann's tortoises created 1985, Village des tortues. Carnoules Turtle Village, Var, France. Website: www.tortuesoptom.org

Toland, E., Bando, M., Hamers, M., Cadenas, V., Laidlaw, R., Martínez-Silvestre, A. and Van der Wielen, P. (2020) Turning negatives into positives for pet trading and keeping: a review of positive lists in animals. *Animals* (Basel) 10(12), 2371.

Vetter, H. (2002) *Turtles of the World Vol. 1, Africa, Europe and Western Asia*. Chimaira, Frankfurt

Vetter, H. (2004) *Turtles of the World Vol. 2, North America*. Chimaira, Frankfurt

Vetter, H. (2005) *Turtles of the World Vol. 3 Central & South America*. Chimaira, Frankfurt.

Vetter, H. (2006) *Turtles of the World Vol. 4, East and South Asia*. Chimaira, Frankfurt.

Warwick, C. and Steedman, C. (2021a) Exotic pet trading and keeping: Proposing a model government consultation and advisory protocol. *Journal of Veterinary Behaviour* 43, 66–76.

Warwick, C. and Steedman, C. (2021b) Regulating pets using an objective positive list approach. *Journal of Veterinary Behavior* 42, 53–63.

Warwick, C., Arena, P., Lindley, S., Jessop, M. and Steedman, C. (2013) Assessing reptile welfare using behavioural criteria. *In Practice* 35, 123–131.

Warwick, C., Steedman, C., Jessop, M., Arena, P., Pilny, A. and Nicholas, M. (2018) Exotic pet suitability: Understanding some problems and using a labelling system to aid animal welfare, environment, and consumer protection. *Journal of Veterinary Behaviour* 26, 17–26.

Yeates, J. (2022) Ch 1 Animal ethics and welfare. In: Rendle, M. and Hinde-Megarity, J. (eds) *BSAVA Manual of Practical Veterinary Welfare*. BSAVA, Quedgeley, UK, pp. 1–18.

Young, P. (2003) *Tortoise*. Reaktion Books, London.

Appendix 1: Example Tortoise Health Record

General Background

Tortoise name	
Species Sub-species	
Age DOB if known	
Gender	
Owned since (date)	
Source	
Enclosure sizes Indoor Outdoor	
Substrate Indoor Outdoor	
Daytime temperature range	
Nighttime temperature range	
Humidity range	
Heat/light sources	
Daylengths	
Water access	
Diet	
Frequency of feeding	
Supplements and frequency of use	
Living alone/companions	
History of disease or illness	
Preventative treatments	
Testing for parasites, bacteria, viruses Results	
Breeding history	

(From Ebenhack, 2012; Chitty and Raftery, 2013)

Appendix 2: Example Monthly Record Keeping of Tortoise Health

Tortoise name	
Species Sub-species	
Age DOB if known	
Gender	

Date	Weight (g)	SLC (mm)	Bone ratio	Behaviour changes, treatments, illnesses

(Based on Ebenhack, 2012; Girlign and Raiti, 2019; Rendle and Megarity, 2022)

Appendix 3: Suitable Food Plants

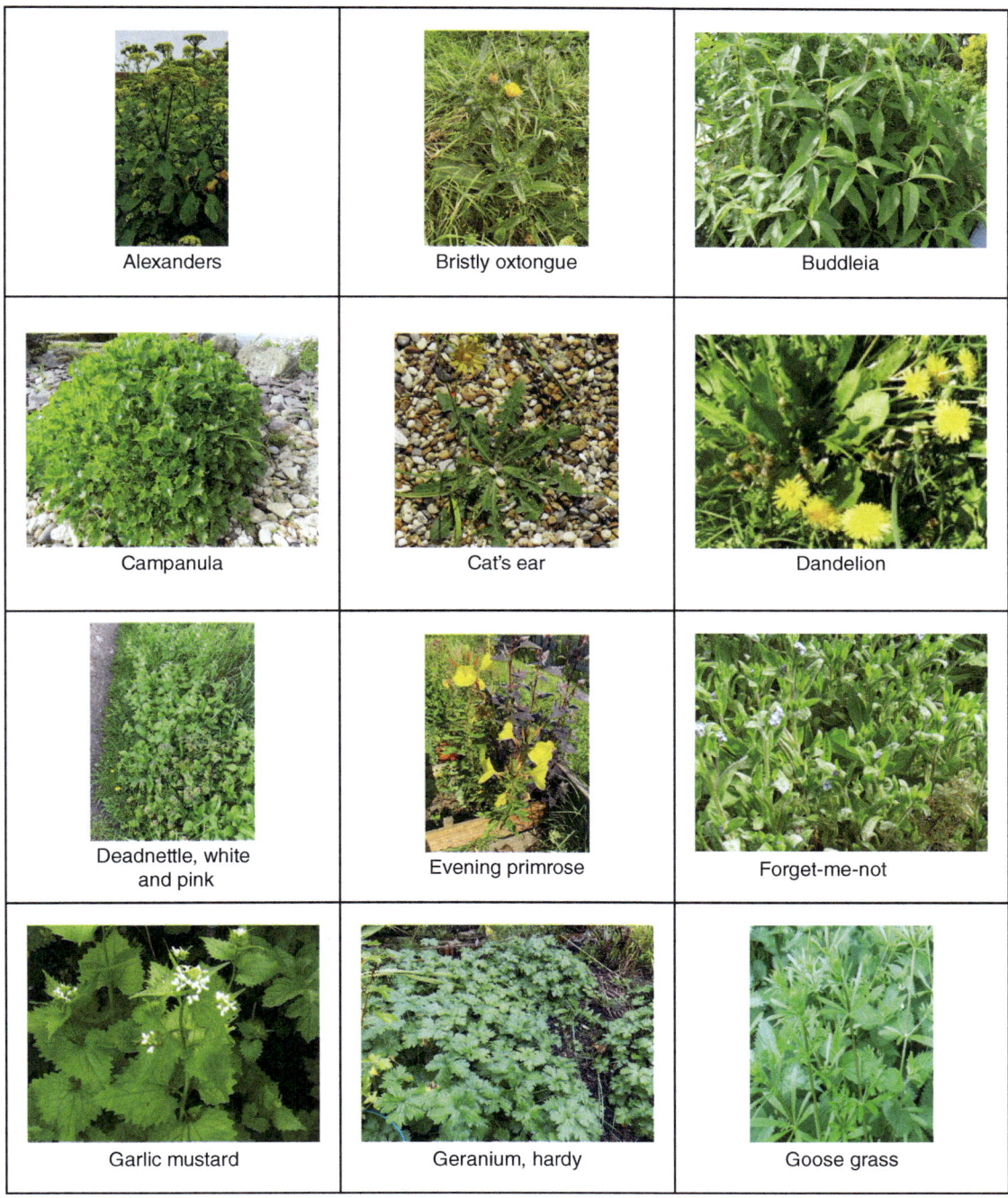

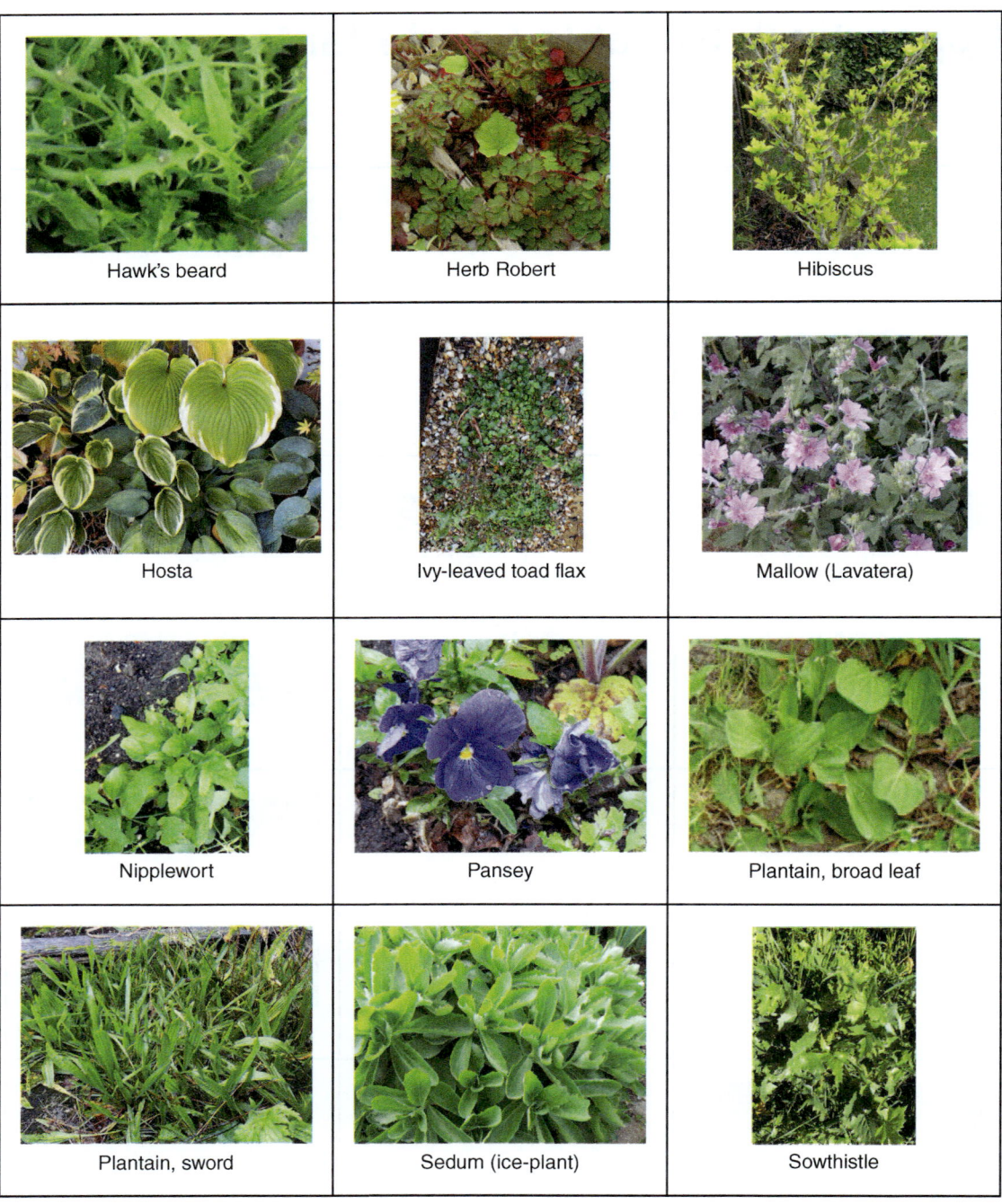

List of Species

Animals

Latin genus and species (sub-species) | **Common name**

Agrionemys horsfieldi — Horsfield's tortoise
Aldabrachelys / Dipsochelys gigantea — Aldabran tortoise
Amystoma mexicanum — Axolotl
Astrochelys radiata — Radiated tortoise
Astrochelys yniphora — Ploughshare tortoise
Basiliscus plumifrons — Emerald Basilisk
Caretta caretta — Loggerhead turtle
Centrochelys pardalis babcocki — Leopard tortoise (Eastern)
Centrochelys pardalis pardalis — Leopard tortoise (Western)
Centrochelys sulcata — African Spurred tortoise
Chamaeleo calyptratus — Veiled Chameleon
Chelonia mydas — Green turtle
Chelonoidis carbonaria — Red-footed tortoise
Chelonoidis denticulata — Yellow-footed tortoise
Chelonoidis nigra — Galapagos tortoise
Chersina angulate — Angulated tortoise
Crocodylus rhombifer — Cuban Crocodile
Dendrobates auratus — Green and Black Poison-dart frog
Emys orbicularis — European Pond turtle
Eublepharis macularius — Leopard gecko
Geochelone elegans — Indian Star tortoise
Geochelone platynota — Burmese Star tortoise
Geoemyda spengleri — Vietnamese Leaf turtle
Gopherus agassizii — California Desert tortoise
Gopherus flavomarginatus — Bolson tortoise
Iguana iguana — Green iguana
Indotestudo elongate — Elongated tortoise
Indotestudo forstenii — Sulawesi/Forsten's tortoise
Kinixys belliana — Bells Hingeback
Kinixys belliana belliana — Bells Hingeback
Kinixys belliana nogueyi — Bells Hingeback Western
Kinixys belliana zombensis — Bells Hingeback Tanzania
Kinixys erosa — Serrated Hingeback
Kinixys homeana — Home's Hingeback
Kinixys lobatsiana — Lobatse Hingeback (Botswana, South Africa)
Kinixys natalensis — Natal Hingeback (Mozambique, South Africa, Eswatini)
Kinixys spekii — Speke's Hingeback (Botswana, South Africa, Eswatini, Zambia, DR of the Congo, Angola)

Lepidochelys olivacea — Olive Ridley's turtle
Malaclemys terrapin — Diamond-backed terrapin

Manouria impressa	Impressed tortoise
Morelia viridis	Green tree python
Pelusios spp.	African Side-necked turtles
Pyxis arachnoides arachnoides	Madagascan Spider tortoise
Pyxis arachnoides brygooi	Madagascan Spider tortoise (Northern)
Pyxis planicauda	Madagascar Flat-tailed tortoise
Rafetus swinhoei	Yangtze Giant Softshell/River turtle
Rhinoclemmys funerea	Black River/Wood Turtle
Sceloporus malatichicus	Malachite spiny lizard
Terrapene Carolina spp.	American Box turtle
Testudo graeca graeca	Spur-thighed tortoise (North African)
Testudo graeca ibera	Spur-thighed tortoise (Turkish)
Testudo graeca nabeulensis	Spur-thighed tortoise (Tunisian)
Testudo graeca soussensis	Spur-thighed tortoise (Moroccan, Souss valley)
Testudo graeca whitei	Spur-thighed tortoise (Algerian)
Testudo hermanni boetgeri	Hermann's tortoise
Testudo hermanni hermanni	Hermann's tortoise
Testudo hermanni hercegovinensis	Hermann's tortoise
Testudo kleinmanni	Kleinmann's tortoise
Testudo marginata	Marginated tortoise
Trachemys emolli	Nicaraguan slider
Trachemys scripta elegans	Red-eared terrapin
Trachemys scripta scripta	Yellow-bellied slider
Trionyx triungis	Soft-shelled turtle
Varanus komodoensis	Komodo Dragon
Varanus niloticus	Nile Monitor lizard
Varanus prasinus	Emerald Tree Monitor lizard

Plants

Latin genus and species (sub-species)   **Common name**

Acacia spp.	Acacia tree
Acer campestre	Field maple
Acer pseudoplatanus	Sycamore
Acer rubrum	Red maple
Aconitum spp.	Aconite, Wolfsbane, Monkshood
Actaea spp.	Baneberry, Sambucus
Aesculus hippocastanum	Horse chestnut
Alliaria spp.	Garlic mustard
Allium spp.	Onion, garlic, leek
Alstroemeria spp.	Peruvian lily
Amaryllis sarniensis	Nerine
Anemone spp.	Windflowers
Anemone hupehensis	Japanese anemone (also wood anemone)
Angelica sylvestris	Archangel
Anthriscus sylvestris	Cow parsley, Queen Anne's Lace, Hedge parsley
Antirrhinum spp.	Snapdragon
Anthurium spp.	Flamingo flower
Apium graveolens	Celery
Aquilegia spp.	Columbine, granny's bonnet
Arnica spp.	Meadow or Silver arnica

Arum maculatum	Lords and Ladies
Arundo donax	Giant Cane or Reed
Asterales campanula	Campanula, Bell flower, Trailing bell flower
Atropa belladonna	Deadly nightshade (also Garden/Jerusalem/Cherry Nightshade)
Borago officinalis	Borage/Star flower
Brassica oleracea	Broccoli/Cabbage/Cauliflower/Kohlrabi/Sprouts
Bryonia dioica	Bryony, white
Calendula spp.	Marigold
Camassia spp.	Wild hyacinth, camas, quamash
Castanea sativa	Sweet chestnut
Cedrus spp.	Cedar
Chelidonium majus	Greater celandine
Cicerbita spp.; *macrophylla, alpina, plumieri*	Blue sowthistle, Alpine sowthistle
Cichorium intybus	Chicory
Cirsium arvense	Creeping thistle, Field thistle, Prickly thistle, Canada thistle
Cissus rotundifolia	Grape or round-leaf ivy
Chenopodium album	Fat-hen/Goosefoot/Good King Henry
Chrysanthemum spp.	Chrysanthemum
Clematis spp.	Clematis
Conium maculatum	Hemlock
Convallaria majalis	Lily of the Valley
Cotoneaster spp.	Cotoneaster
Crepis spp.	Hawk's beard
Crocosmia spp.	Montbretia
Crocus spp.	Crocus
Cyclamen spp.	Sow bread
Cymbalaria muralis	Ivy-leaved toad flax
Cytisus scoparius	Broom
Dactyloctenium aegyptium	Egyptian crowfoot
Daucus carota	Wild carrot
Delphinium spp.	Delphinium
Doronicum orientale	Leopard's bane
Digitalis purpurea	*Foxglove*
Erysimum cheiri	Wallflower
Eucalyptus spp.	Gum tree
Euonymus spp.	Spindle shrub/tree
Euphorbia spp.	Spurge (*Euphorbia pulcherrima* – Poinsettia)
Fraxinus excelsior	Ash tree
Galanthus spp.	Snowdrop
Galium spp.	Goose grass, Cleavers
Plumeria spp.	Frangipani
Gentianales spp.	Gentian
Geranium spp.	Cranesbill, Hardy geranium (not Pelargonium)
Geranium robertianum	Herb Robert, Geranium
Gladiolus spp.	Gladioli
Glechoma hederacea	Gound Ivy
Hedera helix	Ivy
Heliotropium spp.	Clasping/Summer/Blue heliotrope (borage family)
Hellebore spp.	Helleborus
Heracleum sphondylium	Hogweed (common)
Hibiscus spp.	Hibiscus

Hypochaeris radicata	Cat's ear, Cat's ears
Hyacinthus spp.	Hyacinth/Bluebell
Hydrangea spp.	Hydrangea or Hortensia
Hypericum perforatum	St John's Wort
Ilex spp.	Holly
Iris spp.	Iris
Jacobaea vulgaris	Ragwort
Juglans regia	Common or English walnut
Juniperus communis	Juniper (Common)
Kerria japonica	Japanese rose or Kerria
Laburnum anagyroides	Laburnum (Common)
Lamiales buddleja	Buddleia, Butterfly tree
Lamium purpureum; Lamium maculatum	Deadnettle – White. Red or Purple; Spotted deadnettle
Lapsana communis	Nipplewort
Lavendula spp.	Lavender
Leodontodon spp.	Hawkbit
Ligularia spp.	Ligularia
Lilium spp.	Lily
Limonium spp.	Statice/Sea lavender
Linaria vulgaris	Toadflax/Yellow Toadflax
Linum usitatissimum	Flax/Linseed
Lobelia spp.	Lobelia
Lotus corniculatus	Common Bird's foot trefoil
Lupinus spp.	Lupin
Lychnis spp.	Lychnis/Campion
Malva terrestris	Mallow, Tree mallow, Lavatera
Mentha spp.	Mint
Mimosa spp.	Mimosa
Morus spp.	Mulberry tree
Muscari armeniacum	Grape hyacinth
Myosotis spp.	Forget-me-not
Narcissus spp.	Daffodil
Nicotinia tabacum	Tobacco plant/Wolfberry
Oenethera spp.	Evening primrose
Opuntia spp. *(cochenillifera)*	Cactus spp. (e.g. Prickly pear)
Origanum majorana	Marjoram
Origanum vulgare	Oregano
Oxalis acetosella	Wood sorrel
Nerium oleander	Oleander
Paeonia spp.	Peony/Tree peony
Papaver spp.	Poppy
Passiflora spp.	Passionflower
Perea americana	Avocado
Philodendron spp.	Philodendron
Photinia	Christmas berry
Picris echioides (Helminthotheca) echioides	Bristly oxtongue
Pieris floribuna	Forest flame
Pinus spp.	Pine
Pisum sativum	Pea
Phytolacca americana	Pokeweed
Plantago lanceolata	Ribwort, Narrowleaf or English plantain

Plantago major; Plantago media	Broadleaf, Common, Hoary, Rat-tail or Greater plantain
Primula veris	Cowslip
Primula vulgaris	Primrose
Prunus laurocerasus	Cherry laurel
Prunus spinosa	Blackthorn or Sloe tree
Quercus spp.	Oak tree
Ranunculus acris	Buttercup
Rhododendron spp.	Rhododenron, Azalea species
Rheum rhabarbatrum	Rhubarb
Ribes spp.	Flowering currants (Red/White/Black)
Ricinus communis	Castor oil plant
Rosa spp.	Rose (leaves and petals)
Rumex spp.	Dock, broad-leafed and curled
Sambucus nigra	Common elder
Santolina spp.	Santolina, Dwarf lavender
Sedum spp.	Sedum, Ice plant
Senecio jacobaea	Ragwort/Cankerweed/Staggerwort
Senecio vulgaris	Common groundsel
Silene dioica	Red campion
Smyrnium olusatrum, S. perfoliatum	Alexanders, Horse parsley
Solanum tuberosum	Potato
Sonchus oleraceus	Common sowthistle
Spathiphyllum wallisii	Peace lily
Symphytum officinale	Comfrey, boneset, knitbone
Syringa spp.	Lilac
Tagetes patula	French marigold
Tamus communis	Black bryony
Tanacetum parthenium	Feverfew
Taraxacum officinale	Dandelion
Taxus baccata	Common yew
Thymus spp.	Thyme
Tragopogon spp.	Goat's beard, Salsify, Jack-go-to-bed-at-noon
Tricyrtis hirta; T. formosana	Toad lily
Trifolium spp.	Clover
Tulipa spp.	Tulip
Tussilago farfara	Coltsfoot
Valerianella spp., esp. *Valerianella locusta*	Corn salad; Lamb's lettuce
Verbascum thapsus	Mullein
Veronica spp.	Speedwell
Viola spp.	Pansey/Viola
Virbunum lantana	Lantana, Viburnum
Viscum album	Mistletoe
Wisteria spp.	Wisteria
Zantedeschia spp.	Arum lily/Calla lily

Index

Note: page numbers in **bold** type refer to **figures**; page numbers in *italic* type refer to *tables*.
Tortoise names are given with common name first and Latin name in brackets.
Please refer to List of Species for Latin and common names of both animals and plants.

abscesses 89
    ear 97
    leg with 97
    skin 98
accommodation
    African Spurred Tortoises/Sulcatas (*Geochelone sulcata*) 204–205
    Hingeback tortoises (*Kinixys* species) 220
    Horsfield's tortoise (*Agrionemys horsfieldii*) 225–228
    Indian Star tortoises (*Geochelone elegans*) 208
    Leopard tortoises (*Geochelone pardalis*) 202
    Mediterranean tortoises 192–193, **194**
    Radiated tortoises (*Geochelone radiata*) 207
    Red-footed tortoises (*Geochelone carbonaria*) 215–216
    Yellow-footed tortoises (*Geochelone denticulata*) 215–216
additional lighting, UV indexes differences **59**
aestivation 167
African Spurred tortoises (*Geochelone/Centrochelys sulcata*) *3, 4,* 12, 14, 16, 27, 29, 31, 32, 40, 43, 55, 61–62, 77, 81, 111, 123, 126, 150, 202–204, 208–210, 258
    accommodation types 204–205
    natural environment 204
    non-hibernating species 168
    suitable diet 204
aggregation 143
Aldabran tortoise (*Aldabrachelys gigantea*) *3,* **121,** 142
American box turtle (*Terrapene carolina*) 2
amphibians 7
animal–keeper relationships 144–146
    see also tortoise keeper
animal protein 21
anorexia 99
anti-helminth drugs 100
anti-parasitic drugs 100
Arcadia® deep heat projectors 54–56
artificial lighting 16
    additional lighting, UV indexes differences **59**
    artificial lights 50–53
    calcium metabolism and homeostasis 57–59, **58**
    electromagnetic spectrum **49**
    environmental and climate change 56–57
    Ferguson Zones *53,* **54,** 55–56

    LED lighting 53, 59–60
    light intensity 50
    light source, types *51*
    natural sunlight 48–50
    sunlight role in vitamin D synthesis 50
    ultraviolet (UV) light 50
    UV Index (UVI) **49,** 50
    UV radiation, types **49**
    vitamin D3 synthesis 57, **58**
    World Wildlife Fund (WWF) terrestrial biomes *52*
artificial lights 50–53
Axolotl 7

bacterial mycoplasma infections 96–97
    Mycoplasma agassizi 254
Balantidium coli 98
basking/sheltering 80, 122, **145,** 169
bathing 85
Baytril® 19
beak **14,** 88
behaviour 127
    body temperature regulation 122
    cognition and learning 127
        Galapagos tortoises 128–129
        Red-footed tortoises 128
    controlling 120
    definition 118–119
    indicating good health and mental well-being
        basking/sheltering 122
        drinking/bathing/defecating 122
        exploratory behaviour 122
        feeding 119, 122
        mating/breeding 122–123
        social behaviour 123
        territorial behaviour 123
        vocalizations 123
        walking 122
    innate or instinctive behaviours 118
    learning by tortoises 123–128
    naturally occurring tortoise 120–122
    principles when training 125
    techniques used in training tortoises 125–126
    three-stage model, operant conditioning or training using 126–127

Bell's Hingeback tortoise (*Kinixys belliana*) **4**, **216**, **217**
    non-hibernating species **168**
benzimidazoles 100
BIAZA UV Tool 52
biome 53
bladder stones **80**
body temperature regulation 122
body weight during hibernation 179
bone density ratio 84, 171
bone ratio results
    and hibernation *172*
    and meaning *84*
breathing difficulties
    due to pyramiding 76
    hibernation 176–178
breeding tortoises
    control 156–158
    courtship and mating 155
    eggs **157–158**, 158–163, *162*
    ethics 149–151
    female reproductive system 151–154, **152–154**
    home-made incubator **161**
    incubation temperatures and incubations lengths for different species *161*
    incubator **162**
    male reproductive system 151, **152–154**, 154–156
    nest-building and egg-laying in captivity 159–160
    young tortoises **163**
    see also captive breeding; eggs; reproduction
British and Irish Association of Zoos and Aquaria (BIAZA) 48, 51–53, 243
'brrrr-brrrr-brrrr' of male Egyptian tortoise (*Testudo kleinmanni*) 123, 238
brumation *see* hibernation
Burmese Brown (*Manouria emys*) tortoises 24, 69
    feeding 63
    non-hibernating species **168**
Burmese Star (*Geochelone platynota*) tortoise **142**, 209, **209**, 268

calcium 50
    content in enclosures **37**
    in limb bones 106
    metabolism and homeostasis 57–59, **58**
    provided to juveniles 75
calcium:phosphorus ratio 76, 104–105, 237
Californian desert tortoises (*Gopherus agassizii*) 84, 264
cancerous tumours 113
captive breeding 150
    animals 260
    collections 264
    tortoises 8–10
captive environment
    natural environment 25, 26–27
    natural habitats for tortoises 24–25

    terrestrial chelonian species and their natural environments *28*
    tortoise type 25–28
carapace, scutes of **11**
cataracts 89
chelonians (Testudines) 1, 7, *7*
    classification *5*
    distribution around globe 22
    excretion, types *21*
cholesterol and lipid (fat) deposits 89, 113
chronic kidney disease 108
CITES trade database 264
claws **14**
cloaca 20, **22**
cloacal tumour 113
cloudiness 89
coco-coir 42
cognition and learning 127
    Galapagos tortoises 127–129, 134, 141, 143, 146
    Red-footed tortoises 128
colder climates, diet in 68–69
commercial breeding **150**, 262
commercial diets **75**, *75*
constipation 22
Convention on International Trade in Endangered Species (CITES) 150, 181, 199, 205, 258
corticotropin-releasing factor (CRF) 133
courtship
    and mating 156
    rituals 15–16, **145**
Cryptodira 10
cucumber, appetite stimulant 177

daylength 46
Deep Heat Projector® 54
defecates during hibernation 179
defecating 169
defensive reaction 133
deforestation 190
dehydration 69, 77, 85, 99, 108, 109, 177–178
desensitization 125, 127
diets
    adult tortoises 62
    African Spurred tortoise (*Centrochelys sulcata*) 204
    Burmese Brown (*Manouria emys*) 63
    Burmese Star tortoise (*Geochelone platynota*) 209
    calcium:phosphorus ratio 76
    calcium provided to juveniles 75
    in colder climates 68–69
    commercial diets **75**, *75*
    disease in young tortoises 105
    Egyptian tortoises feeding 63
    factors affecting amounts and types of food 70
    favourite foods 64
    feeding process 62

for herbivorous tortoises 66
Hermanns tortoise (*Testudo hermanni*) 193–195
Hingeback tortoise (*Kinixys spp.*) 217–219
Horsfields tortoise (*Agrionemys/Testudo horsfieldi*) 63, 225
Indian Star tortoise (*Geochelone elegans*) 208
Kleinmann's tortoise (*Testudo kleinmanni*) 237
Leopard tortoise (*Centrochelys pardalis*) 63, 199–202
macronutrients and micronutrients 65–66, 67–68
Marginated tortoise (*Testudo marginata*) 193–195
Mediterranean tortoises 64, 193–195, *195*
natural diet 66
nutrient demands 66
nutritional supplements 76
omnivorous tortoises, food for 61, 69
overfeeding 62
plants poisonous to tortoises 66–68
plants to be avoided in enclosures or as food items 74
for poorly fed tortoise 72–76
Radiated Tortoise (*Astrochelys radiata*) 205–207
Red-footed tortoise (*Chelonoidis carbonaria*) 63, 214–215
related disease 102–107
    dietary disease in young tortoises 105
    gout effects 105, **107**
    inappropriate feeding 104
    metabolic bone disease 105–106
    overfeeding 102–104
    vitamin and mineral deficiencies and excesses 104–105, *106*
    vomiting or regurgitation 107
shrubs and flowering plants for grazing, cover and shade 73
Spur-thighed tortoise (*Testudo graeca spp.*) 193–195
suitable plants for tortoise food 69
Sulawesi/Forsten's tortoise (*Indotestudo forstenii*) 121
supplements 76, *77*
tortoises 61–78, **69**
vitamins and minerals, relationship between 68, **69**
water provision 77
water sources 69
'Wild Flowers and Plants Safe for Tortoises to Eat' 69–72, *70–71*
Yellow-footed tortoise (*Chelonoidis denticulata*) 214–215
digestive organs 20, 21
dominance-based hierarchies 146–147
drilling holes in shells 12
drinking 86, 122
drowning 112–113
drying out, hatchlings and juveniles 41
dyads 144–146

ectoparasites causing disease 100
ectothermic/ectotherms 6, 165
    reptiles 6
eggs
    fail to hatch 161
    hatching 161–163, **162**
    incubation 160
    -laying in wild **157–158**, 158–159
    production
        and development 153–154
        incomplete **94**
Egyptian tortoises (*Testudo kleinmanni*) **4**, 29, 156, 231, 231, 232, **232**, 234
    breeding 237–238
    in captivity 233–235, **234**
    definition 230–231
    diet of 237, *237*
    feeding 63
    future for 238–239
    locations map **232**
    natural environment 231–233, *235*
    non-hibernating species **168**
    plants as food and for shelter *233*, **236**
    substrate and furniture type 235–237
electric fencing *see* outdoor enclosures
electromagnetic spectrum **49**
emodepsid 100
EMODE system 263
emotional states
    calmness and comfort signs 138
    definitions 135, *137*
    feelings 133–135
    handling effects and treatment 139
    'happy' tortoise 132–133, **135**
    indicators 132
    pain indicators in Chelonia *138*
    stress, distress, anxiety and fear 135–137
    stress in captive tortoises, signs *137*
    welfare implications 139
endoparasites causing disease
    macroparasites 99–100
    microparasites 96–99, *97–99*
enriched enclosures 37
enrichment 29, 33, 36, 42, 94, 130, 132, 139, 146, **196**, 228
environmental and climate change 56–57
ethical breeding enterprise *see* breeding tortoises
ethics 149–151
European Association of Zoos and Aquaria (EAZA) 238
European Endangered Species Programme (EEP) 150, 238
European pond turtle (*Emys orbicularis*) 2
European Studbook Foundation (ESF) 150, 237–238, 264–265
Exo Terra® 160
exploratory behaviour 122
eye diseases 113

fasting 173
fatality rates 98
fatty liver syndrome 102, 107–108, **109**
fearful behaviours 136
feeding process 62, **119**, 122
    inappropriate 104
female
    cloacal prolapse **115**, 116
    Hermann's tortoise 16
    Marginated tortoise, juvenile growth by weight 83
    reproductive organs **22**
    reproductive system 151–154, **152–154**
    Spur-thighed tortoise (*Testudo graeca whitei*) **94**
    terrapins 143
    tortoises 113–114
Ferguson Zones 53, **54**, 55–56
finch reflex 16
First aid 93, 116
flagellates or ciliates 98
flaking skin 16
fluid-retention 23
follicular stasis **114**, 115
food supply in hibernation 166
F10® products 89
freezing in hibernation 177
freshwater turtles 1–3, **2**

Galapagos tortoises (*Chelonoidis nigra*) **2**, 3, **4**, 15, 18, 31, 151, 154, 202, 209, 257
    cognition and learning 128–129
'garden tortoise' **259**
gender indicator 151
gonadotropin-releasing hormone (GnRH) 95
gout effects 105, **107**
grazing tortoises 61, 66
gut 20

Habistat® 56
habitats and enclosures, creation of 251–252, **252**
'happy' tortoise 132–133, **135**
hatchlings 105
    drying out 41
    and juveniles 85
health and mental well-being, indication
    basking/sheltering 122
    drinking/bathing/defecating 122
    exploratory behaviour 122
    feeding **119**, 122
    mating/breeding 122–123
    social behaviour 123
    territorial behaviour 123
    vocalizations 123
    walking 122

health checks
    daily 79
    for healthy tortoise
        behaviour 82
        drinking 85
        faeces 85–87, **86**
        feeding 85
        length/weight ratio 82–85
        lumps, bumps, swellings 89
        mouth and beak 87–89
        nose, eyes, ears 89
        skin/nails/shell damage 89–91, **91**
        urates 85
    monthly 81
    record keeping 81–82
    use of 91–92
    weekly 79
hearing 120
heart 19–20
heat
    -emitting light sources 57
    sensation 118, 120
    sources 54–56, 112, 160
hepatic lipidosis 107
herbivores 10, 61, 64, 66, 104, 214, 242, **259**
Hermann's tortoises (*Testudo hermanni*) 2, **11**, 16, 29, **167**, **182**, **186**, 186–187, **187**
    basking 80
    ears **121**
    male **145**
    Testudo hermanni boetgeri **188**, 189
    Testudo hermanni hercegovinensis 189, **189**
    Testudo hermanni hermanni 188, **188**
    in wild **266**
Herpes viruses 98
hibernaculum 175
hibernation/brumation 94, 245–247, 259
    body weight during 179
    bone ratio results and 172
    breathing difficulties 178–179
    conditions for 166–167
    defecates during 179
    definition 165–166
    dehydration 177–178
    diseases due to 109–110
    dos and don'ts of 177, *178*
    excessively long 179
    food supply 166
    freezing 177
    hibernating species **167**
    injuries or infections 179
    light intensity 166
    measurements and recommendations 172
    non-hibernating species 166, **168**
    in Northern Europe, timescale for *170*
    period 156
    photoperiod 166

planning for 169
ratio ranges *172*
reason for 166
records 173
regular inspection during 176
species 166, **167**
stages
    preparation 169–172
    slow-down period 172–173
    time and place for 173–176, **174**
    waking up after hibernation 176–177
temperatures 166
thermometer **169**
time for 169
tropical tortoises 25
urinates during 179
Hibiscrub® (Molnlycke) 89
Hingeback tortoises (*Kinixys* species) 156, 216–220
accommodation types 220
diet for 218–220
distribution map of 216, **218**
male and female **219**
home-made incubator **161**
homeostasis 93–94
Home's Hingeback tortoises (*Kinixys homeana*) 216
non-hibernating species 177
Horsfield's tortoises (*Agrionemys/Testudo horsfieldii*) 4, 25, 63, 86, 99, 222–229
accommodation type 225–228
in captivity 225
crowding together **145**
diet for 225
in enclosure **136**
locations map **223**
male and female **152**, **223**
natural environment **224**, **226**
sniffing and head bobbing **145**
human–animal interactions (HAIs) 125, 144–146
humidity levels 42–44, 195
hypervitaminosis 59
hypovitaminosis 98, 113

illnesses and diseases
diet-related 102–107
diseases due to hibernation duration 109–110
drowning 112–113
ectoparasites causing 100
endoparasites causing
    macroparasites 99–100
    microparasites 96–99
eye 113
factors causing different types of 95
injury and damage by predators, other tortoises 110–112
kidney and urinary 108–109
liver 107–108
prolapses 116

reproductive 113–116
shell and skin 100–102
tumours 113
incubation temperatures and incubations lengths *161*
incubator **161–162**
Indian Star Tortoise (*Geochelone elegans*) 24, 207, **209**
accommodation types 208–209
diet for 208
locations **208**
natural environment 207–208
non-hibernating species **168**
indoor enclosures 45, 252–253, **268**
with artificial heat and light **259**
and outdoor set-ups 46
with solid sides **252**
unsuitable **264**
inflammation 23
see also illnesses and diseases
injury and damage **111**
environmental damage 112
infections, hibernation 179
by other tortoises 110–112
by predators 110
innate or instinctive behaviours 123
inspection during hibernation 176
internal fertilization process 21
internal organs affect behaviour 21–22
International Union for Conservation of Nature (IUCN) 150, 205
intranuclear coccidiosis 99
ivermectin 100

Jackson ratio 82, 83, 84, 171
Jungle Dawn LED bar 54
juveniles
growth 83, 195, 198
hibernation/brumation 173, 176
in Moroccan market **182**
safety 163, 192
stress 137
and small adult tortoises 173

kidneys 21
and urinary disease 108–109, **109**
Kleinmann's tortoises (*Testudo kleinmanni*) 3, 4, 27, 29, 31, 55, 156, 230–240
incubation of eggs *161*
male and female **154–155**
mating **155**
size 151
vocalizations 133

lamp index 53
learning by tortoises, behaviour 123–124

least invasive, minimally aversive (LIMA) 125
LED lighting 53, 59
leg abscess 90
legal trade 181
leg-biting 19
    to female 156
Leopard tortoises (*Centrochelys pardalis*) 9, 12, **13**, 29, 44, 77, 151, 199
    accommodation types 202
    feeding 63
    hatchling 150
    male and female **153**
    with nasal discharge **97**
    natural environment 199
    non-hibernating species **168**
    in South Africa 200
    suitable diet for 199–202
lethargy 99
light
    and heat 46
    intensity 50, 166
    source, types *51*
liver 21
    disease 107–108
living fossils 10
Loggerhead juvenile **2**
lung 20

macronutrients and micronutrients 65–66, 67–68
macroparasites 99–100
    parasitic diseases 99
    worms – intestinal parasites 99–100
Madagascan spider tortoises (*Pyxis arachnoides*) **2**
male
    Horsfield's tortoise 80
    Leopard tortoise 13
    reproductive system **152–154**, 154–156
    Sulcata **134**
    tortoises **115**, 116
Marginated tortoises (*Testudo marginata*) 44, **136**, 142, 167, **182**, **189**, 190, 241
    habitat destruction and death **266**
marine turtles 1
mating
    breeding 122–123
    rituals 156
maximum–minimum thermometer **169**, 173, 176, **177**
Mediterranean natural environment 37
Mediterranean Spur-thighed tortoises feeding 63
Mediterranean tortoises 3, 46, 49, 87, 147, **268**
    accommodation need in captivity 192–193, **194**
    day for, in captivity 195–196, **196**
    definition 181
    diet for 193–195, *195*
    Hermann's tortoises (*Testudo hermanni*) **182**, 186, 186–187, **187**

Testudo hermanni boetgeri **188**, 189
Testudo hermanni hercegovinensis 189, **189**
Testudo hermanni hermanni **188**, **188**
map of countries **182**
Marginated tortoises (*Testudo marginata*) **182**, **189**, 190
    natural environment of 190–192, **191**
    Spur-thighed tortoises (*Testudo graeca*) 183
        area distribution 183–184
        Testudo graeca graeca 184, **185–186**
        Testudo graeca ibera 186
    types 182–183
    in wild 197
    see also artificial lighting; captive environment; illnesses and diseases
memory *125*
metabolic bone disease (MBD) 84, 105–106, **107**
Microclimate® 56
microclimates 190
    see also Mediterranean tortoises
microparasites
    abscesses 98
    diseases 96
    effects of 98–99
    flagellates or ciliates 98
    generalized signs 99
    stomatitis inflammation and infection 97–98
    upper respiratory tract disease (URTD) 96–97
modal action pattern (MAP) 128
molecular 'dance' 57
motion detectors 253
mouth
    with internal structures of nose **17**
    rot 87
Mycoplasma agassizii 96

natural diet 66
naturally occurring tortoise, behaviour 120–122
natural sunlight 48–50
nematodes 100
nervous system, behaviour 120
nest-building and egg-laying in captivity 159–160
Nile monitor, hunting **9**
non-hibernating species 166, **168**
North African Spur-thighed tortoise 183
Northern Diamondback terrapins (*Malaclemys terrapin terrapin*) **143**
nutrient demands 66
nutritional deficiencies 14–16
nutritional excesses 102
nutritional supplements 76

obese tortoise **12**
obesity 102
oedema 89

oestrogen levels 152
omnivores 77, 85, 104, 122, 215
    food for 61, 63, **64**, 66, 69, 73
One Health concept 265, **266**
'One Welfare' 265
operant conditioning or training using 126–127
opuntia cactus 75
outdoor enclosures **252**, 253
    predator deterrent in 250
overfeeding 62, 102–104
oxfendazole 87

parathyroid hormone (PTH) levels 57, 105
penis 21, **22**, **116**
    amputation **115**
    prolapse 116
Perspex® **35**, 37, **40**, 193, **226**, 228
roof shelters 35, 37, 40, 193, 226
pet keeping 257–258
    beyond 2020s 265–268
    Five domains and their impacts on *261*
    Five Freedoms and Five Opportunities
        and Provisions 260, *260*
    in 2020s 263–265
    up to 2020s 258–263
pet trading 265
photokeratitis 112
photoperiod, 55
    hibernation 166
physical damage 16
physiological compensation 94–95
pinworms 100
plastron
    physical examination 80
    scutes of **11**
Pleurodira *10*
polycarbonate **38**, **40**, **45**, 193, **226**, 228, **245**
polymerase chain reaction (PCR) tests 99
poorly fed tortoise, food for 72–76
positive reinforcement training (PRT) 123
post-hibernational anorexia (PHA) 109
preferred body temperature (PBT) 29, 31, 32, 122
preferred optimum temperature zone (POTZ) 29–31, 32, 38
    and relative humidity 82
prolapses 115, 116
ProT5 High Output UVB tube 54
puffiness **23**
python, scales and pattern **9**

Radiated tortoises (*Astrochelys radiata*) **2**, 99, **142**, 205, 264
    accommodation types 207
    in Madagascar 207
    natural environment 205

non-hibernating species 168
resting on lawn 134
shell pattern **9**, **206**
suitable diet 205–207
touching and sniffing 142
Readi-Grass® 44
rectal prolapse and treatment **115**, 116
Red-eared terrapin (*Trachemys scripta elegans*) 267
    Red-footed tortoises (*Chelonoidis carbonaria*) **4**, **9**, 25, 62, **63**, 69, **121**, 120, 160
    cognition and learning 127–128
    feeding **63**
    female behaving normally in their enclosures **136**
    male and female **153**, **155**
    non-hibernating species **168**
relaxation in emotional states 133
repetitive behaviours 29
repetitive head and limb flicking 133
reproduction/reproductive 151
    behaviours 81, 120, 143, **145**, 169
    diseases 113–116
        female tortoises 113–114
        follicular stasis **114**, 115
        male tortoises **115**, 116
        stress-related disease in females 115
    organs 21
reptile 6–7
    Emerald tree monitor basking **9**
    groups **8**
    reproduction 7
Reptile Systems® Gold Infrared lamp 56
Reptoboost® 100
residual current device (RCD) 250–251, **251**
respiratory infection 98–100, 109, 112
rhinitis 96–96
roundworms 21, 100
runny nose syndrome (RNS) 18, 96–97, 197, 254

savannah habitat **200**
scales damage 16
scrabbling of limbs 133
seasonal changes 46
secondary hyperparathyroidism 105
semi-aquatic turtles and terrapins 2, 3, 7
senses
    hearing 18
    sight 16–17
    smell 17–18
    taste 19
    touch 18–19
sensitivity to touch 10–12
Serrated or forest Hingeback tortoise (*Kinixys erosa*) **26**, **28**, 216
    non-hibernating species 168
sex identification 151

sexual behaviours 133
    butting 133
    inappropriate 149
shell
    damage 89
    deformities/pyramiding 105
    patterns 142
    and skin disease 100–102, **101**, 103–104
shell-bashing 19
    behaviour 15
shell-butting 156
shortening daylength 49
shrubs and flowering plants for grazing, cover and shade 73
sick or recuperating tortoises 85
signalling and communication 6
single-celled protozoans 98
skin problems 90
smoke detectors 253
sniffing 133
social behaviour 123
social bullying 143
social hierarchy 123
social interactions
    communication 141–143
    environment role 146
    impact on well-being and welfare 146–147
    interactions types 143
    reproductive behavioural interactions 143–144
    types, with human 127, 144–146
Soft-shelled turtle (*Trionyx triungis*) **11**
soft vital organs 19–21
SOPTOM 267
spider tortoise (*Pixys arachnoides*) **2**, 14
    Pyxis arachnoides brygooi egg hatching 162
Spur-thighed tortoise (*Testudo graeca* spp.) **13**, 25, 96, 121, 183–184, **185–186**, 186, 242–243
    adult female weight in 83
    area distribution 183–184
    basking together 145
    eating 80
    eyes 121
    females **134**, **136**, 156
    hibernating species 167
    male resting in enclosure **134**
    relaxed-looking male **134**
staring 133
stimuli 118
stockmanship 146
stomatitis 87
    inflammation and infection in mouth 97–98
    treatment 97–98
straight carapace length (SCL) 82, 84, 151, 171
stress-related disease in females 115
succulents 205–207
suitability 36
Sulawesi tortoise (*Indotestudo forstenii*) **121**

Sulcata tortoises 29, **40**, 44, **43**, 61, **202**, **203**, **262**
    distribution map of **203**
    non-hibernating species 168
    in physical pushing 126
    see also African Spurred Tortoise
sunlight role in vitamin D synthesis 50
supplements 76, 77
Suprelorin®F (Virbac) 95
survival adaptations 119

Tamodine Wound (Vetark®) 89
tapeworms 21
    and trematodes (flukes) 99–100
taste buds 120
techniques used in training tortoises 125–126
temperatures, hibernation 166
terrapin 1, 3, 7, 10, 22
    Red-eared (*Trachemys scripta elegans*) 143, 144
terrestrial tortoises 1–3, **2**
territorial behaviour 123
testosterone levels 156
testudine intranuclear coccidiosis (TINC) infections 89, 254
testudines 7
thermoregulation 12, 15
thermoregulatory behaviours 6
time for hibernation 169
    see also hibernation/brumation
tongue 17, **17**
tortoise(s) 1
    distribution around globe 22–23
    internal structure **20**
'tortoise-friendly' weeds 66
tortoise keeper
    skills and experience
        European Turtle Alliance Conference 2024 **242**
        evidence-based published information 243
        knowledge set 241–247
        Mediterranean tortoise enclosures being created **246**
        Norfolk Tortoise Club (UK) meeting **242**
        planning and preparation 247–248
        practical skills sets *244*, 247
        Red-footed tortoise enclosure being created **245**
        reptile rescue centres 248
        responsibility 248
        Tortoise South East one-day workshop **242**
        useful organizations 243
    and tortoise, health and safety for
        access to water 251
        biosecurity and health 253–254
        electrical things 250, **251**
        habitats and enclosures, creation of 251–252, **252**
        indoor enclosures 252–253

outdoor enclosures 253
pathogens, disease in humans 255
Zoonosis and 254–255
trachea 19, **20**
trading 265
TRAFFIC report 258
tropical dry grassland tortoises
African Spurred Tortoises/Sulcatas (*Centrochelys/ Geochelone sulcata*) 202–204
accommodation types 204–205
natural environment 204
suitable diet 204
Burmese Star tortoises (*Geochelone platynota*) 209, **209**
Indian Star tortoises (*Geochelone elegans*) 207, **209**
accommodation types 208–209
diet for 208
natural environment 205
Leopard tortoises (*Centrochelys/Geochelone pardalis*) 199
accommodation types 202
natural environment 199
suitable diet for 199–202
Radiated tortoises (*Astrochelys/Geochelone radiata*) 205
accommodation types 207
natural environment 205
suitable diet 205–207
species 198–199
tropical rainforest tortoises 15
tropical tortoises from humid forest areas
Hingeback tortoises (*Kinixys* species) 216–220
accommodation types 220
diet for 218–220
distribution map of 216, **218**
male and female **219**
Red-footed tortoises (*Geochelone carbonaria*) 211–213, **212**
accommodation types 215–216
diet for 214–215, **215**
natural environment for 214
origin **212**, 213–214
and Yellow-footed tortoises, difference between 214
Yellow-footed tortoises (*Geochelone denticulata*) 211–213, **212**
accommodation types 215–216
diet for 214–215, **215**
natural environment for 214
origin **212**, 213–214
and Red-footed tortoises, difference between 214
tumours 113
Tungsten or Halide Flood light 54
Turkish Spur-thighed tortoise **183**
turtles 1
painted 264
twokking 18

UK Government Department for Food and Rural Affairs (Defra) 258
ultrasonic pest repellents 253
ultraviolet (UV) light 50
unhappy tortoise **135**, 136
see also 'happy' tortoise
upper respiratory tract disease 98
urates 22, **86**, 108
urinating 169
during hibernation 179
URTD/RNS/rhinitis 179
UVB radiation 48
UV index (UVI) 50, 53
daily fluctuations **49**
information 53
UV radiation, types **49**

veterinary treatment 12
VEVOR® incubator 160
Vietnamese leaf turtle *Geoemyda spengleri* 2
visual discrimination 128
vitamins
and minerals
deficiencies and excesses 104–105, *106*
relationship between 68, **69**
vitamin A excess or deficiency 100–102
vitamin D3 synthesis 57, **58**
vocalizations 123, 133
vomiting or regurgitation 107

walking 122, 169
waste products monitoring 81
water 195
provision 77
sources 69
see also drinking
weighing 80
well-planted enclosure including aromatic plants 38
'Wild Flowers and Plants Safe for Tortoises to Eat' 69–72, *70–71*
World Wildlife Fund (WWF) 52, 52–53
Terrestrial Biomes 52
wounds 16
see also illnesses and diseases
Yangtze Giant Softshell turtle (*Rafetus swinhoei*) 1–3
Yellow-footed tortoises (*Chelonoidis/Geochelone denticulata*) 62, 69, 211–213, **212**
accommodation types 215–216
diet for 214–215, **215**
natural environment for 214
origin **212**, 213–214
young tortoises **11**, 163

Zoological Society of London (ZSL) London Zoo 127, **128**, 146
Zoo Med® 160

Printed and bound by CPI Group (UK) Ltd, Croydon, CR0 4YY
16/01/2025

14627363-0001